OXFORD MEDICAL PUBLICATIONS

Child and Adolescent Psychiatry

Oxford Specialist Handbooks in Psychiatry

Child and Adolescent Psychiatry

David Coghill

Senior Lecturer and Honorary Consultant
Child and Adolescent Psychiatrist
University of Dundee, UK

Sally Bonnar

Consultant Child and Adolescent Psychiatrist
NHS Tayside, UK

Sandra L. Duke

Consultant Child and Adolescent Psychiatrist
NHS Tayside, UK

Johnny Graham

Clinical Lecturer and Honorary Specialist Registrar
University of Dundee, UK

Sarah Seth

Clinical Lecturer and Honorary Specialist Registrar
University of Dundee, UK

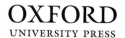

OXFORD
UNIVERSITY PRESS

OXFORD
UNIVERSITY PRESS

Great Clarendon Street, Oxford OX2 6DP

Oxford University Press is a department of the University of Oxford.
It furthers the University's objective of excellence in research, scholarship,
and education by publishing worldwide in

Oxford New York

Auckland Cape Town Dar es Salaam Hong Kong Karachi
Kuala Lumpur Madrid Melbourne Mexico City Nairobi
New Delhi Shanghai Taipei Toronto

With offices in

Argentina Austria Brazil Chile Czech Republic France Greece
Guatemala Hungary Italy Japan Poland Portugal Singapore
South Korea Switzerland Thailand Turkey Ukraine Vietnam

Oxford is a registered trade mark of Oxford University Press
in the UK and in certain other countries

Published in the United States
by Oxford University Press Inc., New York

British Library Cataloguing in Publication Data
Data available

Library of Congress Cataloging-in-Publication-Data
Data available

Typeset by Cepha Imaging Private Ltd., Bangalore, India
Printed in Italy
on acid-free paper by
LEGO S. p. A.

ISBN 978–0–19–923499–8

10 9 8 7 6 5 4 3 2 1

Oxford University Press makes no representation, express or implied,
that the drug dosages in this book are correct. Readers must therefore
always check the product information and clinical procedures with the most
up-to-date published product information and data sheets provided by the
manufacturers and the most recent codes of conduct and safety regulations.
The authors and publishers do not accept responsibility or legal liability for
any errors in the text or for the misuse or misapplication of material in this
work. Except where otherwise stated, drug dosages and recommendations
are for the non-pregnant adult who is not breast-feeding.

Contents

Detailed contents

Foreword

The scope of child and adolescent psychiatry has increased greatly in recent years. The various types of pathology have been described with increasing clarity; the influences of risk and protective factors on mental development are being identified; a growing number of randomized controlled clinical trials have established psychological and pharmacological treatments on a much firmer basis of evidence than before.

One consequence of this increased knowledge is that more people need to know it. Primary health care needs to be involved in the recognition of disorders, the organization of the first steps in care, support and advice to families. An increasing range of professionals are involved in the provision of specialist mental healthcare—not only the old 'trinity' of child psychiatrist, child psychologist and social worker, but also specialist nurses, mental health workers, occupational and speech/language therapists. Specialist education takes clear note of psychopathology in formulating special educational needs.

This book will meet these disciplines' needs for knowledge. It sets out succinctly the current information about the nature of the disorders and the elements of good practice.

Professor Eric Taylor
King's College London
Institute of Psychiatry
2008

Foreword

Preface

When planning and writing this book, we were very conscious that child and adolescent psychiatry has been going through several important transitions. There have been major developments in theory, with increased recognition not only of the important contributions that developmental neuroscience can make to our understanding but also the interactions between biological, systemic, cognitive and psychodynamic models that had previously been treated as mutually exclusive and independent of each other. Clinical practice has also changed considerably, with a welcome emphasis on the provision of evidenced based healthcare delivered by comprehensive multidisciplinary clinical teams working to clinical pathways. At the same time, partly as a consequence of a general increase in referral rates and partly due to the increased recognition of several developmental psychiatric disorders such as attention deficit disorder and the autism spectrum disorders, there has been increased pressures on child and adolescent mental health workers' time, increased caseloads and shifts in work practices. It is for example now relatively uncommon to find a qualified child and adolescent psychiatrist in the UK who has the time or opportunity to be directly involved in delivering psychotherapeutic treatments. Whilst this may indeed be entirely justifiable in terms of cost-effectiveness it is still very important for senior staff to have the skills and understanding to allow them to provide supervision and guidance as to which interventions should be offered in which situations. Changes in the patterns of clinical provision mean that in many areas of child and adolescent mental health paediatricians are making a considerable contribution to the workforce. Clearly the impact of these changes on the training requirements of a broad range of staff need to be taken on board and worked through.

At the same time there have been major changes in the ways that postgraduate medical education is organised and delivered. Competency based training has begun in the UK and whilst it is difficult to predict how these changes will impact in the long term, it does seem clear that trainees are going to be required to take on board increasing amounts of scientifically complex information over shorter periods of time than was afforded to their trainers.

We hope that by taking these considerations on board from the outset that we have achieved our goal of producing a comprehensive book that is both clear and concise. Whilst the handbook was primarily targeted at senior trainees in both psychiatry and paediatrics we hope it will also be of particular interest to junior and senior medical colleagues in both primary and secondary care, and to broader child and adolescent mental health staff including nurses, psychologists, occupational therapists and other allied professions, as well as specialist staff in social work and education.

We have all certainly learnt a great deal whilst putting together this handbook, and we hope it is as helpful and enjoyable for you to read as it was for us to write.

Abbreviations

3Di	Developmental, Dimensional and Diagnostic Interview
ABS	Adaptive Behaviour Scale
ADHD	attention deficit hyperactivity disorder
ADI -R	Autism Diagnostic Interview
ADOS-G	Autism Diagnostic Observation Schedule (Generic)
AIMS	Abnormal Movement Scale
ASD	autistic spectrum disorder
bd	twice daily (dosage)
BMI	Body Mass Index
BP	blood pressure
BPD	bipolar disorder
BPVS	British Picture Vocabulary Scale
CAMHS	Child and Adolescent Mental Health Services
CBT	Cognitive Behavioural Therapy
CD	conduct disorder
CDD	childhood disintegrative disorder
C-GAS	Children's Global Assessment Scale
CGI-I	Clinical Global Impressions—Impairment
CHAT	Checklist for Autism in Toddlers
CMV	cytomegalovirus
CNS	central nervous system
CP	Cerebral Palsy
CSP	co-ordinated support plan
DISCO	Diagnostic Interview for Social and Communication Disorders
DLPFC	dorsolateral prefrontal cortex
DSM-IV	Diagnostic and Statistical Manual of Mental Disorders (4th edn)
ECG	electrocardiogram
ECT	electroconvulsive therapy
EDE	Eating Disorders Examination
EDI-C	Eating Disorders Inventory for Children
EDNOS	eating disorder not otherwise specified
EEG	electroencephalography
EMDR	eye movement desensitization reprocessing
EOS	early onset schizophrenia
EPS	Educational Psychology Service

FAED	Food avoidance emotional disorder
FBC	full blood count
FDA	Food and Drug Agency
GI	gastrointestinal
HALO	Hampshire Assessment of Living with Others
HIV	human immunodeficiency virus
HPA	hypothalamic-pituitary-adrenal
ICD-10	International Classification of Diseases (10th edn)
IEP	Individual Education Plan
IQ	intelligence quotient
LEA	Local Education Authority
LFT	liver function tests
LSD	lysergic acid driethylamide
MMR	mumps, measles and rubella (vaccine)
MRI	magnetic resonance imaging
MTA	multimodal treatment of ADHD
MUPS	medically unexplained physical symptoms
NICE	National Institute for Health and Clinical Excellence
NIMH	National Institute of Mental Health
NOS	not otherwise specified
NYLS	New York Longitudinal Study
OCD	obsessive compulsive disorder
ODD	oppositional defiant disorder
PANDAS	paediatric autoimmune neuropsychiatric disorders associated with streptococcal infections
PCP	phencyclidine
PDD	pervasive developmental disorders
PET	positron emission tomography
PS	Psychological Service
PTSD	post-traumatic stress disorder
RCT	randomized control trial
REM	rapid eye movement
RTA	road traffic accident
SADS	Schedule for Affective Disorders and Schizophrenia
SANS	Scale for Assessment of Negative Symptoms
SAPS	Scale for Assessment of Positive Symptoms
SCOFF	Sick Control One Fat Food (rating scale)
SEED	Scottish Executive Education Department
SEN	special education need
SENCO	Special Educational Needs Coordinator

SIGN	Scottish Intercollegiate Guidelines Network
SLT	Speech and Language Therapy
SSRI	selective serotonin reuptake inhibitor
tds	three times daily (dosage)
TFT	thyroid function tests
TLE	temporal lobe epilepsy
TOWRE	Test of Word Reading Efficiency
U&E	urea and electrolytes
VCFS	velocardiofacial syndrome
VEOS	very early onset schizophrenia
WASH-U-KSADS	Washington University Kiddie Schedule of Affective Disorders and Schizophrenia
WHO	World Health Organization
WISC	Wechsler Intelligence Scale for Children
WORD	Weschler Objective Reading Dimension

Introduction

The history of child and adolescent psychiatry

The first textbook of child psychiatry was written by Leo Kanner and published in 1935. Kanner had previously established the formally organized 'child guidance clinic' in Boston, USA in 1921. This service focused on the treatment of children presenting with delinquent behaviours and was the template for the child guidance movement whereby there was a focus on the use of 'scientific method' to manage behavioural problems.

Kanner's ideas rapidly spread across the Atlantic to the UK and mainland Europe. The first child guidance clinic in the UK was set up in the East End of London by Emanuel Miller, a psychiatrist, and a colleague, a psychiatric social worker, who had trained in Kanner's Boston clinic. This was closely followed by the development of other services. In 1933, when Miller moved to the Tavistock Clinic a children's department was opened, which pioneered a move towards a family-orientated approach to understanding and managing childhood psychopathology.

Child psychiatry became a separate and independent specialty in the UK in the late 1940s and by the time the NHS was established in 1948 there were child guidance clinics in most of the English regions. One negative impact of this process was that these services, which were staffed by psychiatrists, educational psychologists, and social workers, often became rather isolated, and dislocated from the other medical, psychological and social work services. There were limited opportunities for training and research, the recruitment of new staff and trainees was difficult, and services often persisted with outdated and ineffective modes of practice.

Scotland did not follow the child guidance model and here the earliest services were developed either within children's hospitals by paediatricians who had developed an interest in psychiatry or via adult psychiatrists with an interest in young people starting to work down the age range. As a consequence, these services had closer links either to paediatrics or adult psychiatry, and a tendency to be more medically orientated. Here, services were generally staffed by psychiatrists, clinical psychologists, nurses and staff from other professions allied to medicine, such as occupational therapists, and speech and language therapists. Initially, these services focused on child problems with adolescent services developing much later (and often as an independent service running in parallel to the child service).

Academic child and adolescent psychiatry was also rather late in developing compared with its development in other medical specialities in general adult psychiatry and paediatrics in particular. Whilst there were already a few departments in US universities the first academic department of child and adolescent psychiatry in the UK was at the Maudsley Hospital in South London and was led by Professor Sir Michael Rutter. His epidemiological work in the Isle of Wight study remains one of the cornerstones of child psychiatry research. Whilst most medical schools now employ at least one academic child and adolescent psychiatrist the pool of academics in this field is still much smaller than in paediatrics or adult psychiatry.

The lack of a strong academic base coupled with the relative isolation of child guidance clinics, a lack of therapeutic resources, and a reliance on long-term intensive psychodynamic treatments and play therapy, meant that for many years most services were only able to treat a small minority of those children known to have difficulties. As new treatments such as behavioural therapy, the various family therapies, and group treatments became available many services developed in order to integrate these into practice and by the 1980s most services were able to provide a relatively comprehensive treatment package. Around this time there was also an increased recognition of the need for comprehensive assessment and diagnosis practices. More recently, various pharmacological treatments and newer psychotherapies, such as cognitive therapy and interpersonal therapies have been introduced into practice.

In the 2000s there is now a much better developed evidence base and service delivery has become much more highly organized. Services have been refocused away from child and adolescent psychiatry per se to become 'child and adolescent mental health services' (CAMHS). There have been several sets of evidence-based guidance developed in the UK by groups such as SIGN (the Scottish Intercollegiate Guidelines Network) and NICE (National Institute for Health and Clinical Excellence), and a National Service Framework for children's services, which includes detailed sections on CAMHS services has been published in England and Wales.

The purpose of this book is to provide a concise but comprehensive overview of the current knowledge and practice of child and adolescent psychiatry. Our objective was to produce a readable and easy to use book that brings together up-to-date evidence-based material for child and adolescent psychiatrists, psychiatric trainees, paediatricians, clinical psychologists, nurses, other CAMHS workers, and those interested in the field of psychiatric disorders in children and adolescents.

Classification of disorders

Diagnosis and classification

As is the case in general medicine and general adult psychiatry, diagnosis is used in child and adolescent psychiatry to:

- Collect and organize information collected at assessment
- To guide treatment planning
- To inform about prognosis.

Classification systems assist with the standardization of the diagnostic process, and the use of a reliable and effective classificatory system can serve several important functions:

- Their use results in a greater precision in planning treatment at both the individual and population levels
- They are a prerequisite for the conduct of many types of clinical research and facilitate, the communication of research findings
- They allow for the collection of epidemiological data, a process that is central to health-care planning at international, national, and local levels.

Notwithstanding these clear benefits, there has been some resistance to the introduction of standardized diagnostic systems into routine clinical practice in child and adolescent psychiatry. Some clinicians believe that the current emphasis on classification and diagnosis distracts the clinician from developing a holistic understanding of the individual, their strengths and their difficulties. Others feel that the emphasis on categorical diagnoses prevalent in the major classificatory systems is overly restrictive pointing out those disorders such as attention deficit hyperactivity disorder (ADHD) and autism are dimensional constructs with those who currently meet diagnostic criteria simply representing the extreme end of a continuum. From this perspective a criticism of the categorical systems is that the cut-offs have been arbitrarily defined and lack clear validity. Dimensional constructs are less well defined than the major categorical diagnostic systems they are, however, widely used in clinical psychology and systemic practice.

Debates over 'categorical' versus 'dimensional' can become unnecessarily polarized. It is important to have some criteria by which we can choose whether to treat or not treat an individual, and if we are to treat, to decide which treatment is most appropriate. Whilst they are neither flawless nor foolproof, diagnostic systems were designed for this purpose. To use ADHD as an example, whilst it is true that the cut-off for making a diagnosis of ADHD is, to some degree, arbitrary; it was chosen to maximize the chance that an individual meeting these criteria will be suffering from impairment as a consequence of their ADHD symptoms, and that these symptoms and impairments will respond to treatment.

The acceptance of a diagnostic system does not mean that the clinician has rejected the potential importance of dimensionality, which can continue to be helpful, particularly where an individual's difficulties fall near to the cut-off for a particular disorder.

The current diagnostic classification systems used in psychiatry are 'atheoretical' in nature and concentrate on describing phenomenology, whilst not making any attempt to comment on aetiological processes. As a consequence the diagnostic entities generated are 'disorders' not 'diseases'.

The current definitions of disorders in both ICD-10 and DSM-IV include both 'characteristic' and 'discriminating' symptoms:

- Examples of characteristic symptoms include the symptom of over-activity, which is found in several different disorders including ADHD, bipolar disorder and occasionally the agitated form of depression
- Discriminating symptoms, such as the grandiosity associated with bipolar disorder may be of less importance to the patient and their family, but are important in diagnosis as they are not associated with other disorders.

There is often also an assumed hierarchy of symptoms, which are arranged in order of importance (e.g. 'organic' hallucinations and delusions over non-organic psychotic symptoms that are considered over depressed mood, which itself is considered over anxiety).

Most diagnostic systems also stipulate exclusion, as well as inclusion criteria to ensure that diagnostic categories are mutually exclusive without significant overlap. For example, in ICD-10, the exclusion criteria for autism are that the clinical picture is not attributable to:

- The other varieties of pervasive developmental disorder
- Specific developmental disorder of receptive language with secondary socio-emotional problems
- Reactive attachment disorder or disinhibited attachment disorder
- Mental retardation with some associated emotional or behavioural disorder
- Schizophrenia of unusually early onset
- Rett's syndrome.

ICD-10

The two most influential and commonly used diagnostic systems in current psychiatric practice are the 10th revision of the International Classification of Diseases (ICD-10) which was developed by the World Health Organization and the 4th edition of the Diagnostic and Statistical Manual of Mental Disorders (DSM-IV) developed by the American Psychiatric Association. Whilst these two systems have very different histories they now share many more similarities than differences. There do however, continue to be several important differences between them and it is helpful to be familiar with both. As ICD-10 is the predominant classificatory system in Europe it will be discussed in greater detail.

ICD-10 is a comprehensive diagnostic system developed by the World Health organization and intended for use internationally throughout the world. It is a general medical classification system organized in chapters by body system numbered with Roman numerals. The psychiatric disorders are in Chapter V and psychiatric disorders are coded with an alphanumeric code. All start with the letter F, which is followed by two or three Arabic numerals the first representing the main diagnostic group, the second for more special groups etc as required (e.g. F 90.1). Using this system, it would be possible to designate 1000 possible psychiatric diagnoses. About 1/3rd of these are currently used.

The main subdivisions within Chapter V are:
- Organic disorders
- Mental and behavioural disorders due to psychoactive substance use
- Schizophrenia, schizotypal and delusional disorders
- Mood (affective) disorders
- Neurotic, stress-related, and somatoform disorders
- Behavioural syndromes associated with physiological disturbances and physical factors
- Disorders of adult personality and behaviour
- Mental retardation
- Disorders of psychological development
- Behavioural and emotional disorders with onset usually occurring in childhood and adolescence.

The section on 'Behavioural and emotional disorders with onset usually occurring in childhood and adolescence' includes several important sub-sections including:
- Hyperkinetic disorder
- Conduct disorders
- Mixed disorders of conduct and emotions
- Emotional disorders with onset specific to childhood
- Disorders of social functioning with onset specific to childhood and adolescence
- Tic disorders.

It is important to recognize that the diagnosis of psychiatric disorders in children and adolescents is not restricted to those disorders in this last section. Indeed, there are no age limits on the other disorders and, in most cases, no recognition of developmental status, within these criteria. Therefore, for a child to be diagnosed with, for example, schizophrenia, the same diagnostic criteria are required as for an adult. This is both positive and negative. On the one hand, it reinforces the fact that, whilst uncommon, children and, to a greater extent, adolescents can suffer from almost all of the psychiatric disorders more traditionally associated with adults. On the other hand, it fails to take into account the developmental differences commonly seen in symptom presentation between children, adolescents and adults.

As an example of the complexities consider 'grandiosity'. Whilst it is clearly abnormal and probably grandiose for an adult to suggest that they *are* Spiderman, this may not be as clear cut when claimed by an 11-year-old. However, if that 11-year-old insists that not only *are* they Spiderman, but that they *can* fire webs and swing from building to building like Spiderman, and then attempts to jump from the top of a building to demonstrate this, they may well be demonstrating the true grandiosity associated with a bipolar disorder in the same way as is typically seen in adult bipolar disorder.

ICD-10 is presented in three complementary formats:

- The *Clinical Descriptions and Diagnostic Guidelines* ('the Blue Book') gives an extensive description of each disorder followed by criteria for diagnosis with inclusion and exclusion terms. It is intended for use by clinicians in daily practice
- The *Diagnostic Criteria for Research* ('the Green Book') describes a series of more restrictive criteria for each disorder intended to facilitate the selection of groups of individuals whose symptoms closely resemble each other. Compared with the Blue Book, the symptoms are more clearly operationalized and time criteria are stricter. Despite its title, this book is also often a valuable reference for clinicians in day to day practice
- A multi-axial version of the ICD-10 is also available. In addition to the clinical syndromes it contains axes for problems of development, intelligence, somatic disorders, psychosocial problems and the Children's Global Assessment Scale (C-GAS). This book can be extremely valuable in deriving multi-axial diagnoses and formulations, and assisting the clinician to develop a systematic, as well as holistic, description of their patients.

Differences between ICD-10 and DSM-IV

Unlike ICD-10, which is a general medical classification, DSM-IV only encompasses mental disorders. Historically, there were many differences between the previous ICD and DSM systems, however, the latest revisions have many more similarities than differences. An understanding of the differences is helpful when, for example, comparing literature that has used the different systems. The major differences that remain relate to:

- The duration criterion for schizophrenia (6 months for DSM-IV vs. 1 month for ICD-10)
- Different classification systems for eating disorders with DSM-IV differentiating between two types of anorexia (restrictive and binge eating types) and two types of bulimia (purging and non-purging), whilst ICD-10 does not make such distinctions
- DSM-IV makes distinction between conversion and dissociative states, whilst ICD-10 does not
- Despite there being almost identical symptom descriptions for over-activity, impulsivity, and inattention, ADHD is also defined somewhat differently by the two systems. Indeed, the term ADHD does not appear in ICD-10, which refers to 'hyperkinetic disorder'. DSM-IV recognizes three types of ADHD inattentive, hyperactive/impulsive and combined. Hyperkinetic disorder actually describes a severely affected group who comprise only a subgroup of those children who under DSM-IV would be considered to have combined type ADHD. The implications of this issue are discussed more fully in the chapter on ADHD.

A more general difference between the two systems relates to their handling of co-existing disorders. The ICD system is designed as a single diagnosis system with the clinician matching the patient to the pattern that most closely fits. On the other hand, the DSM system encourages multiple diagnoses and has less prominent exclusion criteria. Thus, whilst it is possible to diagnose both ADHD and an anxiety disorder under DSM-IV under ICD-10 the anxiety disorder would be diagnosed and the hyperkinetic disorder would not—assuming that the anxiety is considered the cause.

The development process for DSM-V is underway.

Recommended reading

American Psychiatric Association (2000) *Diagnostic and Statistical Manual of Mental Disorders (DSM-IV TR)*. The Press, Washington DC.

Rapoport JL (1996) *DSM-IV Training Guide For Diagnosis Of Childhood Disorders*. Routledge, New York.

World Health Organization (1992) *The ICD-10 Classification of Mental and Behavioural Disorders: Clinical Descriptions and Diagnostic Guidelines*. WHO, Geneva.

World Health Organization (1993) *The ICD-10 Classification of Mental and Behavioural Disorders: Diagnostic Criteria for Research*. WHO, Geneva.

World Health Organisation (1997) *Multiaxial Classification of Child and Adolescent Psychiatric Disorders: The ICD-10 Classification of Mental and Behavioural Disorders in Children and Adolescents*. Cambridge University Press, London.

Normal child development

Stage theories of psychosocial development

Several of the most influential theories of child psychosocial development have proposed that children pass through several stages as they develop. Whilst it is now widely recognized that none of these theories provide the comprehensive explanations of child development that were originally proposed, they can still be useful in helping us understand aspects of development. These theoretical approaches are discussed in more detail in subsequent chapters and the main stages are described in Table 3.1.

Table 3.1 Stage theories of psychosocial development

	Freud	Erikson	Piaget	Kohlberg
0–1 years	Oral stage	Trust vs. mistrust	Sensorimotor (0–2 years)	Pre-conventional morality: level I
1–2 years	Anal stage	Autonomy vs. shame and doubt		
3–5 years	Phallic stage	Initiative vs. guilt	Pre-operational (2–7 years)	
6 years– puberty	Latency period	Industry vs. inferiority	Concrete operational (7–12 years)	Conventional morality: level II
Adolescence	Genital stage	Identity vs. confusion	Formal operational (over 12 years)	
Early adulthood		Intimacy vs. isolation		Post conventional morality: level III
Middle adulthood		Generativity vs. self-absorption		
Old age		Integrity vs. despair		

Attachment: definition, phases, and theories

Definition

The study of attachment remains one of the cornerstones of developmental psychology. Attachment in this context refers to the strong, enduring, emotional tie that develops over time between an infant and its primary caregiver(s), due to which prolonged separation from the caregiver results in with stress and sorrow. It therefore describes the special affective/emotional relationship normally observed between an infant and its primary caregivers, and which is thought to act as a prototype for all later relationships.

Phases of attachment

The development of attachment is generally divided into four phases:

- **The pre-attachment phase (birth–3 months):** around 4–6 weeks of age the infant develops a preference for other human beings over physical aspects of the environment, demonstrated by behaviours such as nestling, gurgling, and the social smile. Such behaviours are not reserved for a primary caregiver and will be directed at almost anyone
- **The indiscriminate attachment phase (3–7 months):** the infant starts to discriminate between familiar and unfamiliar people, and will smile and respond more to the familiar. They will, however, still allow strangers to hold them without undue distress, as long as they are reasonably caring
- **The discriminate attachment phase (around 7–9 months):** during this phase the infant starts to develop specific attachments. They actively try to stay close to particular people (especially, but not restricted to, the mother), and become distressed when attempts are made to separate them from these 'attachment figures'. This is probably related to the development of object permanence, the ability to hold the primary caregiver in mind even when she is not there and to reliably and consistently distinguish her from others. There is often a strong fear of strangers at this point
- **The multiple attachments phase (9 months onwards):** from this time onwards additional strong emotional ties are made with other major caregivers (e.g. fathers, grandparents and siblings) and with non-caregivers, including other children. The fear of strangers reduces, but the strongest attachment usually remains with the mother.

Theories of attachment

Initial *psychoanalytic and behavioural theories of attachment* emphasized the importance of the caregiver's (usually the mother) role in fulfilling the instinctual needs of the child. These are often referred to as 'cupboard love' theories. Their validity was challenged by a series of experiments conducted by Harlow in the 1950s in which new-born monkeys were separated from their mothers and brought up in relative isolation in individual cages. The cages contained a baby blanket to which the baby monkeys became strongly attached. Separation of these monkeys from their blankets provoked a similar response to that seen when monkeys reared with their mother were then separated from her. The cloth surrogate was also noted to become a 'secure base' from which the infant would explore its environment. Further studies demonstrated that the young monkey prefers the company of a cuddly surrogate mother with no food to a wire surrogate with a bottle.

These findings suggest that the development of attachment is not only about getting nourishment. In a study of Scottish infants Schaffer and Emerson found that the development of a secure attachment was dependent not only on the provision of food, but also on the caregiver being responsive to the infant's behaviours and providing an adequate amount of stimulation by talking, touching and playing with the infant.

Ethological theories of attachment suggest that the infant and the caregiver 'trigger' instinctual social behaviours in the other and therefore develop attachment relationships with each other. The goal of this attachment is to protect the infant from the inevitable dangers that they will encounter and therefore promote survival of the species.

The most comprehensive theory of human attachment was that described by *John Bowlby* in the late 1960s and early 1970s. His initial ideas focused on a single attachment relationship between infant and mother, which he termed monotropy, were heavily criticized and were later retracted. There were, however, several major strengths to his work. In particular, Bowlby developed his thinking from well described empirical observations of children in defined situations. These observations led him to propose three distinct emotional periods on separation from the mother: *protest*, *despair*, and *detachment*. Thus, if a separation between a child and its' mother were prolonged, the child would be seen to become increasingly self-centred, and whilst remaining generally sociable, he/she often seemed to have lost the focus of any deep attachment. Bowlby's work has had many positive effects on how children are cared for, and he was responsible for the move away from large institutions in favour of fostering, adoption, and continuity of carers.

Attachment: research and impact

Research on attachment

Much of the empirical work on attachment has used the *Strange Situation*, devised by Mary Ainsworth in the late 1960s. The Strange Situation consists of 8 separate brief episodes during which a child is placed in several situations in a room accompanied either by the mother, a stranger, both adults, or on their own. Depending on their behaviour in the strange situations children are categorized as having differing qualities of attachment (📖 Table 3.2).

Table 3.2 Types of behaviours seen in 1-year-olds using the Strange Situation

Category	Name	Sample (%)
Type A	Anxious-avoidant	15
Typical behaviour: seeks little contact with mother, randomly angry with her, unresponsive to being held, but often upset when put down		
Type B	Securely attached	70
Typical behaviour: readily explores, using mother as a secure base. Cries infrequently. Easily put down after being held. Confident		
Type C	Anxious-resistant	15
Typical behaviour: cries a lot, is clingy and demanding, upset by small separations, chronically anxious in relation to mother, limited in exploration		

Attachment can also be measured in adults, using the adult attachment interview, a semi-structured interview designed to elicit a subject's recollections about their relationships with their parents and other attachment figures during childhood. The interviewer asks about childhood experiences with parents, significant separations and losses during childhood, and the current state of the child–parent relationship. Scoring of the interview is based on:

- Descriptions of childhood experiences
- The language used to describe past experiences
- The ability to give an integrated, coherent, believable account of experiences and their meaning.

The impact of early attachment on later development

There is growing evidence to suggest that our early attachment experiences create a set of expectations and ideas (an internal working model) that we then bring with us into other relationships, both with peers and other adults.

Several generalizations can be made:

- Securely attached babies tend to be better adjusted as children
- Babies with anxious-resistant attachments are less competent in preschool, have more problems with peers, and are less well liked by teachers
- Anxious-avoidant babies differ the most from secure babies in preschool. They tend to be highly dependent, non-compliant, and poorly skilled in social interactions with peers. They are often described by teachers as hostile, impulsive, quick to give up, and withdrawn
- These differences can be reasonably stable over time, such that adults who experienced attachment difficulties as babies may still find it more difficult to trust others in relationships, etc.
- This stability is, however, not inevitable and studies have clearly demonstrated that the effects of early privation can be reversible
- As temperament and attachment can interact with each other, it is preferable to assess both and address these interactions before making a formulation on a particular child.

Temperament: definition, course, and studies

Definition

Temperamental traits can be seen as inherent, constitutionally-based characteristics that constitute the core of personality and influence directions for development.

- A reasonable working definition of temperament is 'the constitutionally based individual differences in emotional, motor and attentional reactivity and self regulation'
- As used here, the term *constitutional* stresses the biological basis of temperament, which is influenced by genetic inheritance, maturation and experience.

Course of development

Temperamental characteristics demonstrate consistency across situations as well as relative stability over time. However, an individual's temperamental characteristics do change over time—and the outcomes of temperamental traits depend strongly on developmental processes, experience and social context.

- A given set of temperamental characteristics provides multiple possibilities for developmental outcomes
- Different trajectories and outcomes may occur for children with similar temperamental traits, and children differing in temperament may come to similar developmental outcomes via different pathways
- However, the possession of any particular temperamental characteristic will often impact on the probability of any particular outcome occurring. For example, the quiet withdrawn toddler is less likely to develop into an exuberant and very outgoing adolescent (but it can happen).

Early studies of temperament

The most important early contribution to the study of temperament was the New York Longitudinal Study (NYLS)—the first paper from which was published in 1963. Inspired by the differences among their own children, Chess and Thomas set out to study individual differences in what they called *the primary reaction pattern* for infants. They collected longitudinal interview data from parents throughout their child's development. Beginning when the initial sample was three to six months of age, parents were extensively interviewed about their infant's behaviour across a range of specific contexts. Each infant's reaction along with its context was then typed on a different sheet of paper and inductivity sorted into sets that came to represent the nine NYLS temperament dimensions.

These dimensions are:

- Activity level
- Approach/withdrawal
- Adaptability
- Mood
- Threshold
- Intensity
- Distractibility
- Rhythmicity
- Attention span/persistence.

Clusters of temperament were then identified that allowed children to be separated into groups. These included:

- **The 'easy child':** regular/rhythmic, adapts easily to change, mild to moderately intense mood that is usually positive
- **The 'difficult child':** irregular biological functions, doesn't adapt easily/respond well to change, intense mainly negative mood, doesn't persist, easily frustrated
- **The 'slow to warm up child':** mildly intense, negative responses to new stimuli, adapts slowly to repeated exposure. Often shy and needs time and support to adjust.

Later studies of temperament

More recent research on temperament has suggested that several of the nine NYLS dimensions are not independent and overlap somewhat, and it is now agreed that the description of temperamental characteristics can be reduced into fewer categories. The precise number remains under discussion and may well vary across development such that the younger the child the fewer the required domains. The six most frequently described domains are:

- **Fearful distress**, including adaptability, withdrawal and distress to new situations
- **Irritable distress** including irritability, fussiness, distress at limitations, and anger frustration
- **Positive affect**, including the measures smiling and laughter, agreeableness, and co-operation manageability
- **Activity level**, reflecting how active the child is
- **Attention span/task persistence**, including duration of orientating or interest
- **Rhythmicity**, including unpredictability, rhythmicity, and regularity.

Temperament: measurement and impact

Measuring temperament

Several approaches have been taken to measuring temperament in children including caregiver reports, self-reports for older children, naturalistic observations and structured laboratory observations by trained raters. Each method has its own relative advantages and disadvantages. For example, caregiver reports can tap the extensive knowledge base of caregivers who have seen the child in many different situations over a long period of time and are convenient. It is relatively inexpensive to develop, administer, and analyse questionnaires for this purpose. On the other hand, naturalistic observations can possess high degrees of objectivity and ecological validity and laboratory observations allow the researcher to precisely control the context or elicitors of the child's behaviour, but are much more expensive. Current opinion would suggest all methods are useful, should be retained and can be used together.

In addition to these more traditional measures of temperament psychobiological research strategies have also been used to measure temperament. A range of different biological approaches have been used including electrodermal responses, heart rate variability, and vagal tone.

Temperament and adjustment

One of the important reasons for studying temperament in relation to child and adolescent psychiatry is the idea that temperament concepts can help explain the origins of children's individual differences in adjustment. Although the amount of relevant evidence is not large in absolute terms, it is clear that temperament and adjustment do have an empirical relationship.

- Parent ratings of the temperament of children in the preadolescent to early adolescent era are correlated with teacher ratings of classroom adjustment
- Other studies have sought to test the predicative power of temperamental differences on a child's later behaviour. In the NYLS, difficult temperaments at an early age predicted behavioural problems in later life. Predictive correlations in these kinds of studies are modest to moderate in size and the correlations between infancy measures and adjustment in the late pre-school and middle childhood are smaller than the ones between pre-school or middle childhood, and later periods
- Although such predictive studies do not constitute proof that temperament shapes adjustment, they do provide evidence that temperamental characteristics are at least associated with later adjustment.

The development of self-concept

Definition

Self-concept refers to an individual's self awareness and the set of beliefs and attitudes that a person holds about themselves. In the psychological literature the terms 'self' and 'self-concept' are often used interchangeably. Many aspects of self-concept are unique to humans and higher-order primates as these are the only species that have the capacity to see themselves as both *subject* (e.g. 'I', the person looking in the mirror) and *object* (e.g. 'me', the person being looked at).

Components of the self-concept

Self-concept can be separated into three constituent parts:

- **Self-image:** this refers to the ways by which we describe ourselves or what we think we are like. Self-image, in turn, can be subdivided into three sub-domains:
  - *Social roles:* the objective, factual aspects of self-image (e.g. son, brother, parent, friend, boss, student, etc.)
  - *Personality traits:* the more subjective aspects of self, what we think we are like (e.g. reliable, happy, generous, moody, stupid etc.)
  - *Physical characteristics:* e.g. short, tall, fat, thin, blue eyed, brown skinned, etc. These are also part of our body image/bodily self, which also includes bodily sensations, such as cold, hunger, and pain
- **Self-esteem:** this is an evaluative, rather than descriptive term and refers to our feelings of self-worth. Self-esteem can refer to a single overall judgment or can relate to one or more particular areas of one's work (e.g. I am really happy with how hard I am trying at work, but I still feel really inferior to my colleagues). The values attached to different attributes will differ depending on age, culture, gender, social background, etc.
- **Ideal self:** the kind of person we would like to be. Self-esteem will, to a degree, be dependent on the similarities and differences between self-image and ideal self.

Self-schemata

We organize and store this complex information about ourselves in a series of self schemata. However, the complexity and completeness of each schematic will be dependent on the importance of that particular domain to the individual. Most people have a complex self-concept and, therefore, have a large number of well organized self-schemata. These include not only schemata relating to the current self-image, but also those relating to a future possible or wished-for self, which relate to the ideal self. This concept of multiple selves raises the question as to whether any one self is more relevant or real than the others. Whilst social psychologists are comfortable with this notion of multiple selves, personality theorists are less so and have tended to assume that there is a single unitary self.

Theories of self

Symbolic interactionism

Symbolic interactionism stresses the importance of social interactions. It is suggested that because we share common language and are able to think symbolically we can, in principle, see the world not only through our own eyes, but also through those of others. Further it is argued that it is through taking on the roles of others that our sense of self develops. As the theory developed the concept of self-interaction was introduced, stressing the importance of self-talk, self-reflection, and role-taking in the development of the self.

Social constructionist approaches to self-concept

Social constructivists emphasize our tendency to talk about ourselves differently depending on who we are talking with. They suggest that by selecting what to and what not to say we are constantly and actively constructing a self. Self is therefore seen as an ever changing process and one that is dependent on language.

The development of self-concept

The development of an identity is one of the key tasks facing us all. Whilst the development of self clearly starts very early in life it is a continuing life-long process and not one restricted to childhood.

During the first few months of life an infant starts to become able to distinguish itself from its environment, and from other people, and establishes a continuity of self across time. These capabilities are, however, shared by other species, and it is not until the child becomes aware of their own existence and uniqueness that true human self-concept can be said to have developed. Early suggestions of these abilities include the infant's ability to associate the sight of their limbs moving with the associated physical sensations and the sound of their cries with the act of crying.

From here onwards self-concept appears to develop in a predictable pattern over time and throughout life.

- Self-recognition (e.g. of yourself in a mirror) appears at around 18 months
- Autobiographical memory (the ability to recognize that memories constitute a history of the self up until now), the ability to have a concept of a private 'thinking' self and to have a 'theory of mind' (awareness that others have their own thoughts independent of your own) appear to develop around the age of 3½ or 4 years of age
- As the child grows and moves into middle childhood and adolescence the self-concept changes from being described in physical terms to being described from a psychological perspective.

Cognitive development

Definition

Cognitive development describes the way a child learns and learns to think. How one believes this occurs is dependent on which of the many theoretical views of development you give greatest weight to. Whilst several of the previously dominant theoretical approaches remain helpful, many of their fundamental tenets have been challenged and it is generally accepted that none of them provide a complete account of cognitive development.

Theories of cognitive development

Piaget's theory

Central to Piaget's theory was his view of intelligence as adaptation to the environment. He proposed that a young child's intelligence is qualitatively different to that of an older child and was interested in the ways that changes occurred over time (*genetic epistemology*). Piaget proposed that cognitive development occurs through the interaction of innate capabilities and events. He contended that this development progressed through a series of universal, invariant hierarchical stages (📖 Table 3.3).

Table 3.3 Piaget's stages of cognitive development

Stage	Approximate age
Sensorimotor	0–2 years
Typical behaviours: infants learn primarily through their senses and by interacting with objects. Frequent interaction results in the development of object permanence. By the end of this stage there is evidence of the *general symbolic function* including self-recognition, symbolic thought such as language, deferred imitation, and make-believe play	
Pre-operational	2–7 years
Typical behaviours: increased use of internal images, symbols and language; however, thinking continues to be dominated by the look of things, rather than by logical principles or operations. Pre-operational children are egocentric and demonstrate *syncreatic thought* (the tendency to link objects based on what individual instances have in common e.g. ▲→■→■→■→▲), *transductive reasoning* (drawing an inference based on a single shared attribute, e.g. if humans and birds both have two legs, humans must be birds), *centration* (only able to focus on one attribute at a time, e.g. can divide sweets by size or colour, but not size and colour), and *animism* (the belief that inanimate objects are alive)	
Concrete operational	7–11 years
Typical behaviours: logical operations can be performed, *but* only in the presence of actual or observable objects. There is a decline in egocentricity and increasing relativism	
Formal operational	11 years onwards
Typical behaviours: can manipulate ideas and propositions ('second order operations', think hypothetically and display hypothetico-deductive reasoning)	

Whilst Piaget's theories have been hugely influential they have also been challenged on many levels. In particular, children have been shown to be able to perform many tasks earlier than Piaget predicted, as long as the task that is used is designed to be appropriate to the child's developmental level. On the other hand, as many as 2/3rds of adolescents and adults do not appear to achieve formal operational thinking, which itself, does not appear to represent the typical mode of adult thought in many cultures.

Vygotsky's theory

Whereas Piaget emphasized the 'child scientist' Vygotsky saw the child more as an 'apprentice' who learns to think and problem solve through interactions with its parents. Parents provide the *scaffolding* for the child who acquires skills and knowledge through a process of *graded collaboration*. It is suggested that the parent can therefore best help the child learn by giving initial general instruction and then switching to more specific instruction if the child is struggling. The *zone of proximal development* defines those skills and cognitive functions that have started to develop, but which are still in the process of becoming fully mature.

Bruner's theory

Bruner was influenced by both Piaget, with whom he agreed that abstract thinking grows out of action, and Vygotsky in emphasizing the importance of language, interpersonal communication and the role of adults in helping the child develop. Bruner proposed three *modes of representation*; the initial *enactive* mode (representing the world through actions), the subsequent *iconic* mode (building up mental images of things we have experienced) and the *symbolic* mode (whereby language itself becomes an influence on thought allowing the child to 'go beyond the information given'). For Bruner the most important shift is from iconic to symbolic, which occurs at around the age of 6–7 years.

Information processing approaches

Information processing theorists believe that there are psychological structures in the mind that explain behaviour, and that are independent of both social relationships and cultural environment. We solve problems by using a series of component tasks. Information from a stimulus, for example, is attended to, perceived, and encoded. It is then held in working memory, where it may or may not be manipulated. This information is then compared to or combined with other information held in memory, plans for a response are made, a response is selected, and then actioned. Self-monitoring is essential for these processes to become increasingly efficient and there is evidence that the degree of self-monitoring increases greatly at school age. Many of the more complex processes in this chain are considered to form the *executive functions* (sometimes described as the conductor of the brain's orchestra). Recent evidence suggests that the executive functions, many of which are dependent on intact pre-frontal cortical functioning, continue to develop through adolescence and in to early adulthood. Executive functioning deficits have been associated with many psychiatric disorders including schizophrenia, depression, attention deficit hyperactivity disorder (ADHD), and autism.

Moral development

Definition

Moral development is defined as the development of our understanding of the rules and principles that distinguish right from wrong.

Theories of morality

Freud's psychoanalytic theory

This theory focuses on the affective components of morality and, in particular, the tensions between guilt and moral anxiety, on the one hand, and pride or self-esteem, on the other. According to Freud our *psychic apparatus* consists of the *id* (governed by the *pleasure principle*), *ego* (governed by the *reality principle*) the *superego*, which itself comprises the conscience (the 'punishing parent') and the ego-ideal (the 'rewarding parent'). Freud proposed that it is only after the development of the superego, which represents the internalization of parental and social moral values that we can truly be described as moral beings. For boys this is represented by the end of the Oedipus complex at which point he identifies with his father ('the aggressor'). For girls the picture is less clear, but Freud suggested that due to her fear of losing the mother's love and a need to keep the mother 'alive' inside her she internalizes her becoming the 'good' child her mother would want (*anaclitic identification*).

Cognitive-developmental approaches

Piaget

Piaget noted that as they get older, children start to co-operate to a greater degree and with greater mutual respect. They start to participate as equals in the administering and following of the rules of a game and start to take a particular interest in the rules themselves. Piaget called the morality of younger children *heteronomous* (subject to the rules of others) and that of older children *autonomous* (subject to their own rules). He believed that the shift occurred as a consequence of the transition from egocentric to operational thinking, which occurs at about 7 years. The 2-year lag between this and the shift in morality is explained by the requirement of an additional shift from *unilateral respect* (unconditional obedience to parents/adults) to *mutual respect* (disagreements between equals can be resolved by negotiation with each other). Although it is now believed that children's understanding of intention is much more complex than Piaget suggested, his age trends have stood both the test of time and cross-cultural investigation.

Kohlberg

Kohlberg studied a group of boys between the ages of 10 and 16 years, with initial in depth interviews and 3 yearly follow-ups. He investigated moral reasoning by eliciting their responses to a series of 'moral dilemmas'. From their responses he defined 6 stages of moral development, spanning 3 basic levels of moral reasoning (Table 3.4).

Table 3.4 Kohlberg's six stages of moral development

Level 1 Preconventional morality	(Middle childhood)
Stage 1	Punishment and obedience orientation

Typical behaviours: rules are kept in order so that punishments may be avoided. The consequences of an action determine whether it was good or bad. Others' points of view are not considered

Stage 2	Instrumental relativist orientation

Typical behaviours: the 'right' action is one favourable to oneself but some consideration is given to the needs of others and fairness

Level 2 Conventional morality	(13–16 years)
Stage 3	Interpersonal concordance or 'good boy–nice girl' orientation

Typical behaviours: able to put oneself in another's shoes. Able to value the intentions of others as well as socially accepted standards. Being moral is being good in your eyes *and* those of others

Stage 4	Maintaining the social order orientation

Typical behaviours: a respect for authority and maintaining the social order for its own sake and society must be protected. Laws are unquestionably accepted and obeyed

Level 3 Post-conventional morality	10–15% adults are at stage 5, stage 6 is rare
Stage 5	Social contract–legalistic orientation

Typical behaviours: laws are established by mutual agreement and can also be changed by the same process. Individual rights can over ride laws of society in certain situations. Life is more sacred than the law so the law should not be accepted at all costs

Stage 6	Universal ethical principles orientation

Typical behaviours: moral action is determined by our own inner conscience operating in concordance with certain universal moral principles. Society's rules are arbitrary and may be broken when they conflict with universal moral principles

Eisenberg
Eisenberg was less concerned with misdeeds and more concerned with prosocial behaviour. Many of the predictions derived from her theory have been supported. She used stories that involved the subject making a choice between self-interest and helping another person. She found that pre-school children were concerned with the implications of choices themselves, rather than with moral conscience (*hedonistic reasoning*). Gradually, as a child develops, concern is given to others, even if this conflicts with self-interest. Initially, this occurs without any clear evidence of self-reflection, however, as the child develops they start to use stereotyped images of good and bad to justify behaviour ('it is good to help') and later demonstrate clear self-reflection, sympathetic responding, and role taking. At the highest level internalized values are more strongly stated e.g. 'she would help out because it would benefit society'.

Social learning approaches (e.g. Bandura)

The social learning theorists attempted to reinterpret certain aspects of Freud's psychoanalytic theories in terms of classical and operant conditioning. Many of their experiments concerned aggression and investigated the individual's ability to behave in a moral way, or refrain from violating moral rules in conditions of temptation, even when there was no one else there. Their subjects observed a model who behaved in a particular (often aggressive) way. They observed that the learner's behaviours were modified even where no rewards are given. Whether or not the subjects imitated the models behaviour was, to a degree, dependent on the consequences of the behaviour both for the model and the learner. Reward was only important in that it affected performance (but not the learning). In reality, social learning theory is not a developmental theory as it does not account for possible changes due to development, rather than learning. Bandura later proposed that as a child develops they also learn how to self-reinforce and self-monitor, which is the social learning approach's equivalent of the super-ego. This comes to represent an internalized societal standard and can result in mature moral behaviour.

Peer relationships

The development of peer relationships

Children seem to be interested in their peers from an early age. In one study, two 12–18-month-old infants (accompanied by their mothers) who were sharing a playroom with each other spent much of the time in close proximity to their mothers frequently touching them, but also spent more time looking at each other than they did looking at either their own or the other child's mother.

Although this suggests at least some interest in peers at this age it is not until around 2–3 years of age that children really start to develop a competence in acting socially with their peers. By this age, which often coincides with entry into nursery school–there is a sharp increase in social skills.

At this age children at play tend to behave in a range of different ways. They can be 'unoccupied', an 'onlooker' or if engaged in play can be 'solitary', in 'parallel' activity with others (playing alongside, but not with others) or in 'associative' (interacting by doing similar things) or 'co-operative' (acting together in complementary ways) play. The first four types of play decrease as the child develops whist associative and co-operative play increase with age. Most research has reduced these types of play down to three—'solitary', 'parallel', and 'group'. Preschool children in free-play typically spend equal amounts of time in each type of play with the balance shifting towards group play as they get older. The size of the groups generally starts at 2–3 children and increases in older preschoolers. These trends continue in the early and middle school years with group size continuing to increase, especially for boys, as they start to get interested in team games such as football. Groups tend to be rigidly split along gender lines until mid adolescence. By the ages of 10–11 boys are tending to play in large mixed age groups whilst girls are in smaller same age groups. In adolescence there are further changes with the formation of large same sex 'cliques' or 'gangs', which again change as heterosexual relationships become more important in later adolescence. In late adolescence, we see 'crowds' that comprise groupings of several interacting cliques. Young people then tend to shift towards couples which are loosely associated with other couples.

Types of peer relationships

Different children have different types of predominant peer relationships each of which is associated with different characteristics.

Popular children

Popular children have good interpersonal skills, are low in aggression, and are not withdrawn. Popularity may be affected by the type of peer group one is in. It may be difficult to be popular if you differ in some salient way, e.g. ethnicity, intelligence, interests from most of the others in the group. Physical attractiveness is also a predictor of popularity.

Rejected children

This group has been studied more than the others. Being a rejected child is a fairly stable characteristic such that 30% of children rejected at one point in time continue to be rejected 4 years later, whilst another 30% were 'neglected' at this second time point (📖 below). By contrast those who were 'neglected' at the start tended to be 'average' at 4 years. Rejected children spend less time in co-operative play and social conversation, and more time fighting and arguing. They tend to play in smaller groups, and with younger or less popular companions. There are at least two subtypes of rejected children; 'rejected-aggressive', and the less common 'rejected-submissive'.

Controversial children

Children in this group tend to be somewhat aggressive, but not clearly disliked. They can be highly socially skilled and highly aggressive, and often use aggressiveness to gain status in the peer group.

Neglected children

Much less is known about this group. Although it is often assumed that they should be lonely this is not what they say when asked. They do however seem to be low on sociability and there is a degree of social withdrawal. It has been argued that this may arise from a combination of a type C (anxious-resistant/ambivalent) attachment status and high behavioural inhibition as a temperamental trait. Over-protective or over-solicitous parenting may also play a part.

Friendships

A friendship is usually defined as a close relationship between two people as indexed by their association together, their psychological attachment or their mutual trust. Whilst friendships and peer relationships are associated they are not synonymous with each other. It is, for example, common for a rejected child to still have one close friendship. The relationships between friends are characterized by their tendency to exhibit four particular features not seen in non-friend relationships:

- Reciprocity and intimacy
- More intense social activity
- More frequent conflict resolution
- More effective task performance.

Children themselves define friendships differently at different ages. Whilst there are several different descriptions of these changes, most share a common thread. Bigelow and La Gaipa asked 480 Scottish and 480 Canadian children to write essays on best friends and extracted several common stages (📖 Table 3.5).

Table 3.5 Stages of understanding friendship

Reward-cost stage	Around 7–8 years
Shared common activities, living nearby, similar expectations	
Normative stage	Around 9–10 years
Shared values, rules and sanctions	
Empathic stage	Around 11–12 years
Understanding, self-disclosure, shared interests	

Adolescence: definitions and tasks

Whilst adolescence was traditionally seen as the period of transition between childhood and adulthood, it is today more often considered to be a time of multiple transitions. The age of onset of puberty, often seen as the start of adolescence, has come down over time. In addition, adolescents have experienced a greater degree of self-determination, at an earlier age, in recent years. This increased freedom has brought increased risks of teenage pregnancy, sexually transmitted disease, homelessness, and substance misuse. Whilst some aspects of adolescence occur earlier now than they did in the past, the termination of adolescence has also been delayed with, for example, marriage taking place 6 or 7 years later and increased opportunities to delay earning an income by taking further education courses.

Developmental tasks of adolescence

There are a wide range of tasks, which need to be addressed for the young person to successfully negotiate adolescence. They must:
- Adjust to a new physical sense of self
- Adjust to new intellectual abilities
- Adjust to increased cognitive demands at school
- Develop expanded verbal skills
- Develop a personal sense of identity
- Establish adult vocational goals
- Establish emotional and psychological independence from their parents
- Develop stable and productive peer relationships
- Adopt a personal value system
- Develop increased impulse control and behavioural maturity.

It is important to recognize that adolescents do not move through these tasks separately and that, therefore, a young person is likely to be dealing with several of them at any given time.

Puberty and body image

The bodily changes seen in adolescence are, to a large degree, related to the onset of puberty. At no other time since birth does an individual undergo such rapid and profound physical changes. Puberty is marked by sudden rapid growth in height and weight. Also, the young person experiences the emergence and accentuation of those physical traits that make him/her a male or female. After puberty the young person looks less like a child, and more like a physically and sexually mature adult. The effect of this rapid change is that the young adolescent often becomes focused on his or her body. Whilst all adolescents experience the same bodily changes, the sequence of these changes varies considerable within individuals. Also the timing of onset varies greatly. In general, puberty seems to be a more difficult change for girls than for boys. This is related to the subjective meaning and socio-cultural significance of puberty. Thus, puberty brings boys closer to their physical ideal (increased muscle mass and lung capacity → greater strength and stamina), whilst girls move further from theirs (increase in body fat with rapid weight gain, menstruation).

The timing of puberty is also important. Girls, on average, enter puberty 2 years earlier than boys. An early onset of puberty is likely to be advantageous for boys and disadvantageous for girls, whilst the opposite is likely to be true for delayed onset puberty, which will disadvantage boys.

Adolescence: theories of adolescent development

Hall's theory: adolescence as storm and stress

This early theory of adolescence argued that each person's psychological development recapitulates the biological and cultural evolution of the human species. Adolescence is characterized as a period of storm and stress mirroring the volatile history of the human race over the last 2000 years. Evidence used in support of this hypothesis includes:

- The presence of intense and volatile emotional reactions during adolescence
- A perceived increase in psychiatric symptoms in those (particularly girls) with early onset adolescence
- An increase in delinquent behaviour seen in early maturing girls.

There are, however, many caveats and exceptions to these findings.

Erikson's theory: identity crisis

Erikson proposed that development progressed through a genetically pre-determined sequence of psychosocial stages, each of which is character-ized by a struggle between two conflicting outcomes - one positive and the other negative. Healthy development is dependent on the conflict being resolved in favour of the healthy outcome. In adolescence the main challenge is that of forming a stable sense of personal identity. In many tra-ditional cultures there are clear rites of passage into adulthood; however, in Western societies these processes have been withdrawn in order to allow a young person to take time to make appropriate adjustments. Whilst there are many benefits in this, it can also make transition more dif-ficult, as it places the responsibility firmly with the young person to create their own identity. Erikson initially coined the term *identity crisis* to account for the loss of identity experienced by some soldiers as a result of combat experience. He extended it to include those 'severely conflicted young people whose sense of confusion is due ... to a war within themselves'.

Erikson also used the term *role confusion* to describe a failure to inte-grate the self into a coherent whole. He said that role confusion would result in problems with:

- **Intimacy**, with a fear to commit to a close relationship
- **Time perspective**, with difficulties in planning for the future
- **Industry**, with a young person experiencing difficulties in channelling them self into work
- **Negative identity**, with the young person engaging in delinquent behaviours.

Marcia's theory: identity statuses

Marcia extended Erikson's work by proposing four statuses of adolescent identity formation. He suggested that the formation of a mature identity is dependent on the individual successfully negotiating several *crises* and arriving at a *commitment* in the choices made. The four statuses are:

- **Diffusion/confusion:** the least mature status, whereby the individual has not started to think about issues seriously or formulated any goals
- **Foreclosure:** the individual has avoided the anxieties and stresses involved in dealing with the crises by prematurely committing themselves to a safe 'adult' role. As no alternative paths have been explored the result is a rather shallow and fragile identity
- **Moratorium:** the individual is actively searching for solutions to the crises. Several different approaches will be tried
- **Identity achievement:** the individual has successfully managed their crises and has made commitments towards a future with clear goals and a strong personal identity.

Sociological approaches to adolescence

Sociologists have emphasized the importance of *role change* in adolescent development. Such changes include the move from primary to secondary school, from secondary to college or university, moving into work, etc., all of which require a change of peer group and expectations. There is also a shift from a reliance on adults to one on peers for support and advice. This introduces the *generation gap*. Relationships with parents have to be renegotiated from child–parent to young adult–parent. Whilst the difficulties in adolescent–parent relationships are often highlighted, in both the social sciences and the popular media, most evidence suggests that adolescents generally report positive changes in their relationships with their parents. Indeed, sociologists emphasize that most adolescents do very well and point out that the previous theories tended to address problematic issues which are faced by only a small minority of young people.

Coleman's *focal theory* proposes that most adolescents are able to cope with the stresses of adolescence by managing them one issue at a time and by being allowed to spin this process out over a number of years. Those who attempt to address more than one issue at a time are the ones who would be predicted to experience the greatest difficulties. It has also been suggested that problems are more likely for those where important changes (such as puberty) occur too early in life, happen more suddenly than expected or occur at the same time. These young people will require greater support to manage their transitions.

Brain development

The human brain continues develop during childhood, adolescence and into early adulthood. Although our understanding of the relationships between brain development and behaviour is still somewhat limited, it is clear that this continuing developmental process places various constraints on an individual's performance. It is therefore essential that psychological development is seen within the context of brain development.

Key events in brain development

The development of the nervous system is complex, and involves several coordinated and synchronized processes, which occur both pre- and postnatally.

- The first key event is the formation of the neural tube which is complete by week 4 of gestation. The neural tube is a specialized fold of ectodermal tissues, which forms the basis of all neural development
- Between 4–12 weeks the neural tube differentiates into several components with the forebrain at one end and the spinal cord at the other
- The hollow centre of the tube in the region that will become the brain will itself become the ventricles
- There are proliferative regions around these ventricular areas from which, between 12 and 20 weeks, neurons multiply and migrate along a scaffolding of glial cells to the cortical regions
- Following this migration there is a period of rapid programmed cell death, which reduces the number of neurons by 50% between week 24 of gestation and week 4 postnatally
- Neurons are initially un-myelinated and myelination starts at about 29 weeks. Initial myelination takes place in the brain stem and proceeds, thereafter, in an organized pattern moving from posterior to anterior and inferior to superior. Also proximal pathways myelinate before distal, sensory before motor and projection fibres before association fibres. Whilst most myelination occurs during early childhood several areas including the cortical axons continue to myelinate into the second and third decades of life
- A further important process is the proliferation and organization of synapses (synaptogenesis). This begins around the 20th week of gestation with synaptic density continuing to increase rapidly after birth. At 2 years of age the brain has around 50% more synapses than in adulthood
- Synaptogenesis is followed by a regionally specific elimination of connections. This again occurs at different rates in different brain regions, e.g. it is complete for the visual cortex by 4 months after birth, but does not peak in the prefrontal cortex until 4 years of age. The net effect of these changes is a rapid growth in the brain in the first 2 years of life at the end of which time it is 80% of its adult weight and by age 5 years it has reached 90%. However, recent studies have emphasized that there continues to be a high level of remodelling of both grey and white matter into the third decade of life.

National Institute of Mental Health (NIMH) paediatric brain imaging project

This project set out to map the developmental trajectories of brain development. Sequential brain magnetic resonance imaging (MRI) brain scans were taken from a large number (around 1000) of healthy subjects and a similar number of children from different diagnostic groups. Scans were taken every 2 years and there is now published data covering the age range 5–22 years. Whilst brain size differences must not be interpreted as imparting any direct functional advantage or disadvantage they do suggest the timings of developmental changes and highlight areas where development is continuing. The NIMH group have described the total and regional changes in brain volume over time. Key findings include:

- Total cerebral volume peaks at 14.5 years in males and 11.5 in females with the brain being 95% of this peak by 6 years
- Male brains are approximately 9% larger than female brains
- Lateral ventricular volume continues to increase across the age span
- Cortical grey matter volume follows an inverted U developmental course. The volume, however, peaks at different times in different regions, e.g. for boys the frontal lobe grey matter peaks at 12.1 years and the temporal lobe at 16.2 years. When mapped in more detail there are distinct patterns of development seen within these specific brain regions. For example, the dorsolateral prefrontal cortex (important for impulse control and decision making) is particularly late to reach adult thickness
- There are gender specific differences in the amygdala and hippocampus grey matter with amygdala volume only increasing with age in males and hippocampal volume only increasing in females
- In contrast to the grey matter, white matter volume increases throughout childhood and adolescence (indeed, reports from other groups suggest it does not decrease until the fourth decade of life)
- Underlying all of these findings is a very high level of inter subject variability.

There are still many unanswered questions regarding human brain development, however, increasingly sophisticated neuro-imaging and electrophysiological techniques are likely to continue to present new opportunities and advances in the future.

Recommended reading

Bjorklund DF (2005) *Children's Thinking*. Wadsworth/Thomson Learning, Belmont.

Damon W, Lerner RM. (2008) *Child and Adolescent Development: An Advanced Course*. John Wiley & Sons, Hoboken.

Giedd JN (2004) Structural magnetic resonance imaging of the adolescent brain. *Ann NY Acad Sci* **1021**: 77–85.

Giedd JN, Blumenthal J, Jeffries NO, Castellanos FX, Liu H, Zijdenbos A, Paus T, Evans AC, Rapoport JL. (1999) Brain development during childhood and adolescence: a longitudinal MRI study. *Nat. Neurosci.* **2**: 861–3.

Smith PK, Cowie H, Blades M. (2003) *Understanding Children's Development*. Blackwell Publishing, Maldon.

Abnormalities of child development

Psychiatric aspects of premature birth

Premature birth is associated with a number of risk factors for physical health problems, which can have a direct or indirect effect on mental health. Very preterm birth (before 33 weeks' gestation) is significantly associated with psychiatric morbidity.

Aetiology

Physical effects

Premature birth carries a significantly increased risk of developing neurological damage and subsequent chronic physical illness.

- Chronic physical illness increases the risk for mental health problems by a factor of two
- The presence of chronic neurological disorders increases the risk for mental health problems by a factor of five.

Psychological effects

The attachment process may be disrupted depending on severity of complications, and the length of separation between mother and child due to protracted admission to a special care baby unit.

Parental mental health

Increased rates of anxiety, depression, and post-traumatic stress disorder (PTSD) have been reported in parents following premature birth. Parental mental health problems are associated with an increased incidence of mental health difficulties in children and adolescents.

Maternal stress and anxiety, and drug, alcohol and cigarettes use during pregnancy increase the risk for premature birth and have also been associated with increased risk of child psychiatric problems.

Specific difficulties and disorders associated with prematurity

Childhood

- Lower IQ
- Developmental disabilities, learning difficulties
- Sensory and co-ordination difficulties
- Communication difficulties and peer relationship problems
- Behaviour problems
- Increased incidence of attention deficit hyperactivity disorder (ADHD).

Adolescence

- Lower mood and lower self-esteem
- Increased risk of depression in adolescence
- Anxiety.

Attachment disorders

Definition of attachment disorders

The key features of attachment disorders are a pattern of abnormal social functioning that is apparent during first 5 years of life and is associated with a significant disturbance in emotional functioning. These patterns persist into later childhood and adolescence in spite of changes in the child or young person's environment. Two patterns of attachment disorders are described.

Disinhibited attachment disorder (ICD-10 and DSM-IV)

It is hypothesized that children with attachment disorders have not developed appropriate attachment behaviour. Disinhibited attachment disorder is associated with an 'institutional' style of care in early life, with care being provided by a number carers and the absence of a specific primary care giver. Opportunities to form social relationships do not appear to compensate for the absence of a primary care giver. Developing a good relationship with a carer in later childhood does not appear to decrease indiscriminate approaches to strangers.

These children show an indiscriminate sociability or apparent friendly approaches to strangers, which is seen both in the presence and the absence of the primary care giver. There is an abnormal quality to these interactions in that there is a lack of reciprocity and that they do not appear to meet the child's emotional needs.

The approach of a stranger does not trigger normal attachment behaviour (i.e. seeking proximity to a trusted adult with a subsequent decrease in anxiety, and increase in focused and purposeful activity).

The incidence of disinhibited attachment disorder is not well characterized, but is relatively low in the general population. Significant rates of disinhibited attachment disorder are, however, reported in children raised in institutional care from birth.

Inhibited Attachment Disorder (DSM-IV) or Reactive Attachment Disorder (ICD-10)

These children fail to respond appropriately to social interactions, and display a fearfulness and hypervigilance that is not responsive to reassurance. Contradictory or ambivalent social responses may also be present.

Parental abuse, neglect, and severe maltreatment are highly significant aetiological factors. The severity and duration of abuse or neglect influences the severity of the disorder.

The prevalence of inhibited attachment disorder is low and not all children who experience significant abuse and neglect will develop an inhibited attachment disorder. The degree of risk is influenced by predisposing and protective genetic and environmental factors.

Course and prognosis

Children with attachment disorders have significant difficulties with interpersonal relationships, and are at greater risk of developing mental health problems in adolescence and adulthood. Duration of inadequate care is linked to outcome. Children who are placed with appropriate carers before age 2 have a better outcome.

Focus of assessment of attachment disorders

- The quality of social interactions
- The level and frequency of indiscriminate or inappropriate social interactions
- Pervasiveness of inappropriate interactions and behaviours across social settings
- Evidence of appropriate attachment behaviour
- Behaviour when distressed
- Structured assessments using narrative approaches may also be used, e.g. Manchester Attachment Assessment.

Interventions

The focus of interventions with this group of children is to ensure a secure nurturing care setting that provides consistent behavioural management and emotional responses.

Infants and young children often have the capacity to alter their behaviour in response to sensitive and emotionally responsive parenting. There is less evidence for significant change in older children.

Children with severe attachment disorders may require placement in a therapeutic residential unit.

Parents/carers may benefit from consultation using a psychodynamic framework facilitate understanding of the child's behaviour and facilitate change.

Children with co-morbid anxiety disorders or PTSD will benefit from appropriate psychological therapy. The benefit from individual psychotherapy for attachment disorders without co-morbid psychiatric disorders requires further research.

Differential diagnosis

- **Pervasive developmental disorders (PDD) or autistic spectrum disorder (ASD):** for a diagnosis of attachment disorder, children need to have had the capacity to develop normal social interactions and relationships, but failed to do so because of inadequate care in early life. Therefore, a diagnosis of PDD or ASD needs to be excluded
- **PTSD:** children who have experienced early single episode trauma may show signs of inhibited attachment disorder, hypervigilance and social withdrawal
- **ADHD:** impulsivity in social interactions may present as indiscriminate sociability
- **Anxiety disorders and selective mutism**.

Personality disorders

Definition

Diagnostic criteria for personality disorder require the person to be over 18 years of age. Diagnosis of a personality disorder requires there to be evidence of difficulties in interpersonal functioning, resulting in social impairment, which are not explained by mental illness and are persistent across time.

Personality development

Childhood temperamental traits that significantly impact on the development of adult personality include:
- Emotionality
- Activity
- Sociability
- Impulsivity.

Adult personality develops from temperament traits that are:
- Present from childhood
- Primarily genetically determined, but are modified by environmental influences and life experiences.

Adult personality disorders impact on interpersonal functioning in a wide range of ways including:
- Abnormal cognitions, perceptions, and interpretation of self, others, and events
- Unstable affect control with emotional lability and inappropriate emotional responses
- Poor impulse control
- A lack of empathy.

While it is inappropriate to diagnose personality disorders in children and adolescents, problems in these areas of functioning may often be identified, particularly in adolescents, and may be significant factors in the development of personality disorders.

Emerging personality disorder in children and adolescents

Due to the criterion that they may only be diagnosed over the age of 18 years, personality disorders have not been studied in any great depth in children and adolescents. There is, however, some literature describing the predisposing factors in childhood and adolescence for antisocial personality disorder, psychopathic personality disorder, and borderline personality disorder.

Antisocial personality disorder

Early onset conduct disorder has been linked with persistence of antisocial behaviour into adolescence and the development of antisocial personality disorder in adulthood. In adolescents with latter onset conduct disorder, antisocial behaviour tends to decrease with age and a significant number of these adolescents do not go develop antisocial personality disorder.

Psychopathic personality disorder

Psychopathic behaviour, lack of empathy, and callousness in childhood, which persists into adolescence, particularly when accompanied by low anxiety levels about poor quality of social relationships, is associated with the development of psychopathic personality disorder in adulthood.

Borderline personality disorder

Borderline personality disorder is associated with abuse, neglect, frequent changes in carer, and inconsistent intrusive parenting in childhood and adolescence.

Treatment

There is no available evidence for treatment of personality disorders in children and adolescents.

Prognosis

Diagnosis of personality disorders in adulthood is associated with continuing problems and an increased risk of co-morbid psychiatric disorders.

Gender identity disorders

Definition: gender identity disorder (ICD-10)

A child or adolescent needs to demonstrate:
- A persistent and intense distress about assigned sex
- A desire to be, or insistence that one is of, the opposite sex
- Persistent preoccupation with the dress and or activities of the opposite sex
- Rejection of their own sexual anatomy, usually in older children.

Symptoms need to be present before puberty for a diagnosis to be made. DSM-IV requires, in addition to the above criteria, that there is also evidence of significant impairment in functioning.

Epidemiology

The incidence is 1% prepubertal children with an average age of presentation of between 4 and 5 years of age.

Referral rates are higher for boys. It is unclear whether this reflects the true picture or is the consequence of a referral bias. As a result, there is more information available on gender identity disorders in males than females.

Aetiology

There is some early evidence for a biological basis with recent research focusing on possible subtle hormonal or immunological influences during pregnancy.

Social reinforcement of cross-gender behaviour in preschool children may also be a contributing factor.

Differential diagnosis

- Physical inter sex conditions
- Congenital adrenal hyperplasia, in genetic females
- Partial androgen insensitivity, in genetic males.

Treatment in childhood and adolescence

- Psychoeducation for parents and children about gender identity and roles is a key element of any intervention
- Behaviour modification is used to promote gender neutral and same sex activities and relationship in children. This approach is more effective in children than adolescents
- Individual therapy may be of benefit for children
- Adolescents may benefit from group therapy exploring issues of psychosocial and psychosexual roles and development
- Surgical and/or physical interventions are not generally indicated.

Outcome

The majority of gender identity disorders remit in later childhood or adolescence. Persistence of symptoms appears to be higher in those referred for assessment.

Outcome in adolescence

Gender identity disorders are associated with mental health problems, specifically emotional difficulties, low self-esteem, and peer relationship problems.

Outcome in adulthood

A significant number of males are bisexual or homosexual. A minority will continue to have persistent gender dysphoria.

Specific developmental disorders of speech and language

Normal speech development requires

- An ability to hear properly
- Receptive language skills, i.e. an ability to understand what has been said
- The cognitive ability to process information
- Expressive language skills, i.e. the ability to generate a verbal response at cortical level
- Articulation skills, i.e. the ability to put a response into words.

Skill deficits in any of these areas contribute to developmental disorders of speech and language.

Specific developmental disorders of speech and language

Specific speech articulation problem

- A specific problem in the oral-motor component in the production of speech sounds, for example, stammering, stuttering or cluttering
- There are no deficits in other social or language skills
- Anxiety is associated with a decrease in fluency of speech production.

Expressive language disorder

- A delay in the development of appropriate language production, in the presence of normal language comprehension skills
- The child demonstrates the desire to communicate and uses non-verbal communication strategies
- The child has good imagination, appropriate play skills, and engages in imaginary play.

Receptive language disorder

- A delay in understanding spoken language
- Usually associated with an expressive language delay
- The content and process of these children's thoughts are difficult to assess, and a diagnosis of ASD should be excluded.

Acquired aphasia with epilepsy (Landau–Kleffner syndrome)

- A rare condition with rapid deterioration in expressive language skills with the preservation of other cognitive skills
- Epilepsy may pre or post date language deterioration.

Assessment

Where there are concerns regarding a child's or adolescent's speech and language development, or verbal and non-verbal communication skills, a referral should be made to a speech and language therapist for assessment.

The assessment of speech and language disorders should include assessment of both hearing ability and global development.

Where speech and language development is in keeping with a child's overall developmental stage, a diagnosis of specific developmental disorder of speech is *not* appropriate.

Psychiatric co-morbidity

Children with speech and language disorders have increased incidence of:
- ADHD
- Oppositional defiant disorder (ODD)
- Conduct disorder (CD).

They are also at increased risk of developing emotional disorders secondary to peer relationship problems and bullying. Low self-esteem in adolescence is also common.

Differential diagnosis
- Deafness
- Global developmental delay
- Selective mutism
- ASD
- Structural brain deficits.

Sensory impairment

Sensory processing disorder

Sensory processing disorder is a disorder of the brain whereby an individual has problems organizing, interpreting, and responding to sensory information, specifically hearing, touch, smell, vision, taste, and movement.

Children with sensory processing disorders misinterpret sensory information. This will often trigger an emotional or motor response, which can interfere with the focus of attention.

Sensory processing disorders can be further divided into over or under responsive sub groups.

Sensory avoidant or over-responsive subtype

Misinterpretation of sensory information is perceived as a threat, and triggers anxiety, which may be severe. This, in turn, can result in a sensory defensiveness with an aggressive response or a withdrawal response to misinterpreted information. For example, a boy who misinterprets someone lightly brushing past him in an unthreatening manner as an aggressive attack, and as a result becomes angry and responds aggressively.

Associated features are:
- Anxiety in noisy environments
- Avoidance of new things
- Dislike of certain clothes.

Sensory seeking or unresponsive subtype

Sensory seeking children may have a high threshold for sensory perception. They seek high levels of sensation to trigger sensory pathways.

Associated features include:
- Over-activity when seeking sensation
- High pain threshold
- Enjoyment of high levels of stimulation, e.g. loud noise
- Engagement in dangerous activities.

Co-morbidity
- Motor skills problems
- Fine motor and gross motor skills deficits
- Balance, sequencing movement and bilateral integration difficulties
- Neurodevelopmental psychiatric disorders
- ADHD
- ASD.

Assessment and interventions

For children with significant difficulties, assessment should be undertaken by a paediatric occupational therapist. Interventions include individual occupational therapy treatment and provision of psychoeducation and management techniques for child, parents, and school.

Hearing impairment

1.2 in 100 children and adolescents have permanent bilateral hearing impairment.

Significant hearing impairment is associated with:
- Decreased academic achievement
- Social isolation particularly in adolescence
- An increased incidence of:
  - Emotional disorders
  - Disruptive behaviour disorders.

Psychiatric co-morbidity is more common when hearing impairment is associated with other cognitive deficits.

Intervention

- Appropriate academic input, opportunities for social interactions and relationships are important
- Psychological interventions need to be delivered thoughtfully, taking into account that hearing impaired children and adolescents have a more limited emotional vocabulary compared with their non-hearing impaired peers
- The use of an interpreter is often a key component to therapy
- Dedicated psychiatric services for children and adolescents with hearing impairment are desirable, but difficult to access. Therefore, all child and adolescent mental health professionals should be prepared to work with hearing impaired children.

Visual impairment

Significant visual impairment is associated with an increased risk of:
- Disruptive disorders in children and adolescents
- Social isolation particularly in adolescence
- Anxiety and PTSD due to difficulties in observing and, therefore, processing potential risks and threats
- Emotional disorders in adulthood.

Psychiatric co-morbidity is more common when visual impairment is associated with other cognitive deficits and significantly increased in children with learning disability.

Learning difficulties are present in approximately 1/3 of children with significant visual impairment.

The incidence of ASDs is higher in children and adolescents with visual impairment than that in peers without visual impairment. However, as there are also common features between the two, in particular poor eye contact, careful assessment is required to ensure that co-morbid ASDs are accurately identified (but not over identified).

Recommended reading

De Clercq B, De Fruyt F. (2007) Childhood antecedents of personality disorder. *Curr Opin Psychiat* **20**: 57–61.

Newman L, Mares S. (2007) Recent advances in the theories and interventions with attachment disorders. *Curr Opin Psychiat* **20**: 343–8.

Social and family effects

Parenting

Although on the face of it, the task of child rearing seems to have become more complex in the last three decades, in reality, the desired outcomes have remained unchanged. The goal is still to bring up children to take their places as successful, productive and healthy members of their society. In that sense, the skills required of parents remain the same today as always. What is indisputable is that family composition, certainly in western developed societies, has changed significantly over the past 20 or so years. Where once the nuclear family of mother, father, and children with grandparents usually living nearby was the norm, the permutations now include step-families, often with multiple parents and grandparents, same sex parents, single parents, adoptive and foster parents, and institutional care. Certainly, although children have always been brought up in differing situations, the traditional nuclear family is now 'home' for a minority, rather than a majority of children.

Parenting within families has also changed with a majority of mothers now in employment from a child's early years and a variety of child care arrangements substituting for parents for at least part of the child's day. This may include grandparents, other relatives and friends, but is just as likely to be child care provided by Local Authorities or commercial enterprise.

Nevertheless, children are supremely adaptable and, providing the quality of care is sufficient, the precise arrangements appear to be less important to the ultimate outcome, although research in this area continues.

What constitutes good parenting?

The answer to this question will depend greatly on where you are reading this. Different cultures have a bewildering variety of practices that they consider acceptable parenting. Good parenting can be seen as a dialogue that develops between a child and their parents and there is no 'one size fits all'. Children differ in temperament as parents differ in personality. There are, however, some general pointers and the following are some of the necessary features for successful parenting.

- Attention to the child's physical needs for food, warmth, shelter, health care, safety, etc.
- Warm, accepting affection, and empathy
- Being available to the child
- Affirming the child's worth
- Being consistent
- Modelling good social interaction
- Encouraging play and learning
- Providing social opportunities
- Encouraging the development of individual identity
- Setting appropriate limits
- Supporting the child, although not unrealistically
- Working together as a parenting couple even if not co-habiting
- Treating children as individuals.

What happens when parenting goes wrong?

Parents do not always get it right. The skills of parenting are learned, rather than being instinctive, and all parents carry with them the learning they have acquired from the previous generation, which may not always have been a helpful experience. Occasional lapses in good parenting and even some quite serious situations can be coped with provided the overall context is one of clear, affectionate bonds within a predominantly sound parenting framework. When parents provide chaotic or coercive parenting or are neglectful, there are serious consequences for a child's development depending on their age at the time.

- Early neglect or seriously deficient parenting leads to attachment difficulties, which can persist into adult life
- Abuse at any age is traumatizing and has consequences on adjustment, anxiety, post traumatic stress disorder (PTSD), and tendency to depression
- Emotional neglect or humiliation has serious effects on self-esteem and potentially predisposes to frank psychiatric disorder
- Chaotic parents leave their children feeling uncertain and can produce children who are quite anxiously controlling
- Parents who are too laissez-faire in their approach run the risk of having children who are domineering and disliked by other children. In extreme cases this can develop into conduct disorder
- Children who lack affection, but are given material reward come to associate this with love, and find the giving and receiving of genuine affection very difficult
- Poor parenting is an important factor in a general loss of resilience.

The importance of good parenting has now been recognized in national policy by many governments and a variety of initiatives have been put in place to try to identify children at risk and to provide remedial action. There are now good evidence-based interventions that provide good outcomes in young children, although equivalent programmes for adolescents are less effective.

Family conflict and divorce

Dissolution of marriage is affecting increasing numbers of children (147,000 under the age of 16 in the UK in 2001). Almost a half of the children in the UK will experience the divorce of their parents. (Census 2001, Office of National Statistics)

Children and young people whose parents divorce experience a sense of loss and often bewilderment that can be very long lasting. Their sense of loyalty is often divided between their parents and feelings of guilt and blame are common. A period of adjustment is normal and it should be remembered that for many children they are experiencing other associated losses as well, including the loss of income, school, friends, and even perhaps siblings who go to live with the other parent. They may also have to become accustomed to a new step parent figure in their life who brings with them children of their own. Nevertheless, if separation and divorce are handled sensitively, without acrimony on the part of the parents, the adjustment may be relatively smooth and can be managed with as little hurt as possible. In fact, chronic family and marital discord is much more damaging for children and young people, and can lead to a variety of psychiatric and psychological sequelae.

Consequences of family discord

- Increased behaviour problems
- Poor social skills
- Low self-esteem
- Aggression
- Depression
- Exposure in early childhood can lead to distance in relationships, violence in adult relationships, psychological distress, and poor self-esteem
- Long-term predictor of delinquency, depression, and alcohol problems in girls.

Separation and loss

The effects of separation and loss on a child are dependent upon their age and stage of development. Thus in the circumstances of loss by death, the understanding of the meaning will be very different for a child of 5 and an adolescent of 15.

The early research based on the work of Bowlby described three stages in a child's response to separation from their primary care giver. These have now been widely accepted.

Separation

Stages of response to separation

- **Protest:** the child is obviously distressed and protests loudly about the separation. This is seen at its most obvious in children age 6 months to 5 years
- **Despair:** where the child becomes quieter and may appear withdrawn, but chronically distressed, often with periods of quiet persistent sobbing
- **Detachment:** the child appears to accept that the person is not coming back and often will reject their caregiver on reunion.

This does not mean that separation is inevitably damaging for a child and this research has led to identification of factors, which will mitigate towards a poor or a good outcome. This has led to many changes in practice in child care particularly in hospitals and care situations, where separations are happening on a regular basis.

Factors likely to increase harm in separation situations

- Family discord
- Death of, or permanent separation from a parent
- Loss of normal routines
- Strange environment
- Painful experiences, such as hospital procedures
- Being looked after by strangers—hospital again.

Factors likely to help in separation situations

- Keeping routines as normal as possible
- Contact with familiar people, especially primary care giver
- Familiar objects such as a favourite toy
- Other familiar things such as food and drink, music, etc.
- Preparation for the separation at an age appropriate level.

Even adolescents can find separations difficult and all children tend to regress under stressful situations. It is, therefore, sensible to take these factors into account whatever the child's age.

Losses

Very few children or young people manage to get through their growing years without experiencing some loss. Whilst these losses might not appear to be particularly significant in adult terms, the views of children can be very different as has been demonstrated in life events research. Significant losses for young people include:

- Bereavement
- Loss of a pet
- Loss of friends with family moves or moves of school
- Loss of a favourite object such as a toy or worn out clothes
- Moving school at transition times and losing contact with primary school teachers
- Breaking up of a romantic relationship for adolescents
- Physical illness especially if leading to loss of function.

This is by no means an exhaustive list. Children and young people demonstrate the same responses to loss as adults with different behaviours depending on age. Unresolved grief can have a seriously handicapping effect on a child's development and losses should be dealt with sensitively by adults. It has been clearly demonstrated that children cope best when:

- Their feelings are taken seriously and validated
- They are allowed to express their feelings
- Adults listen to them carefully and address what they really feel and not what adults think they do
- The adults around them are coping well and if their immediate carers cannot, that someone else steps in to assist
- Adults don't try to 'make everything all right'.

Care outside the family: general issues and residential care

In 2005 in England and Wales, 55 in every 10,000 children were 'looked after' by public authorities. This amounted to 60,900 children. Of these almost 34,000 were boys and just over 27,000 were girls.

Age breakdown of care for children (England & Wales, 2005)
Under 1 year 2800
Age 1–4 8700
Age 5–9 12,900
Age 10–15 26,500
Age 16+ 10,800

Breakdown of care: subsequent placements
Foster care 41,700
Children's home 7000
With parents 5700
Placed for adoption 3100
Other 3300

The placement of children in residential units or residential schools has markedly reduced over the last three decades, and some form of family care is now the preferred option. Much of the rationale for this is based on the work of Bowlby and others that has emphasized the need for children to have consistent care givers. Whilst there remains an explicit aim to rehabilitate as many children as possible with their biological families, this is not always possible.

Residential care

- This is now often in schools where education and care is provided on the same site
- Encompasses secure residential care for young people who persistently offend or place themselves at risk
- Considered the 'high tariff' end of the care system
- The majority of children are older (more than 10 years old)
- More boys than girls
- Is often at a significant distance from families and communities
- Can be isolating for young people
- Constantly changing with a fluid group of residents and a changing staff group
- Long-term placements are uncommon often due to high costs
- High profile cases of abuse of children in residential care have been reported in the past decade
- Often poor amenities
- Institutionalization is a common consequence
- Often poor after care
- Poor outcomes in comparison to those who have never been in care, with problems in relation to psychiatric disorder, education, employment, parenting, and relationships.

Care outside the family: foster care and adoption

Foster care

The term 'foster care' covers a wide range of different family situations. Sometimes foster care is a transit from one situation to another, other times it is more long term. Foster families are quite diverse in composition and many consist of families with more than one foster child.

Care placements can be short or long term, emergency or planned, temporary, sometimes up to years when looking for an adoptive family, or permanent; placement can be with strangers or with other family members, so called 'kin care'. One clear characteristic of foster care is that it does not carry the permanence of adoption. It can be terminated by a period of notice on either side and often ends abruptly with placement breakdown.

Characteristics of foster care

- Care is provided by assessed carers in their own homes
- There may be other foster children or the family's own biological children
- Carers are usually paid an allowance, which may increase with the perceived 'difficulty' of the child
- Younger age group than residential care
- Training is available for carers
- Long-term placement is more common in foster care than in residential care
- May have sibling groups placed together or separately
- Perceived as less costly than residential care, but often requires a great deal of community support (which may or may not be provided)
- The best placements are very child orientated, non-coercive, warm, and with good discipline structures
- Embedded in the community with children usually attending local schools.

Good foster care can be very successful for children who cannot live with their families, especially if the carers are able to tolerate the child's need to maintain contact with their birth family. Sadly, many children do not experience this and poor outcome is associated with:

- Repeated breakdown of placements
- Frequent moves of carer
- Repeated failure of attempts to rehabilitate with biological family
- Abusive experiences in care
- Educational breakdown.

Adoption

Adoption is a legal process by which a child moves permanently from one family to another and acquires all the rights of a child of that family as if they had been born into it. (📖 p. 442). Historically, adoption was seen as a mechanism by which couples who could not have children, or who could afford to bring up more children than their own, created a family, usually by adopting babies who were born to young mothers or those who could not look after them. The adoption landscape has changed dramatically over the last decades with more single mothers keeping their babies and those children who are now placed for adoption often being older with a history of family breakdown, special needs, or abuse and neglect.

Issues to consider in adoption

- **The best interest of the child:** care is given to match children to adoptive parent, and this can be a lengthy and involved process. Age, social class, ethnicity, culture are all taken into account
- **Open adoption:** where the child may continue to have contact with their birth family is more usual with older adopted children who may have clear memories of their family of origin. It requires special skills and sensitivity on the part of the adoptive parents
- **Children with special needs:** good outcomes are seen with adoptive mothers who are more experienced and are committed from the start. Good mental health and religious belief in the adoptive parents are also associated with a positive outcome
- **Right to trace birth parents:** most adopted children are curious about their birth parents, and some seek more information and even a meeting. This can be a difficult time and many need support from other agencies to complete the task successfully. In England and Wales, adopted people now have the right to see their birth certificate at age 18. In Scotland this right has always existed from the age of 16 up. (📖 p. 443)
- **Assessment of suitable adoptive families:** can be a lengthy process and is often experienced by these families as intrusive. Families need support through the process, and also between approval and matching with a suitable child. However, it is often after the adoption that families need most support, while they adjust to the changes that a new child brings.

Bereavement

The process of dealing with bereavement is well documented in adults and can be observed in older children and adolescents when faced with the loss of a person to whom they were close, especially a parent or close family member. From the age of around 5 years depending on development, children have a growing awareness and understanding of the concept of death, and by the time they are 8 years old, most children who are not learning disabled have a good understanding of the permanence of death.

Younger children will, of course, be less able to verbalize their feelings, and have less social awareness of the reactions and feelings of others. Their cognitive function is immature and their reactions have to be seen in the light of this.

Like most adults, the process of grieving and coming to terms with such a loss is a normal reaction and generally takes place without the need for professional intervention, particularly if the young person is well supported in a sympathetic way by the remaining adults in their family and close circle.

Vulnerable groups of children who may develop problems with grieving

- Younger children, under 10 years old
- Where the bereavement has been traumatic and/or sudden
- Children with learning difficulties
- Family or personal history of psychiatric disorder
- Where their supportive adults are not coping and may not be able to care for them
- Children who are already vulnerable through deprivation, loss, or previous trauma
- When the bereavement is part of a larger traumatic experience in which they have been involved, such as a road traffic accident.

Treatment options

- Family work to help parents support their children better
- Treatment of any co-morbid disorder such as post-traumatic stress disorder (PTSD) or depression
- Individual counselling can be helpful for older adolescents.

Resilience

As has been noted, not all bereaved children develop problems. Resilience in the face of stress comes from a combination of genetic and environmental factors, and is an important predictor of whether or not children and young people will cope well with bereavement.

Ethnicity and culture

Children and young people are an integral part of the societies in which they live. These societies are increasingly multi-national and multi-cultural, particularly in developed countries where economic migration has increased dramatically. In the UK there is a history of immigration from the former Commonwealth countries. In Europe, the expansion of the European Community with freedom of labour has meant that many parts of the community are now also multi-lingual.

Many young people face the additional challenges of being second or third generation immigrants, whose parents and grandparents are perhaps less adjusted to the culture of their adopted homeland than they are themselves. This can bring tensions within families, as well as between cultures.

Children and young people can be subjected to the same stresses and discrimination as adults in a multi-ethnic society and it is important to address these issues when assessing children's mental health.

Concepts of mental illness and psychiatric disorder are interpreted differently across different cultures and children can miss out on essential health care because of this.

Issues of ethnicity and culture

- Racism: affects children's self-esteem and, at its worst, can lead to depression and self-harm
- Discrimination on the grounds of race, colour, and religion is experienced by children and young people in many inner city areas. In rural areas, the problems tend to be less obvious, but may still exist
- Young Afro-Caribbean males are more likely to be involved in violent attacks, both as victim and perpetrator, and 5 times more likely than white youths to be stopped by the police
- Under-achievement in school is commoner in the Afro-Caribbean population with black youths being more likely to be excluded from school in inner city areas
- Some cultures seem to be more able and/or more willing to integrate than others
- Women first generation immigrants often struggle to integrate and can therefore be remote from their children's experiences in school and community
- Psychiatric disorder is sometimes recognized late or hidden
- Culture has an impact on the presentation of psychiatric disorder
- Rates of psychiatric disorder in children and young people do not vary greatly across cultures.

Refugees

- There are in excess of 20 million refugees worldwide
- Most of these are in Africa and Asia
- There are around 6 million in Europe
- A significant number of child refugees have no adult carer with them.

Although many of the issues discussed in the section on ethnicity and culture also apply to refugees, there are additional problems which include:

- Poverty
- An acute sense of dislocation and disorientation with feelings or isolation
- Language differences
- High levels of post traumatic symptoms
- High levels of mental health problems (although around half of refugee children *do not* have a psychiatric disorder)
- Distress is often expressed in culturally specific ways
- Physical illness, including HIV/AIDS particularly in populations of African origin
- Repeated moves
- Living in refugee camps
- Poor housing.

Protective factors for refugee children and young people

- Remaining within a family group
- Support of a same culture community
- School
- Integrating into a community
- The support of health and social services from their own community where possible. Many refugees are highly skilled professionals.

Specific risk factors for mental disorder

- Having been involved in a war zone
- Being a child soldier especially if coerced into this role
- Experiencing the traumatic loss of family
- Continuing uncertainty about the future
- Psychiatric disorder in their parents.

Parental mental illness

The effects of maternal depression on the child have been well studied particularly in the early years of life. However, less is known about the specific effects of other major mental illness, although they too can clearly have a devastating experience on a child's wellbeing. There is, for example, an increasing awareness of the impact of parental substance misuse, and government policy has developed particularly in the wake of tragic deaths of children from ingesting their parents' drugs and other medication.

Up to a quarter of adults with mental illness will be living with a child under the age of 16; many are also the child's main carer. Many children and young people will experience the repeated illness of their parents with episodes of hospitalization, self-harm, and attempted or threatened suicide. In addition, the symptoms of psychiatric illness can themselves be difficult for a child to understand. Assessment of the impact on children must view things from the child's point of view taking their age and development into account.

With the reduction in hospital beds for psychiatric patients and the growing emphasis on care in the community, many children are having increased daily contact with quite seriously ill parents and other adults.

The experience of being in close contact with an adult who is suffering from a mental illness is different for each child and depends on the nature of the illness, the child's age and developmental stage, their intellectual ability, their exposure to florid symptomatology, and their experience of previous episodes. Adult psychiatric services naturally are more concerned with the treatment of their patient and often it is not until quite late on in an episode of care that the needs of any children are taken into account. The solution is then sometimes to refer to a child and adolescent mental health service, but it is important that services work together to manage these difficulties.

Where the care of a child comes into question, it may be necessary to involve the social services to support the family or indeed to provide a temporary period of alternative care if the family is unable to meet the child's needs. This sometimes raises conflict between child and adult services and patient confidentiality may become an issue. However, current legal guidance is clear that the needs of the child are paramount and should be addressed by all concerned.

Because of the heritability factor in many major mental illnesses, older children who have some understanding of this may fear that they themselves will become ill and may develop anxiety symptoms, which they then interpret as mental illness.

Effects of parental mental illness on their children

- Lack of availability of the parent either through illness, drug treatment or hospitalization. Children can be bewildered and believe that they have done something to upset their parent
- Unpredictable behaviours, or sudden and unexpected bizarre parental behaviour leading to fear and anxiety in the child
- Neglect and/or abuse either driven by symptoms or through inability to put the child's needs first
- Chaotic home organization and decision making
- Inability to make sense of parents' symptoms
- Distancing from parents due to repeated experiences of being ignored or neglected
- Long-term consequences on attachment, vulnerability to psychiatric disorder, conduct problems
- Tendency for some children to develop a caretaking role for their parents, which then interferes with their own development.

Not all parents with mental illness or substance misuse problems fail to provide 'good enough' parenting, and indeed many children are resilient enough to survive their parents' illness intact. Protective factors include:

- A good experience in the first 3 years of life
- Good parental functioning between episodes of illness
- Clear and honest age appropriate explanations of the illness and what is being done to treat. Misguided misinformation such as 'mummy's gone on holiday' should not be given
- Good support networks within the family
- Good school adjustment
- Early intervention if problems arise
- Perinatal mental health services for women at risk and their children.

Additional issues in substance misusing parents

- Poverty due to spending on drugs/alcohol and unemployment
- Higher levels of domestic conflict and violence
- Increased risk of child abuse and neglect
- Generally, more chaotic lifestyle and parenting
- Drug users are normally multi-substance using and the effects on the parents may be unpredictable and variable
- Involvement with the police because of illegal activity
- Higher risk of drug and alcohol misuse in children of substance abusing parents
- More frequent child care issues with child protection involvement
- Parental physical health problems.

Recommended reading

British Association for Adoption and Fostering. Available at: http://www.baaf.org.uk/index.shtml (accessed on 7 April 2008).

Reder P, McClure M, Jolley A. (2000) *Family Matters*. Routledge, London.

Rutter M, Taylor E. (2002) *Child and Adolescent Psychiatry*, 4th edn. Blackwell, Oxford.

Schaffer HR. (1998) *Making Decisions About Children*, 2nd edn. Blackwell, Oxford.

Pre-school problems

Sleep disorders

These are common during the preschool years (around 1/3rd of 0–3-year-olds), and are very variable in origin. Contributing factors include:

- Temperamental differences (good vs. bad sleepers)
- Parenting practices or living arrangements, e.g. poor bedtime routine, bed or room sharing
- Specific risk factors such as learning disability or attention deficit hyperactivity disorder (ADHD).

Assessment should:

- Differentiate true disorders from variations of 'normal' sleep (particularly in younger children)
- Aim to differentiate primary from secondary sleep problems, for example, wakening secondary to nocturnal cough in asthma
- Determine onset, timing, and impact of sleep difficulties enabling the clinician to differentiate parasomnias from dyssomnias and rule out differential diagnoses.

Normal sleep variations and younger children

Around 1/4 of 1-year-olds will still be night-waking several times per week and many will still be waking occasionally at 5 years. Breast-fed children wake more. The point at which night-waking becomes a problem may be to some extent dependent on parental attitude and tolerance.

Parasomnias

Parasomnias are defined as an intrusion into sleep without a reduction in sleep length. In the preschool age group these will usually be *night terrors* or variants of *somnambulism* (sleepwalking). The main differential diagnosis of parasomnias are the nocturnal epilepsies, which may require video electroencephalogram (EEG) assessment if suspected.

Night terrors

The child will appear afraid, inconsolable, and often moaning or whimpering repetitively. They will usually be either unresponsive or only partially responsive to attempts to intervene or communicate. Characteristically, the child will remember nothing of the event in the morning. Night terrors usually occur in the first few hours after going to bed [a non-rapid eye movement (REM) parasomnia]

Nightmares, or frightening hypnogogic episodes, which are REM parasomnias, are distinguishable from night terrors by:

- Their occurrence later in the night
- The child being consolable and responsive to the parent.

Management

Anticipatory awakening. Night terrors will often occur at a surprisingly similar time each night and waking the child 15–30 min prior to this is usually effective after a few nights.

Somnambulism

Many children sleepwalk at some point, a few habitually, including those who may leave the house or do odd things. Episodes usually peak at 5–7 years. There is no specific treatment.

Dyssomnias: insufficient (or excessive*) sleep

Upper airway obstruction/apnoea

Apnoea is defined as at least 5 seconds of lack of airflow, despite breathing effort. In the pre-school child, it is most commonly caused by tonsillar hypertrophy, but can also be caused by also structural abnormalities and obesity. May be a contributing factor to the development of daytime sleepiness, mood swings, and inattention.

Circadian rhythm sleep disorders

This is a broad term that describes a mismatch in the established sleep–wake cycle (jet lag is an example of a circadian disruption). These difficulties are common in learning disability. Milder circadian rhythm disruption may arise from chaotic bedtime routines or children who stay up playing on computers or watching TV, especially when off school and allowed to sleep in.

Circadian rhythm disorders are important in that they may respond to treatment with melatonin if re-establishment of a consistent bedtime routines fails.

---

* *Hypersomnia* is rare and associated with Kleine–Levin syndrome, whilst *narcolepsy* does not typically present until puberty.

Sleep disorders: management

Behavioural management/sleep hygiene

In younger children with night-waking, extinction techniques, such as controlled crying, are usually employed. Positive reinforcement/star charts can useful in the over 3's to reward a child who stays in bed.

Basic 'Sleep Hygiene'

'Sleep hygiene' is a collection of common-sense tactics to address with the parents:

- Maintain strict routine of both bedtimes and getting up times
- Engage in calming activities at bedtime, such as playing relaxing music, or 'special time'—a dedicated, non-rushed period of time spent playing a quiet game or reading stories
- Avoid or reduce daytime naps, especially in older children
- Avoid stimulating activities, foods, or drinks in the evening
- Discourage TVs and computers in rooms
- Ensure that the bedroom is conducive to sleep—dark enough, quiet enough, cool enough.

Controlled crying

There are various versions of controlled crying all based on the same theme of gradually extending the time the child is left to cry before entering the room and comforting him/her, before leaving.

Depending on the child's nature and the parents' anxiety levels, this may vary from allowing the child to cry for between 5 and 30 min, and then increasing by greater or lesser intervals each time.

The vital ingredient to this and other techniques, such as controlled comforting, is *consistency*. If the intervention is carried out with loving care, but begun early and maintained firmly, there is no evidence of a negative effect on the child in later years. That said, controlled crying is most certainly easier said than done for most parents.

Medication

Benzodiazepines should be avoided due to the risks of paradoxical over-excitement and tolerance.

Antihistamines, such as chlorpheniramine have a mild sedative effect and have an occasional place in the temporary respite of secondary dyssomnias, such as those occurring during an inter-current illness, e.g. chickenpox.

Melatonin is indicated in marked circadian rhythm disturbances which often occur against a backdrop of learning disability, ADHD, anxiety, etc. Melatonin is available as an 'over the counter' food supplement in the USA and as an off-licence prescription in the UK. There is mounting evidence supporting it's safety, but more trial data is needed. It is recommended to start with 1 mg 30 min before bedtime, increasing as necessary every few days. The maximum safe dose is not known, but doses of 3–9 mg are common in clinical practice.

Feeding issues

These are common during the pre-school period and often appear to be somewhat fuelled by parental anxieties. Children whose parents are concerned about feeding are, however, usually entirely physically healthy and growing normally.

Picky eaters/food refusal

These are more likely to occur in children aged between 6 and 36 months, and those who:
- Have 'difficult' temperaments
- Have had less opportunity to try novel tastes and textures in the early weaning period
- Have parents who may be overly invested in 'the right amount' to feed or perfect nutritional content.

Management generally involves degree of change in parental behaviours.

Colic

Colic is common affecting around 1/3rd of infants. It is associated with intense bouts of crying with flushing and leg-flexing, which often occur after feeding, and between the ages of 4 weeks and 4 months. Colic appears to be self-limiting, its causes are unknown and whilst there are many folk remedies there are no evidence-based treatments.

Gastro-oesophageal reflux

Many young children regurgitate small amounts of food, associated with both a short-term insufficiency of the gastro-oesophageal sphincter and supine posture, both of which improve as development proceeds and, as such, do not require treatment. However, more severe forms of gastro-oesophageal reflux can lead to problematic recurrent vomiting with associated morbidity, including failure to thrive and aspiration. Severity is usually indicated by frequency of vomiting and weight trajectory; centile chart plotted weight gain decreasing sufficiently to cross two centile lines is a common rule of thumb.

Management ranges from milk thickeners and posture advice (propping up the head of the cot) to medication and surgery in severe and intractable cases.

The main differential diagnosis is the projectile vomiting associated with pyloric stenosis, particularly in boys.

Pica

Pica is the consumption of things that aren't food. It should be distinguishable from normal 'mouthing' by around the age of 2 years of age. Pica is more common in autism and learning disabilities, and can be an early indicator of these. On the other hand, it may simply indicate poor levels of supervision.

Advice for picky eaters

- Attempt to reduce parental anxiety with basic advice, e.g. 'Children are very efficient at processing their intake, and will usually thrive despite failing to meet a "textbook" quantity or quality of intake each day' and 'Missing an entire meal is not dangerous to a child's health, and children go through phases of needing lesser or greater intake'
- Remove the mealtime focus on the child, and avoid protracted games like 'aeroplanes'. Try to eat as a family in order to reduce this focus and encourage vicarious learning, and encourage eating with peers at nursery, etc.
- Positive rewards are much more effective than harsh discipline, e.g. force feeding (often when the child takes a breath from crying) will very effectively increase the trauma that the child associates with mealtimes in general and worsen the problem
- Make one meal only, but use small self-feedable pieces of relatively neutral foods in achievable quantities
- Continue to offer previously refused foods. Refused one week doesn't mean refused the next
- Encourage appetite at mealtimes by reducing snacks and particularly drinks between meals.

Enuresis

Enuresis is the involuntary passage of urine, and is common in preschool children:

- 90% of 2-year-olds are not dry at night
- 20% of 3-year-olds and 5% of 10-year-olds are not dry at night.

Enuresis is most often addressed by health visitors in the pre-school age group and community paediatricians in older children, but also occasionally comes to the attention of Child and Adolescent Mental Health Services (CAMHS). It is highly familial and, although not clinically serious, causes a great deal of stress, and incurs relatively high costs from ruined clothing and mattresses.

Approaches to treatment

Establish first:

- Primary (never dry) vs. secondary (follows a period of continence)
- Nocturnal, diurnal (daytime), or both.

Nocturnal enuresis

- This is more common in boys after age 5 years
- Primary causes:
  - Idiopathic
  - Familial
- Secondary causes/associations
  - Idiopathic
  - Familial
  - Urinary tract infection
  - Constipation
  - Psychiatric disorder such as ADHD
  - Structural abnormality (rare, includes myelomeningocoele and spina bifida occulta).

An association with stressful life events and deep sleeping are often described anecdotally, although these are not as well supported by the literature.

Diurnal enuresis

- More common in girls after age 5 years
- Causes:
  - Behavioural
    - —over absorption in play,
    - —(and /or) 'leaving it too late'
  - small/'irritable' bladder
  - pelvic floor insufficiency
    - —particularly if stress or 'sneeze' incontinence occurs.

Assessment

Begins with further investigation of primary (is there a positive family history?) or secondary causes as described above. Routinely renal function [palpation, blood pressure (BP), urinalysis], urological function (examination for hypospadias, urine culture), GI function (palpation for loaded colon), and lower spine (examination of sacrum and lower limb neurology) are conducted.

Management

Enuresis in pre-school children is initially managed using educational and behavioural techniques although medication may be considered if these approaches are unsuccessful.

Management of wetting

Nocturnal enuresis

- **Education and reassurance:** the problem is common, often familial, frequently self-limiting, and not intentional. This may be all that is required in preschoolers
- **Practical advice:** reduce evening fluid intake, lift to the toilet at parental bedtime, use of mattress covers, avoidance of pull-up nappies (which can prolong the problem)
- **Behavioural:** reduce punishment, increase positive reinforcement (and self esteem), star charts, token rewards, etc.
- **Alarms:** pad and buzzer. These consist of a sensor in the pants that sounds an alarm when wet. This conditions the child to connect the urge to void and the signal to wake.

Medication

- **Oral or intranasal desmopressin** (antidiuretic hormone analogue): this allows short-term dryness which enables attendance at camps/ sleepovers, etc.
- **Tricyclic antidepressants** are effective at reducing wetting (secondary to antimuscarinic effect) and are used occasionally in older children/adolescents.

Diurnal enuresis

- **Behavioural:** regular visits to the toilet, positive reinforcement
- **Physical:** bladder training (learning to drink increasing amounts and holding on for increasing amounts of time), pelvic floor exercises.

Encopresis and soiling

Encopresis is the repeated and involuntary passage of normal faeces into places not appropriate for that purpose. It is usually accepted that for diagnosis this should have been taking place for longer than 6 months in a child over 4 years of age. It is relatively common, occurring in around 1% of children, and is more common in boys than in girls.

A complex and difficult area, not least because of the reaction it provokes from family and friends. It is often poorly understood, but should not be under-estimated.

Categorization of encopresis

- Retentive
- Non-retentive
- Aggressive.

It is likely that this is an over-simplification and the clinical presentation can range greatly, including:

- Involuntary liquid overflow in chronic constipation
- Repeatedly passing normal stools into underwear (which then may be hidden)
- Overtly demonstrative and hostile smearing of faeces in the home or school
- A mixture of the above.

Aetiology

Combinations of causes are common

Constipation

Constipation is present in the history in the majority of encopretic children. Many cases of soiling will be secondary to the loss of control that constipation engenders, including liquid stool bypassing a loaded rectum. Anorectal malformations such as Hirschprung's disease should be considered.

Continuous soiling

There is a failure to correctly achieve cleanliness because of poor parental supervision, learning disability, or dyspraxia. The child may be unable to co-ordinate cleaning themselves, leading to smearing in underclothes and around the toilet.

Personal stressors

A complicated, and unhappy, subset of encopretics often includes boys with very stressful personal circumstances, including significant family problems.

Management of encopresis (and constipation)

- Simple 'continuous' encopresis, may respond to closer supervision/ training
- Constipation is best treated by preventio; by eating a balanced diet, and prevention of dehydration, particularly during episodes of viral illnesses and holidays. Some cases of encopresis may have originated as constipation several years prior to presentation
- If constipation is present, the rectum will be loaded. It needs to be emptied and *kept empty*, using laxatives. Laxatives may be *stimulants*, such as sennokot or osmotic *softeners*, such as lactulose or lubricants,

such as liquid paraffin (caution if risk of aspiration) and will usually
be required in addition to the usual sufficient fluid and fibre intake.
Treatment needs to continue for long enough to allow the dilated and
insensitive rectal smooth muscle to return to function

- Bowel imaging pre-meds, such as picolax and gastrograffin are often
tried as an in-patient strategy for acute impaction, prior to enemas,
which are clearly potentially traumatizing for young children
- Reduction of punishments for soiling and from increased positive
reinforcement of successes accompanied by strict regular toileting
(post prandially to take advantage of the gastro-colic reflex)
- Relaxation training can help children who inadvertently constrict their
external anal sphincter, whilst straining. A book (or hand-held games
console) at toileting time helps with this
- Specific stressors and social difficulties should be addressed wherever
possible, whilst specific therapies are helpful for entrenched cases, such
as externalizing strategies like 'sneaky poo'.

Prognosis

The majority of encopretics who are constipated will do well with correct
bowel management. Poor prognosis is associated with chronic cases with
systemic family or social problems.

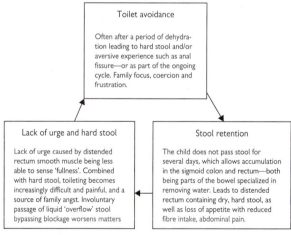

Fig 6.1. The vicious cycle of constipation.

Recommended reading

Kotogal S. (2003) Sleep disorders in childhood. *Neurol Clin N Am* **21**: 961–81.

Cathey M, Gaylord N. (2004) Picky eating: a toddler's approach to mealtime. *Paediat Nurs* **30**: 101–7.

Loeining-Baucke V. (2002) Encoporesis. *Curr Opin Paediat* **14**: 570–5.

Chapter 7

School issues

As with the legal systems the education systems differ across the UK with respect to both legislation and policy. This chapter will focus on the most common educational issues that are referred to Child and Adolescent Mental Health Services (CAHMS); however, it would be advisable to contact the relevant local education authority to clarify details of practice in the local area.

Most CAHMS in the UK will see children from age 5 to 16/18 years of age if they are still within full-time education (typically excluding colleges or university). The majority of patients will therefore be in some form of educational placement. In the UK children are required to receive education from the beginning of the term after their 5th birthday until a date around their 16th birthday. Although, some children with birthdays that fall later in the year will not yet be 5 when they start school.

Absence from school

Truancy

The *deliberate* failure to go to school, often associated with conduct problems in the child or young person. There may be a history of low educational achievement and disruptive behaviour. These children and young people may be referred to CAHMS services, particularly if the onset of this behaviour is recent.

School refusal

School refusal refers to a persistent absence from school as a consequence of the young person finding it difficult to go to school, rather than deliberately avoiding school. School refusal is often linked with an emotional disorder. Assessment and treatment of school refusal is dealt with in more detail in Chapter 19 on anxiety disorders.

Child and adolescent psychiatrists may be asked to comment on the nature of school refusal, and the current or predicted response to treatment. In England and Wales, children and adolescents may be referred to court under the Children Act 1989, and an educational supervision order may be made. Parents may also be prosecuted for persistent non-attendance of their child at school, although this is rare and may reflect a lack of parental co-operation with treatment.

Below are some of the features that distinguish truanting from school refusal based on mental health problems:

- Children who truant usually try to conceal their non-attendance
- School refusers typically miss weeks or months at school- whereas children who truant usually miss several lessons or a day at a time
- Truants usually express a dislike for school and have a poor level of achievement, while school refusers are usually good students
- Truancy is more often associated with a diagnosis of oppositional or conduct disorder, rather than with an emotional or anxiety disorder
- Children who refuse to go to school typically demonstrate fearful, avoidance behaviours, e.g. clinging to parents, not getting dressed, or somatic symptoms in response to going to school.

Suspension or exclusion from school

Temporary suspensions or exclusions from school have been increasing over recent years. The reasons for this are hotly debated, with some suggesting that the push towards 'inclusion', and the expectation that all children and young people have a 'right' to be educated in mainstream is a factor, while others believe that the increasing focus on standards and competition within education has meant that teachers have less time or inclination to cope with disturbed pupils in class.

The number of children officially excluded increased from about 3800 in 1991 to 12,500 in 1995 (figures exclude Scotland). The rate of unofficial exclusions is likely to be even higher.

The most common reasons for exclusion are violent or aggressive behaviour to peers or teachers. Boys are almost five times more likely than girls to be excluded. Rates are highest among Afro-Caribbean pupils.

Bullying

Bullying is defined as one child directing aversive behaviour towards another child that is physically or emotionally harmful or intimidating.

- Bullying is repetitious and characterized by relationships with an asymmetrical power hierarchy (i.e. the bully has more power than the victim does)
- The most typical pattern of bullying is a boy bullying another boy or girl, but some girls will bully other girls and, very occasionally, boys
- Most bullying takes place during primary and early secondary school. Bullying can occur both in and out of school, but is most prevalent in school settings
- Bullies are aggressive to their victims, but also generally aggressive to other children and even to adults. Bullies are more likely to exhibit impulsiveness, and lower levels of empathy and anxiety than non-bullies. Many bullies are on the trajectory of antisocial behaviour development
- Bullies can use a variety of verbal/physical and psychological techniques to accomplish their bullying acts
- Bullying boys use physical intimidation, while bullying girls use verbal or psychological intimidation. Boys' physically aggressive behaviours decline as they get older, but their verbally aggressive behaviours increase. Girls' verbal and psychological intimidation stays fairly stable across developmental periods
- Some children end up being both bullies and victims. These children have significant psychological disturbances, exhibit a variety of externalizing and internalizing psychological problems and are often referred for psychiatric services.

Although there may be differences throughout the UK, local education authorities and all individuals' schools, whether in state sector or not, are required to have an anti-bullying policy. This typically defines the strategies in place and should be accessible to all.

Special educational needs

The Education (Additional Support for Learning) (Scotland) Act 2004, came into force in Scotland in November 2005. This places the education authorities under a duty to give extra help in school to all children and young people identified as having 'additional support needs'.

Additional support needs vary broadly. Within the act, whilst there is no standard definition or list of criteria, it recognizes that there are a very wide range of difficulties that may cause barriers to learning. These include not only learning problems, but also emotional and behavioural difficulties, bullying, or family/care circumstances.

Under the act the education department must have a co-ordinated support plan (CSP) for all children and young people identified as having additional support needs, this replaces the previous Record of Needs system. The CSP should include a description of the individual's additional support needs, the support required, educational objectives, and details of who will provide them.

It requires social work services, any other local authority, health services, further and higher education institutions, and careers services to assist the education authority, if requested, to identify and support children's and young people's learning needs.

Parents/carers have a number of rights under the act, including requesting that the education authority make an assessment of their child's needs, and being involved in decisions about plans made for their child, together with the right to appeal decisions.

In addition, the act introduces a new independent mediation service to facilitate communication between parents, school, or the education authority.

The act is an attempt to move towards a system that is tailored not just to learning needs, but addresses a wider range of needs that an individual may have, and will give greater support through school years and help preparing for leaving school.

In the rest of the UK the provision of a system for supporting children and young people with special education needs is the responsibility of the school's Special Educational Needs Coordinator (SENCO).

The SENCO collaborates with the head teacher and the school's governing bodies to help determine special education need (SEN) policy and provision within the school.

SENCOs have a number of duties including:
- Overseeing day-to-day operation of the school's SEN policy
- Liaising with and advising fellow teachers
- Liaising with external agencies including the local education authority, educational psychology services, health and social services, and voluntary agencies
- Liaising with parents of children with special educational needs.

Educational psychology services

Educational psychology services in England and the rest of the UK are part of the Local Education Authority (LEA). A few LEAs do not have an educational psychology service of their own as such, but instead 'buy into' a neighbouring LEA's service. The majority of educational psychologists working in Scotland are employed by the Local Authority Educational Psychology Service (EPS) or Psychological Service (PS).

Educational psychologists have moved away from a medical model, where the perceived problem was within the child, towards an ecological model, which focuses on the interaction of children with their environment, curriculum, peers, teachers, and other relevant adults. The potential scope of work undertaken carried out by educational psychologists is extensive, covering mainstream and special sectors, and relating to learning, behaviour, and development. Their work has broad aims, including enhancing social inclusion, promoting the social and emotional well-being of young people and families, and raising achievements.

Work is carried out with children and young people, parents and carers, educational establishments, education management, as well as a range of agencies, such as social work services and health service.

Although health professionals cannot usually refer directly to educational psychologists for assessments or interventions, good practice and multidisciplinary working would suggest liaison with educational psychologists when they are involved and advice to schools where it is felt that the involvement of an educational psychologist would be helpful.

Educational psychology services differ across each region of the UK, and often between localities. In Scotland the functions of the Educational Psychology Service were defined by the Review of Provision of Educational Psychology Services in Scotland, (Currie Report, SEED, 2002) and include:

- **Consultation to service users and educational establishments** in relation to children and young people with additional support needs
- **Assessment:** this may be based on direct or indirect involvement with the child or a combination of both, and aims to limit the effects of barriers to learning and to promote inclusion of the child or young person
- **Interventions:** solution-orientated and motivational approaches, promoting inclusion and alternatives to exclusion, contributions to whole establishment interventions (raising achievement, anti-bullying, contributions to curricular innovation and initiatives), contributions to devising behaviour management, and individual education plans and working with small groups
- **Training** to a range of service providers and educational establishments regarding the learning, behaviour, and development of children and young people, as well as an understanding of the systems they are working in, including the local and national contexts and policy, and legislative frameworks support training
- **Research** to evolve an evidence base for educational practice, inform policy and strategy, explore new ideas and to evaluate and encourage reflective practice.

In England and the rest of the UK the Government recognized in the Green Paper *Meeting Special Educational Needs: a Programme of Action published in November 1998*, that statutory assessments are a necessary and key function, but educational psychologists also have a crucial role in providing a range of services and outlined their main areas of work as:

- **Early intervention**
  - Work with parents
  - Early years work
  - Advice to schools on pupils prior to admission
  - Joint home visits/liaison with parents
- **Code of Practice work**
  - Advice and support to teachers and pupils as part of statutory assessments
  - Observation and assessment of children with learning and communication difficulties
  - Consultation on curriculum planning and differentiation for individual or groups of pupils
  - Planning IEPs with the SENCOs and teachers
  - Working with teachers to devise appropriate strategies for addressing individual pupil needs
  - Advice on strategies for working with individual pupils
- **Behaviour support**
  - Reviews with school staff working with children at risk of exclusion
  - Observation and assessment of children with behavioural difficulties
  - Counselling and therapeutic work.
  - School-based project work, particularly in behaviour management and social inclusion
- **Wider school development**
  - Consultation and problem solving with the head teacher over whole school issues
  - Consultation and problem solving with the SEN co-ordinator over groups of pupils
  - Contribution to multi-agency planning
  - Consultation and problem solving with school staff
  - Contribution to school development
  - Target setting at group or school level
  - School-based multi-agency planning meetings
- **Training**
  - Guiding Learning Support Assistants on pupil learning and targeted teaching.
- **Other areas of work**
  - Assessment of exam conditions
  - Critical incident response.

Recommended reading

Black D, Wolkind S, Hendricks JH. (1991) *Child Psychiatry and the Law*. Gaskell, London.

Further information about educational psychology service in England and Wales is available at: http://www.everychildmatters.gov.uk/ete/agencies/psychology/ (accessed 7 May 2008).

Scottish Executive Schools Directorate. Further information about Additional Support for Learning is available at: www.scotland.gov.uk/Topics/Education/Schools/welfare/AS (accessed 7 May 2008).

Mental retardation

Cognition and intelligence

Concepts and IQ

In terms of Latin derivation, cognition is to *know*, whilst intelligence is to *understand*. The overlapping nature of these concepts together with the complex nature of human ability, knowledge, emotion, and experience mean that any attempt to classify these constructs will necessarily involve over-simplification; an apt reminder that individuals should not be simply categorized according to a single number, as often happens with IQ.

Measurement of intelligence is usually a reference to a quantitative assessment of subgroups, or combinations of subgroups, of cognitive abilities—the scores of which are most commonly combined and quantified as IQ—intelligence quotient. Although no longer calculated as a quotient, the term has stuck.

Terminology: learning disability or mental retardation?

Whilst terminology to describe those with compromised intellectual abilities is clearly required, it is also important to recognize some of the complexities associated with this process. Diagnostic labels can be both a cue for prejudice and exclusion, and the key to accessing support and care, with a resultant maximizing of potential, reduced frustration, and increased self esteem.

The stigma surrounding sub-average intelligence has resulted in frequent adjustments of the accepted descriptive terms over the years. Throughout the 20th century, such terms have included: idiocy, imbecility, feeblemindedness, mental subnormality, mental handicap, and finally to a current mixture of terms that are generally equivalent to each other, including mental retardation (general term, ICD-10), mental impairment (UK legal term), and learning disability (general UK-based term)

Whilst the UK commonly uses learning disability, the most widespread term used remains mental retardation, which will be the term used in this book. The main reason for not using learning disability here is that it can cause confusion, as when used in the US it does not refer to those with global difficulties, but relates to more specific educational problems, such as dyslexia. Newly-emerging terms include developmental disability and intellectual disability.

Diagnosing mental retardation: IQ and adaptive functioning

A broad approach to diagnosis is important, as exemplified the WHO criteria, which describe 'impairment of skills manifested during the developmental period which contribute to the overall level of intelligence… assessment should be based on whatever information is available, including clinical findings, adaptive behaviour and psychometric performance'.[1]

The American Association on Intellectual and Developmental Disabilities describes a tri-dimensional definition for mental retardation, requiring:
- Significantly sub-average functioning (on psychometric testing) *plus*
- Two or more deficits in adaptive functioning from the following list: communication, self-care, home living, social skills, community use, self-direction, health and safety, functional academics, leisure, and work.

Measuring IQ

The Wechsler Intelligence Scale for Children (WISC) is the measure most commonly used in children in the UK (the adult scale is used in over 15s, a preschool version is available for the under 7s.) This and the other commonly used measurement tools:
- Correlate well with each other
- Are standardized and reliable
- Have strong predictive validity (heritable, predict employment status).

The WISC includes multiple subtests administered by a trained rater to provide verbal and performance sub-scores, which are combined to give an overall score.

IQ categories are derived from the application of the total score to a Gaussian distribution of the population, with the cut-off for the lower end of normal being 2 SD under the mean IQ of 100, i.e. 70. Below this, IQ is categorized thus:

IQ 70–79   Borderline mental retardation
IQ 50–69   Mild mental retardation
IQ 35–49   Moderate mental retardation
IQ 20–34   Severe mental retardation
IQ <20   Profound mental retardation

The main criticisms of this system are a perception of it penalizing certain social and ethnic groups, leading to the search for 'culture-fair' IQ assessment tools, and also the arbitrary nature of the cut off points—this emphasizes the need to look carefully at other areas, such as adaptive functioning.

Measuring adaptive functioning

Supplemental to a general comprehensive assessment of the individual's situation are scales such as the Adaptive Behaviour Scale (ABS) and the Hampshire Assessment of Living with Others (HALO). No scale can take into account the full context of each individual, which remains the task of the assessing team—ideally including members with a variety of skills and perspectives.

Mental retardation: epidemiology

Prevalence

As predicted by the definitions and the fact that the cut-off of IQ of 70 is 2 SD below mean (which should therefore include the lower 2.28% of IQ), most population studies give a prevalence of 2–3% for mild mental retardation. However, subgroup analysis reveals that:
- Mild mental retardation is more common in lower socioeconomic classes
- Mild mental retardation is more common in some ethnic groups.

Further caveats are that many of those with IQ scores below the IQ cut-off point of 70 are, for various reasons, not impaired to a degree such that they require any additional support. There are, however, a similar number of those with IQs above 70 who suffer severe impairments.

As such, when a requirement for impairment is added to an IQ lower than 70, the prevalence of mental retardation is nearer to 1%.

Severe mental retardation has a prevalence of around 0.3 to 0.5%, which varies less according to subgroup, as all of those in this group are significantly impaired. This prevalence is, however, much higher than would be expected from the normal distribution curve cut-off for IQ 20–34, as result of the higher incidence of organic disorders in this group.
- Of the mental retardation population, 85% are in the mild category
- Diagnosis is affected by age:
  - Peak diagnosis is at school age, with some no longer meeting impairment criteria by adulthood having achieved a sufficient level of functioning
  - More severe mental retardation is diagnosed in much earlier childhood.

Associated prevalences

- Epilepsy in 15–30% of those with severe or profound mental retardation
- Cerebral palsy or similar motor disability in 20–30%
- Sensory impairment in 10–20%

Mental retardation: aetiology

Knowledge of causation raises the possibility of treatment in some, while in others it allows prediction of specific difficulties, including common co-morbidities.

Mental retardation is usefully conceptualized by Rutter et al.[3] as having 3 main types of cause:

- **Organic:** more common in more severe mental retardation, although it is not always possible to predict level of IQ by cause
- **Polygenic**
- **Socio-cultural**.

In around two-thirds of mild mental retardation, and one-third of severe mental retardation, no cause is found. Trisomy 21 and fragile X are by far the commonest diagnosable organic causes of mental retardation.

Organic causes of mental retardation

- (Adapted from Rutter et al.[3])
- **Prenatal genetic**
  - *Chromosomal:* trisomy 21, fragile X, 47 XXX
  - *Genetic:* inborn errors of metabolism and 'syndromes', e.g. Prader Willi
- **Prenatal environmental**
  - *Infections:* rubella, toxoplasmosis, CMV, HIV
  - *Toxins:* Alcohol
  - *Maternal severe illness:* diabetes, septicaemia
- **Prenatal multifactorial**
  - *Brain development disorders:* epilepsy, CP, hydrocephalus
- **Perinatal**
  - *Maternal illness:* e.g. pre-eclampsia
  - *Foetal distress:* e.g. birth hypoxia
  - *Prematurity:* e.g. respiratory distress syndrome, periventricular bleeds
- **Postnatal**
  - *Trauma:* road traffic accident (RTA)
  - *Infection:* meningitis, encephalitis
  - *Endocrine:* hypothyroidism
  - *Neoplasm:* brain tumour
  - *Iatrogenic:* irradiation
  - *Toxin:* lead poisoning.

Caveats to this list are the relatively small contribution of perinatal factors, which are more often markers, rather than a direct cause of mental retardation related disease, and the likelihood of organic causes that so far remain unidentified and undetected.

Most cases of severe and profound mental retardation will co-occur with neurological and/or psychiatric diagnoses, which may confuse the exact organic origins of the mental retardation.

Polygenic causes of mental retardation

Roughly 50% of the variation in IQ is accounted for by heritability. Mild mental retardation is also thought to be strongly heritable when confounding factors are controlled for, although the relationship is weaker for more severe mental retardation.

Socio-cultural causes of mental retardation

IQ testing unavoidably risks assessing experience in learning, as well as actual inherent ability. Twin studies have shown that rearing environment can result in differences of around 10 IQ points overall.

Data suggests that the sociocultural influences on intelligence come from a range of sources. Likely candidates include both direct causes, such as neglect and a lack of stimulation, and indirect causes, such as diet. Of recent interest with regard to the latter have been breast milk and fatty acid content, and dietary iron content.

Multifactorial causes

Overall, it is of course unlikely that all mental retardation will fit neatly into these 3 categories. Overlapping genetic, environmental, and socio-cultural risks are likely to be relevant to many cases.

Mental retardation: psychiatric co-morbidity and effects on the family

Psychiatric co-morbidity

Co-existing psychiatric diagnoses are much more common in mental retardation than in the non-mental retardation population (overall prevalence of co-morbidity estimated at 30–70%) and, within these, pervasive developmental disorders and attention deficit hyperactivity disorder (ADHD)-type diagnoses are particularly common.

This increased prevalence is generally due to shared risk in many of the organic and psychosocial causative factors, and because of the risk of psychiatric illness secondary to the various lifetime difficulties that mental retardation may cause.

In terms of management, most co-morbid disorders respond in generally similar ways in the mental retardation group compared to the non mental retardation population, (but see management section on pharmacotherapy).

Specific disorders and mental retardation

- **Pervasive developmental disorders (PDD)**
  - A mnemonic that probably remains useful in autism spectrum disorders is that around 66% of those with autistic spectrum disorder (ASD) will have an IQ of less than 66
  - The triad of impairments seen in most PDDs is also seen in the majority of those with severe mental retardation
  - The stereotypies and self-injurious behaviour seen in PDD are commonly a source of difficulty in mental retardation, even in the absence of a PDD diagnosis
- **ADHD:** in particular the hyperactive subtype is commonly seen in mental retardation. Indeed, it was in this group of children that stimulant medications were initially used
- **Challenging behaviours**
  - These are usually related to degree of mental retardation and are an important determinant of placement
  - Can sometimes be re-framed and made more understandable if seen as non-verbal/behavioural consequences of an inability to communicate problems, views, or emotions. For example, sexual urges in an adolescent boy with moderate mental retardation
- **Affective disorders:** These are difficult to diagnose in many types of mental retardation, and may manifest as new onset or increasing levels of challenging behaviours, rather than meeting full criteria designed for affective disorders in a non-mental retardation population
- **Anxiety disorders:** Particularly common part of a mild mental retardation. Often co-morbid with PDD, in response to difficulties in coping with mainstream elements of daily living

- **Psychotic disorders:** Should, as with normal intelligence, be suspected where there is a new onset of bizarre behaviour in late adolescence. Content is dependent on cognitive ability, and so may involve very repetitive hallucinations or simple delusionary constructs, or positive symptoms may be absent entirely
- **Eating disorders:** Such as pica and comfort-vomiting or rumination.

The effects on the family

There are various types of impact that frequently result as a consequence of caring for a child with mental retardation, all of which are moderated by a family's particular abilities and methods for coping with stress, and other protective and vulnerability factors.

- **Impact of the 'bad news'** (often in the first days or weeks after delivery): Worsened by delay and uncertainty (for example, when 'soft' dysmorphic features are found at the newborn check), and when confirmed often then associated with stages of response similar to bereavement
- **The nature of the caring task**
  - Parenting any child is an exhausting process at times. Where children with mental retardation are cared for at home, as is increasingly the case, the unremitting nature of the task and the extra burden of care have a marked impact, in terms of assisting with mobility, feeding, self-care, dressing, toileting, administering medication, etc.
  - Depending on availability of resources and services, support for a child cared for at home may range from respite periods in a residential unit to full time support staff at home
- **The impact of challenging behaviours and co-morbid psychiatric illness** is frequently greater than that due to the increased routine care required
- **The extended timescale of responsibility/lifecycle factors**
  - When a child becomes an adult, the care required often remains or becomes greater, and frequently the provision of services for adults with mental retardation lags behind that for children
  - Carers will themselves have less stamina as they get older, and as supportive siblings grow up and leave home.

Mental retardation: assessment

Assessment for mental retardation may vary according to circumstances, e.g. in young infants when there is reason to suspect a specific cause, such as Down syndrome, testing may be necessarily less comprehensive if there is strong clinical suspicion based on examination alone. However, frequently a combination of behavioural or emotional symptoms may cause an older child to present, which usually requires a much wider ranging assessment.

- Comprehensive assessment for mental retardation is ideally multidisciplinary, and many areas have specialist developmental assessment centres employing a range of professionals, often on a sessional basis such as:
  - Developmental or neurology-specialist paediatricians
  - Psychologists
  - Psychiatrists
  - Speech and language therapists
  - Occupational therapists
  - Audiologists
  - Optometrists
- A typical assessment should include:
  - Use of age and culture appropriate IQ testing, by appropriately skilled staff
  - Formal assessment of adaptive skills
  - Investigation of family, pregnancy, perinatal, developmental, health, social, and educational history
  - Assessment of psychological and behavioural functioning
  - Physical examination with an emphasis on neurodevelopment
  - Speech assessment
  - Auditory assessment
  - Investigations, as indicated by the history and physical examination, such as karyotyping, brain imaging, electroencephalogram (EEG), urinary amino acid analysis, blood organic acids and lead level and biochemical tests for inborn errors of metabolism.

Psychiatric assessment of mental retardation

The role of the psychiatrist in assessment of children and adolescents with mental retardation often overlaps with that of others in the team. However, identification of psychiatric illness is often one of the key roles for the doctor. Symptoms that are a consequence of, or inherent to, the particular degree of mental retardation present in an individual, need to be distinguished from those that indicate the presence of psychiatric disorder. However, even in this task it is likely that normal rules, such as the meeting of full formal diagnostic criteria be may neither applicable to mental retardation population nor in the best interests of the individual.

Psychiatric assessment is further complicated by variability in the degree of mental retardation present and the presence of associated disorders, such as motor problems or epilepsy. In general, all these issues will act to worsen the picture of any co-existing illness; in particular the more severe end of the mental retardation diagnosis will entail a pre-existing degree of frustration, difficult behaviour, and self-injury, increased stress and expressed emotion in family or care staff. Individuals may be already receiving neuroleptic drugs, despite a lack of a diagnosis that usually determines such treatment.

Assessment of specific disorders with mental retardation

Any psychiatric disorders can co-exist with mental retardation and, therefore, all should be considered. Look for patterns such as sudden change from baseline functioning and age of presentation:

- Eating and sleeping problems in young children
- New onset ADHD symptoms in older children
- Mood changes, socialization, sexuality and self-harm in adolescents.

ADHD
Increased rates compared with the general population. Developmentally inappropriate levels of over-activity, inattention, and impulsiveness need to take into account degree of developmental delay. Inattention may be a result of inappropriate academic expectations.

Disruptive behaviour disorders
Occur in around one-third of mild mental retardation. Failure to understand situations and boundaries may manifest as oppositionality.

Mood disorders
Occur more frequently in mental retardation. A change in mood with no clear environmental trigger should prompt consideration of mood problems.

Anxiety and related disorders
May be manifest in observable behaviour more than in self-report, e.g. avoidance. Lack of understanding and conceptualization in situations may make phobias or reactions to trauma complex or exaggerated. The mental retardation group may be more prone to exposure to traumatizing situations.

Obsessive compulsive disorder (OCD), stereotypies and self-harm
Both may manifest as repetitive actions that reduce anxiety. OCD behaviours are more likely to involve washing or arranging things, stereotypies are usually specific motor patterns, such as hand wringing and rocking. Stereotypies may take self injurious forms, e.g. biting of limbs or head banging.

Psychosis
Psychosis is no more common in mental retardation, but may manifest as sudden worsening in social/intellectual functioning. Self-discussion or creation of imaginary friends, may be normal behaviour in the mental retardation population and needs to be distinguished from hallucinations.

Eating disorders
Anorexia nervosa is extremely uncommon, but pica, regurgitation, and under-and over-eating are frequently seen.

Mental retardation: approaches to management

Location of intervention

It is now the exception for an individual with mental retardation to be a permanent resident in a care 'institution', with most services embracing the principle of normalization, allowing children with mental retardation to be cared for in their own homes and schools.

Prevention

Many causes of mental retardation are preventable or reducible by
- Primary prevention which may be medical (e.g. folic acid supplementation) or societal (e.g. use of bicycle helmets in children)
- Secondary prevention, such as treatment of underlying condition to minimize degree of mental retardation (e.g. CSF shunting in hydrocephalus)
- Tertiary prevention by intervening early in all aspects of the problem, to minimize impairment and maximize potential (e.g. optimizing communication with appropriate aids).

Treatment overview
- Address the specific daily difficulties associated with mental retardation
- Treatment of co-morbid medical conditions including epilepsy, deafness, contractures
- Treatment of co-morbid psychiatric conditions
- Therapies for PDD-type impairments such as stereotyped behaviours.

Psychosocial treatments

Aims are to:
- Alter patterns of maladaptive behaviour allowing understanding of the disability and associated feelings
- Recognition of strengths, resolution of internalized conflicts, and development of realistic expectations for self
- Training to recognize, manage, and communicate emotions
- Training to recognize the effect of one's own behaviours upon others
- Development of age appropriate social skills, and learning to constructively handle developmental crises and challenges.

The formats of these treatments depend on the abilities of the individual, e.g. communication abilities, etc., but may take the format of individual, group, or family interventions, and involve play, music, and art.

Pharmacological treatments

Whilst there is no clear reason to expect an alternative or idiosyncratic response to medication in those with mental retardation, the mental retardation context of effects or adverse effects of drugs means that extra caution is required, with application of the 'start low, go slow' adage. Usually, the main risk is of over-sensitivity to certain drug effects, e.g. erratic fluid intake risking lithium toxicity.

Reported drug risks in mental retardation include:
- Anticholinergics causing cognitive impairment and delirium (e.g. in Trisomy 21)
- Benzodiazepines causing paradoxical over-excitement

- Gabapentin causing aggression and choreoathetosis
- Lithium causing cognitive dulling and risk of toxicity
- Methylphenidate causing social withdrawal and tics.

Emergency treatment of challenging behaviour in mental retardation

A common exposure for mental health professionals to the mental retardation population is an on-call request for assessment, in the setting of an episode of particularly difficult challenging behaviour.

Before transfer, restraint, or sedation, which may be truly necessary in some cases where there is significant risk to the safety of the patient or others, it is important to first assess the situation from the patient's point of view and to thoroughly consider acute medical causes. The outburst of aggression may, indeed, be an attempt to communicate need, albeit in an 'exotic' fashion.

Issues to consider

Some services rely on closely adhering to rules or achieving skills in a relatively cold and controlling manner, so called 'affectionless control', with overly high expectations of behaviour

Medical causes to consider

- Constipation
- Infection
- Medication side-effects (akathisia from neuroleptics or disinhibition from sedative/hypnotics can be expressed in aggressive and self-injurious behaviours).

If acute use of medication is unavoidable, neuroleptics or benzodiazepines may have a place, with low doses of drugs and choices of previously useful compounds being advisable.

Specific learning disability: language development and disorders

Specific learning disabilities are diagnosed where testing in a specific aspect of functioning reveals scores that are significantly lower than would be expected from the level of general intellectual ability.

Language development and disorders

The development of language is the acquisition of skills that allow the production and understanding of language, including making the correct sounds, learning vocabulary, and the structure of grammar, as well as learning the complex social patterns that surround communication.

Language disorders in children are relevant to child psychiatrists because of their relationship with a range of emotional and behavioural problems in childhood, and also because they are commonly overlooked or misunderstood.

DSM-IV and ICD-10 both classify language disorders similarly, distinguishing problems of:

- Specific speech articulation (problems with speech sounds, but normal language skills otherwise)
- Expressive language (expressive spoken language deficits, but normal comprehension)
- Receptive language (understanding of language being the principal problem, but expressive language is also affected by extension).

The ICD-10 category F80: specific developmental disorders of speech and language describes the situations whereby normal patterns of language acquisition are disturbed from early in development. These problems are not attributable to neurological or speech mechanism abnormalities, sensory impairments, mental retardation, or environmental factors. They are often associated with problems such as difficulties in reading and spelling, abnormalities in interpersonal relationships, and emotional and behavioural disorders.

Aetiology

- Whilst most speech and language disorders that arise during childhood are of unknown aetiology, many are suspected to result from abnormalities of early development, some of which being a consequence of genetic predisposition
- Environmental causes, both prenatal and postnatal, also have a role in a minority of presentations
- The role of lack of experience of language, such as that caused by insufficient exposure to language in children due to recurrent ear infections, having deaf parents, or other reasons, is currently unresolved, but is unlikely to be an important factor in the majority of cases.

Assessment

When more detailed assessment beyond parental report is required there are standardized age-appropriate assessment tools available, which supplement careful clinical observation, such as the MacArthur Communicative Development Inventory.

Assessment should aim to:

- Distinguish specific language problems from general developmental delay
- Distinguish specific language problems from disorders, such as those on the autistic spectrum, or acquired language loss syndromes, such as Landau Kleffner
- Diagnose and/or account for hearing loss.

Management

- There is some debate over age of intervention, as a significant number of early problems with speech and language resolve with time
- **Structured** interventions focus on the child in the clinic with practice being encouraged in weak areas
- **Naturalistic** interventions aim to improve the child's use of language through experience at home or nursery
- **Signing** is an important part of management in very impaired children.

Specific learning disability: reading and reading disorders

Learning to read, write, and do maths are just some of the many complex tasks negotiated in childhood, but for some, one or more of these specific areas remains a lifelong problem, despite few or no other cognitive or learning difficulties. These individuals are also at increased risk of co-existing psychiatric disorder, in addition to the disadvantage posed by their problem. This section will focus on reading deficits.

The ability to read is the result of the successful combination of a variety of sequential cognitive processes, including:

- Letter recognition and visually differentiating similar-looking letters
- Understanding the sequencing of words
- Ability to recognize sound patterns within words
- Ability to know the meanings of words.

Reading disability and dyslexia

Definitions

Reading disorders are classified in ICD-10 within F81 specific developmental disorders of scholastic skills and are separated into:

- Specific reading disorder (also termed developmental dyslexia)
- Specific spelling disorder
- Specific disorder of mathematical skills.

The main feature of specific reading disorder is described in ICD-10 as being: 'A specific and significant impairment in the development of reading skills that is not solely accounted for by mental age, visual acuity problems, or inadequate schooling. Reading comprehension skill, reading word recognition, oral reading skill, and performance of tasks requiring reading may all be affected.'[1]

The term dyslexia is subject to a dizzying variety of nosologies, and for the purposes of this book can be restricted to Lyon et al's description as being characterized by 'difficulties with accurate and/or fluent word recognition, poor spelling and decoding abilities'. The cut-off point required to define what is 'abnormal' has been difficult to pin down in what is frequently regarded as a spectrum-based condition.

Epidemiology

Prevalence figures vary from 5 to 17.5%, depending on the precise definition and assessment models used. Longitudinal studies suggest a long-term continuation of the problem, whilst improvements may be made, the gap between the individual with dyslexia and average peers usually remains.

Co-morbidity

Specific reading disorders have been particularly linked to disruptive behaviour disorders, such as ADHD and conduct disorder, and also to emotional disorders. It is likely that this reflects specific links and is therefore more than just a response to the disability.

Aetiology

Multiple aetiological theories exist, with a consensus emerging for the phonological theory as an explanation for the majority of dyslexia:

an inability to co-ordinate the segments of spoken words known as phonemes. Even with knowledge of the word's meaning, it cannot be recognized on the page.

This inability is found to strongly run in families and linkage analysis has identified several vulnerability loci that may represent a multifactorial route to the disorder. These genetic factors are thought to have a far greater influence than environmental causes and, whilst acquired dyslexia has been described, it is usually the result of gross anatomical changes, rather than teaching or parenting deficits.

Functional imaging studies have reliably shown a disruption of left occipitotemporal activity in individuals with dyslexia who are engaged in a reading task.

Assessment

Some authorities may screen for dyslexia in children, whilst others may just maintain an awareness of the problem as a potential cause for a child struggling at school, particularly as the abilities to decode and segment words emerge at around 4–6 years.

A number of more in-depth tools are available, usually to psychologists working within education, if suspicions are raised about a child's reading ability, such as:

- An instrument to measure reading ability, such as WORD (Weschler Objective Reading Dimension), a single word reading test in common use in British schools
- Test of Word Reading Efficiency (TOWRE) measures word reading rate and accuracy
- An instrument to measure overall cognitive ability, such as the WISC IV.

Management

The underlying principles of management of specific learning disabilities are the implementation of early school-based specific educational support, with advice as to how to help at home.

In dyslexia there are a number of preventative and remedial approaches to this, including:

- Early instruction in how the most common sounds are spelt
- Phonemic awareness tasks, include rhyming, encouraging differentiation between similar words and segmenting words
- Help in practicing and retaining learned sound-spelling relationships.

Additionally, children are increasingly provided with supports such as scribes or computers in examinations, allowing their understanding and knowledge to be tested without the handicap of a specific learning problem.

References and recommended reading

1 World Health Organization (2005) *International Statistical Classification of Diseases and Health Related Problems*. ICD-10 2nd edn. World Health Organization, Geneva.

2 American Academy of Child and Adolescent Psychiatry. (2008) *Practice Parameters for the Assessment and Treatment of Children, Adolescents and Adults with Mental Retardation and Co-morbid Mental Disorders*. Available at: http://www.aacap.org/galleries/PracticeParameters/Mr.pdf (accessed 20 April 2008).

3 Rutter M, Taylor E. (2005) *Child and Adolescent Psychiatry*, 4th edn. Wiley Blackwell, Oxford.

4 Lyon GR, Shaywitz SE, Shaywitz BA (2003) A definition of dyslexia. *Ann Dyslexia* **53:** 1–14.

Lewis, M. (2002) *Child and Adolescent Psychiatry: A Comprehensive Textbook*, 3rd edn. Lippincott, Williams and Wilkins, Philadelphia.

Shaywitz SE, Shaywitz BA. (2005) Dyslexia (specific reading disability). *Biol Psychiat.***57:** 1301–9.

Taylor S, *et al.* (2003) Practical Child Psychiatry: The Clinicians Guide. Blackwell BMJ Books, London.

Assessment

Purpose and structure of assessment

A thorough assessment and understanding of presenting difficulties forms the basis for any treatment interventions offered for children, young people, and their families or carers. As psychiatric problems rarely occur in isolation with co-morbidity the norm, it is essential that any assessment is sufficiently comprehensive to present a clear and complete formulation of the presenting problems.

We would therefore consider assessment to have 3 major components:
- Identification of problems, history, signs, and symptoms
- Evaluation/synthesis
- Care/treatment planning.

The information gathering stages in an assessment

The psychiatric history and examination of child and adolescent mental health problems bears many similarities to that of adults. However, there are several differences in detail and emphasis. The general processes include several stages.

Clinical interview with the parent(s)/carers
- Clarify presenting complaints with systematic evaluation of psychopathological symptoms and description of how problems developed over time
- Developmental history
- Pre- and post-natal factors
- Early developmental history (e.g. milestones, language, attachment, sleep, feeding problems, early temperament)
- Medical history (especially tics and epilepsy, and psychosis for adolescents)
- Medication (especially anticonvulsants, antihistamines, sympathomimetics, steroids)
- Family history, functioning, problems coping styles, warmth and hostility, social networks, and other resources.

Interview with the child/young person
- Functioning in the family, the school and the peer group
- Emotional problems and self-esteem
- Self-report rating scales may be useful as supplement especially for emotional symptoms in those 9 years and older
- Behavioural observation during clinical examination is very useful when problems are seen, *but* absence during assessment does not mean they are not there. Also look for social disinhibition and evidence of language disorder
- In general, the child should be seen more than once during the assessment process.

Systematic screening for psychiatric symptoms/disorders
- This will usually be conducted as part of a joint interview with parents and the child/young person
- Some clinicians believe that it is sufficient to concentrate on those problems that are brought as the presenting complaint. However, in view of high levels of co-morbidity found in patients with psychiatric

disorders we strongly suggest that all cases are screened for the presence of a full range of co-existing disorders and that, where screening suggests the possible presence of such a disorder this possibility is fully explored. Commonly co-occurring conditions are described in each of the specific disorder chapters
- This may require several clinicians, with complementary skills and experience, collaborating in the assessment.

Preschool or school information
- Invaluable if parents consent
- Narrative report of behaviour and behaviour problems seen within school setting
- Academic functioning
- Social functioning
- Situational variation, such as with different teachers, or between home and school
- Classroom observation may be helpful, but is not always required or feasible.

Psychometric tests
- Assessment of IQ can help to determine academic performance versus academic potential and should be considered when there is a suggestion of problems with classroom performance or progress. When time or resources are scarce, a short Weschler Intelligence Scale for Children (WISC) or equivalent (e.g. British Picture Vocabulary Scale, BPVS II) is better than no assessment
- Tests of attention, executive functioning, etc., have progressed recently, but remain research, rather than clinical tools at present
- There are *no* psychometric tests that are diagnostic for any psychiatric disorders.

Physical examination
- General assessment of physical health is important, particularly in certain conditions such eating disorders
- Height, weight, head circumference should *always* be recorded
- Any evidence of breakdown in care or neglect
- Vision (Snellen chart) and hearing (clinical screen and audiogram if indicated)
- Neurological examination (including fine and gross motor control, and motor and vocal tics)
- Stigmata of congenital disorder, e.g. foetal alcohol syndrome or effects, Williams syndrome, neurofibromatosis.

Investigations
Not routine, but guided by physical examination.
- EEG if history suggestive of seizures
- DNA assessment (fragile X) in global developmental delay
- Audiogram when significant hearing loss cannot be ruled out
- Brain scanning and neuropsychological assessment not generally indicated, unless there is particular reason to suspect a structural brain lesion. Functional brain imaging remains a research tool.

Problem clarification

Types of problems

There are 4 main domains of symptoms that present to child and adolescent psychiatry.

- Emotional symptoms
  - Anxiety
  - Fears
  - Affective symptoms
  - Sleep and appetite
  - 'somatic equivalents' of emotional symptoms
- Conduct problems
  - Defiant behaviour, often associated with irritability and temper outbursts
  - Aggression
  - Antisocial behaviour, such as stealing, fire setting, truanting
- Developmental delays
  - What is normal?
  - Areas of particular relevance to child and adolescent psychiatry
  - Attention and activity regulation
  - Speech and language
  - Play
  - Motor skills
  - Bladder and bowel control
  - Scholastic attainments, especially reading, spelling and maths
- Relationship difficulties
  - Children's relationships change with development
  - Aloof indifference
  - Passivity
  - Disinhibition
  - Over familiar
  - Difficulty relating to most social partners or specific type of relationship.

Rating scales

Rating scales can be a helpful adjunct to clinical assessment (recommended reading). They should not, however, be used as a substitute for careful clinical questioning and examination. A large number of rating scales are now available, which measure many aspects of child and adolescent psychopathology. Rating scales and questionnaires can be grouped into either generic or disorder specific. There are a number of major factors that need to be taken into consideration when using rating scales.

- It is not possible for an individual rating scale to capture the complexities of child and adolescent psychopathology
- The need for multiple informants to provide a comprehensive picture of a child's' functioning (however, when different informants disagree on their rating scale answers/scores, this can be difficult to reconcile or interpret)

- The impact of age and developmental changes on rating scale scores (e.g. a healthy 5-year-old will score higher on measures of over-activity than a healthy 10-year-old)
- The tension between the dimensional and categorical aspects of psychiatric disorders
- The importance of the psychometric properties (e.g. reliability, validity, sensitivity, specificity) of a rating scale. This will impact on the usability of the scale as a screening tool, outcome measure, etc. For example, with a rating scale that has a sensitivity of 80% and a specificity of 70%, 20% of the 'cases' identified will be 'false positives' and 30% of those identified as being 'non-cases' will actually be cases ('false negatives').

Rating scales can be classified as either generic or disorder specific. A comprehensive list of rating scales is beyond the scope of this book but further information can be found in the suggested reading at the end of this chapter. Many rating scales are produced under license and are available at a cost.

The Strengths and Difficulties Scale is a generic rating scale of emotional, behavioural, and prosocial problems validated in a number of different population for children aged 4–16 that is quick to complete, with versions for parents, teachers, and the individual to complete. It is also freely available at www.sdqinfo.com

Interviewing children and adolescents

In conducting individual interviews with children and adolescents it may be useful to think of the process in 4 stages, each of which should blend into one another.

- Enabling the child to separate from the parents
- Developing trust and rapport with the child
- Discussion with the child or young person, including any paper and pencil tests or other type of assessments
- Conclusion of discussion with appropriate safe closure before return to the parents

General considerations

- Prior to the interview be clear about its purpose and your objectives. This will vary in different situations, e.g. in anxiety and depression children will often provide the most accurate account of symptoms. However, in attention deficit hyperactivity disorder (ADHD) and disruptive behaviour disorders parents are often the best informants with respect to symptoms, but a child can tell you how the symptoms impact on them and how they feel
- Establishing a rapport
  - There is no one correct way
  - Think about introductions and demystifying the interview process
  - Give age appropriate explanations
- Consider the context of the interview
  - Privacy issues
  - Minimal distraction
  - Age appropriate toys or drawing equipment
- Who should be present
  - This depends on the age and wishes of the child and purpose of the meeting
  - In general younger children may want or need a parent or carers present older children and teenagers may be more variable, but should all be given the option of speaking with a clinician on their own
  - Utilize active listening skills—not only listening to what is being said, but also develop and awareness of non-verbal cues
- Approach
  - Friendly and non threatening
  - Guided by child/young person's responses
  - Means of communication—this does not need to be solely based on words, drawing, play, and toys can be used to communicate.

Age specific considerations

(📖 Black (1993) and Lask (2003) for further details)

Pre-school

- Children younger than 4 are rarely seen in Child and Adolescent Mental Health Services (CAMHS) services, and when they are seeing them without their parents may not be helpful.
- Parent reports of how a child is behaving or may behave in situation, such as separation, may be more helpful
- Observation of play and interactions with parents will be useful in this age group

- With older pre-school children, once the child and parent has relaxed it may be possible to have a short separation. It is, however, important to let them know that their parents will be nearby
- Always explain what you will be doing, e.g. drawing or playing with some toys, and what you will not be doing, e.g. taking blood or giving injections, as their previous experience of going to see healthcare professions may be very limited.

Early school age

- Early school aged children are usually more familiar with separating from parents
- As with younger children, play and observation of behaviour is important as they will be unlikely to understand or be able to report in detail about their internal emotional world
- When meeting with the child make sure that there are appropriate toys and drawing materials for the age and gender of the child
- Let the child take the lead in the playing as this will allow assessment of several important aspects of development:
  - How easily does they child separate from the parent?
  - How long does it take the child to relax with you?
  - What toys do they choose?
  - What are the themes of the play and are these appropriate for the child's stage of development?
  - Is the concentration span appropriate?
  - Is the child over-active, impulsive, or very distractible?
  - What is the child style of social communication?
  - Do they avoid eye contact?
  - Do they include you in their games?
  - Do they show imagination in their playing or drawings?
  - Are there any odd movements evident?
- Even in an unstructured brief play session it should also be possible to make an approximate assessment of the child's cognitive capacity, which can then inform further assessment.

Middle childhood

- Most children from around 7–8 years of age should be able to tolerate separation for parents more easily, but it is important to keep in mind any factors such as anxiety or previous experience that might impact on this. About 15–20 min is usually sufficient at least for the initial meeting
- It is important to let the child know that what they talk about with you will be private and that, whilst it is often helpful to be able to discuss some issues with parents, you will not be telling their parents exactly what they have said if they don't want you to
- It is however important to also explain the limits of this confidentiality. A statement such as 'I will need to let your parents know if anyone is hurting you or you are planning to hurt anyone else or yourself' is usually a sufficient explanation at this age
- The individual assessment should have a mixture of playing and talking. The order of these is a matter of judgment but a brief period of 'warming-up' may be helpful talking about other things, e.g. hobbies, pets or friends

- The following stylistic points should be considered in this age group:
  - Grammatical structure should be relatively simple and appropriate for the child's age and development
  - Use short words
  - Only ask single questions and make single statements/comments
  - Using open questions may cause anxiety or be misunderstood better to start with a broad open statement about the area you what to ask about e.g. 'I wanted to talk about what has been happening at school' then move to more direct, closed questions
  - At this age children's concept of time are not well developed so provide clear time points, such as holidays or birthdays
  - Re-capping or summarizing with the child regularly to check that you have understood is helpful
  - If strong emotions or views are expressed it is important to acknowledge these and to balance being supportive, whilst not appearing to endorse unacceptable behaviour 'It sounds like you have been getting angry at school a lot'
- When assessing mental state, the child may be less able to report on more abstract concepts, but it should be possible to gain an idea about feelings of sadness or anger
- Don't shy away from asking questions about self-harm or suicidal thought—these are a necessary part of the assessment. It may be helpful to ask some general questions about sad feelings before moving to more specific questions, such as 'have you ever hurt yourself' or questions that may be a marker of distress or wish to escape from intolerable feelings or situations, such as 'have you ever thought about running away'
- Facilitating statements and using the experience of someone else may be helpful, e.g. 'I saw another boy who also had problems at school and didn't want to go to school, have you ever felt like that?'
- In ending the interview, provide the child with a brief summary of what you have understood from them are the problems and go over what information you will feedback to their parents.

Adolescents

- With adolescents, it is possible to examine a broader range of emotions and behaviours, and as adolescents will be more able to report of their own internal mood states and feelings a more comprehensive mental state assessment is possible
- As with younger children, it is important to be clear about confidentiality and a more detailed explanation of the rules and boundaries of confidentiality may be necessary for adolescents than younger children
- It is important to ask about risk taking behaviour such as smoking, substance use and sexual relationships. This should be carried out in a non-judgmental manner, encouraging openness, and allowing exploration
- If talking is difficult it may be helpful to provide facilitating questions or statements or to reflect on any non verbal communication such as 'you look quite angry/sad at the moment'

- It is important for the adolescent to know that you do not expect that they will see the problems in the same way as do their parents, and that you are genuinely interested in their views and are not just going through the motions
- Again, when ending the interview summarize the problems discussed to check that both of you have understood what has been said and review what information will be given to the parents.

Genograms

Genograms are diagrammatic representations of family structure and relationships, and are a practical way of capturing and presenting information about family structure. They enable structural, relational, and functional information about a family to be viewed both horizontally across the family context and vertically between generations.

Although genograms have been widely used by clinicians and therapists over the years it was not until the 1980s that there was a generally agreed format.

Genograms:
• Can aid collaborative working between families and therapists
• Encourages a family to reflect on its history
• Aids identification of patterns, similarities and differences, themes, and major life events.

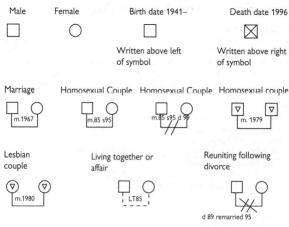

Male   Female   Birth date 1941–   Death date 1996

Written above left   Written above right
of symbol   of symbol

Marriage   Homosexual Couple   Homosexual Couple   Homosexual couple

m.1967   m.85 s95   m.85 s95 d 99   m. 1979

Lesbian   Living together or   Reuniting following
couple   affair   divorce

m.1980   LT85   d 89 remarried 95

Standard symbols for children
For birth order start with oldest child on the left

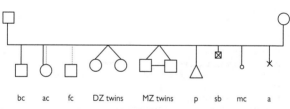

bc   ac   fc   DZ twins   MZ twins   p   sb   mc   a

Ages inside symbols; D.O.Bs above left of symbol

Key bc = biological child; ac = adopted child; fc = foster child; DZ twins = Dizygotic twins; MZ twins = Monozygotic twins; P = pregnancy; sb = stillbirth; mc = miscarriage; a = abortion

Fig. 9.1 Standard symbols for genograms.

Assessing family functioning

An assessment of family functioning is an essential component of a comprehensive assessment. As with all aspects of assessment it is very helpful to have a structure to guide this assessment and there are several available. One of these the McMaster's Dimensions of Family Functioning is described in more detail. It allows a structured and systematic way of assessing important aspects of family functioning and includes the following dimensions.

Problem solving
- Who identifies the problem and do others agree?
- Do family members discuss the problem in a way that increases the likelihood of it being solved?
- Are different ways of resolving the problem considered?
- Is the agreed action taken?
- Does the family make sure that the action agreed upon is taken?
- Is the progress as a result of the action noted?

Communication
- Is this
  - Clear or masked?
  - Direct or indirect?
  - Congruent or incongruent?
- Is it received in a way that
  - Validates
  - Ignores
  - Disqualifies.

Roles
- Who allocates roles?
- Are they allocated to the appropriate person?
- How accountable is a person for the successful undertaking of their role?
- Roles fall into five groups
  - Systems management and maintenance
  - Resource provision
  - Nurturance and support
  - Sexual gratification
  - Life skills development.

Affective responsiveness
Are family members responsive to the emotional needs of others in the family or out of touch, excessive or muted?

Affective involvement
Varies greatly between an exclusive, all encompassing closeness to virtual absence of involvement.

Behaviour controls

- **Rigid controls:** narrow limits, little negotiation, no flexibility, not reflecting the context
- **Flexible controls:** broad range, negotiable, clear, but taking account of contextual changes
- **Laissez faire controls:** 'anything goes'
- **Chaotic controls:** random, unpredictable shifts across the range of control styles.

Diagnosis, formulation, and report writing

The purpose of assessment is to be able to evaluate the nature of a child's difficulties, where possible explain how and why they have developed and, if necessary, decide on the most appropriate package of care/treatment. Having gathered information it is necessary to combine this, and synthesize it into a diagnosis and a comprehensive and meaningful formulation. In addition to history and symptoms, it is also important to consider and describe the impact of these difficulties for the child and the family; these may be described under a number of headings.

- Social impairment
- Family life
- Classroom learning
- Friendships
- Leisure activities.

In addition, how much do the problems cause distress for the child and family

Diagnosis

Diagnoses should be made using either the ICD-10 or DSM-IV diagnostic systems. One benefit of the ICD system is the possibility of using the multi-axial system, which allows for a more complete description of the child/young person's problems. The multi-axial system includes axes for:

- Primary psychiatric disorder
- Problems of development
- Intelligence
- Somatic disorders
- Psychosocial problems
- Children's Global Assessment Scale (C-GAS).

Formulation

An ideal formulation will contain all the information required to make a comprehensive treatment plan. It 'explains' the diagnosis and hypotheses about the factors that have resulted in the development and perpetuation of the child's problems. There are several ways to construct a formulation many of which are complementary.

- Five key questions in making a formulation (SIRSE)
  - *Symptom:* what sort of problem is it?
  - *Impact:* how much distress or impairment does it cause?
  - *Risks:* what factors have initiated or maintained the problems?
  - *Strengths:* what assets are there to work with?
  - *Explanatory model:* what beliefs and expectations do the family bring with them?
- Biopsychosocial model of causation
  - Biological
  - Psychological
  - Social factors

- 3Ps approach to formulation
  - Predisposing factors- biological and environmental
  - Precipitating factors- parenting style, other environmental factors
  - Perpetuating factors.

Report writing

Many reviews and audits of child mental health work have identified problems with the routine recording of information in the case files. This often starts with the recording of information from the assessment process. Furthermore, many traditional child psychiatric reports were written in unstructured prose, which often made them difficult to read and the information contained within them difficult to interpret.

We have found that a more structured approach, both to report writing and record keeping can be of great assistance when reviewing a case at a later date. Again, there are several formats. The headings below are those used by our service to write-up end of assessment reports.

- Reason for referral
- Nature of assessment undertaken
- Presenting problems
- Current level of functioning
- Brief family history
- Obstetric, developmental, medical and psychiatric history
- Clinical findings:
  - Symptoms and impairments
  - Appearance and behaviour
  - Mental state examination
  - Rating scale scores
  - Investigations
  - Clinical Global Impressions—Impairment (CGI-I)
  - CGAS
- Diagnosis (multi-axial)
- Formulation (3Ps)
- Treatment and management plans.

Example formulation and genogram

James is a 12-year-old boy who lives with his Mother and 3 siblings. He presents with 6-month history of attention problems, aggressive behaviour, and mood swings. His parents report that he has always liked routines and has never been good at talking about his feelings. He is at risk of being excluded from school due to aggressive behaviours toward peers.

His parents separated 3 months ago after 15 years of marriage; there was a history longstanding marital discord and possible domestic abuse. The children stay with their father every second weekend. Both parents have new partners. The father feels that there is little wrong with James and that his mother gives in too easily to the children. None of James's siblings have had mental health input from CAHMS services, but his 15-year-old sister had input from Speech and Language Therapy (SLT) in primary school. Despite their disagreements, both parents attend the initial appointment and are willing to work together.

	Predisposing factors	Precipitating factors	Perpetuating factors
Biological	Genetic; sensory difficulties; temperament	Inflexible responding styles	Possible language problems? Family history
Psychological	Attachment difficulties and maternal postnatal depression	Stress with forthcoming move to secondary school	Poor problem-solving skills
Social	Inconsistent boundaries/limits within home	Parental separation	Different parenting styles. Overcrowding in house

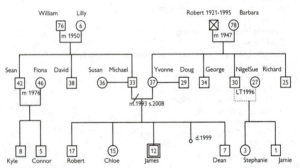

Fig. 9.2 Example genogram.

Recommended reading

McGoldrick M, Gerson R, Shellenberger S. Genograms (1999) *Assessment and Intervention*. W.W. Norton and Company Inc, New York.

Black D, Gower S. (1993) *Seminars in Child and Adolescent Psychiatry*. Gaskell, London.

Lask B, Taylor S, Nunn K. (2003) *Practical Child Psychiatry, The Clinician's Guide*. BMJ Books, London.

The pervasive developmental disorders

The pervasive developmental disorders (PDD): definitions

The PDDs comprise a group of 5 diagnostic categories that includes disorders of specific aspects of developmental functioning, namely social interaction and communication, but that are also often characterized by stereotyped or restricted interests and behaviours.

- There are clearly many other disorders of normal development, ranging from dyspraxia to hyperkinetic disorder, which are not included within the PDD label. As such, PDDs should perhaps be called pervasive disorders of social development
- In being *pervasive*, these disorders present with impairments in a range of day to day situations, rather than just at specific times.

Rutter and Schopler (1992) define PDDs as occurring in: 'Children and adults who have severe lifelong difficulties in social and communication skills beyond those accounted for by general delay'.

This definition allows PDD to encompass diagnoses of 5 types, some of which are relatively common, whilst others are rare and will often not be seen by most clinicians. These are (in the order listed in DSM-IV):

- Autism
- Rett's syndrome
- Childhood disintegrative disorder (CDD, Heller's disease)
- Asperger's syndrome
- PDD: not otherwise specified (NOS).

Note:

- The value and use of the category of 'PDD' remains subject to some debate. Whilst it is potentially helpful as an overarching concept in an area where multiple similar and overlapping terms are frequently used there is also the possibility that its use can become unfocussed and over inclusive
- Autism is the most commonly diagnosed of the PDDs, and as with Rett's and Heller's it is quite easily recognizable
- Whilst the use of the diagnosis of Asperger's is becoming increasingly widespread in child and adolescent mental health services (CAMHS), the relationship between Asperger's and what are commonly referred to as the Autistic Spectrum Disorders remains subject to debate
- PDD-NOS may be of use in cases where a child is exhibiting social or communication difficulties, but where there is insufficient evidence, at the time, to allow more specific diagnosis; it may also be a way of categorizing those diagnosed with ICD-10 atypical autism.

This chapter will focus mainly on autism and Asperger's—the other PDD's are included for completeness, but as they are relatively rare they will not be covered in any detail.

PDD: not otherwise specified (PDD-NOS)

The PDD-NOS diagnosis allows a diagnosis to be made in sub-threshold cases, where there is marked impairment of social interaction, communication, and/or stereotyped behaviour patterns or interest, but where the full features for autism or another explicitly defined PDD are not met.

As such, PDD-NOS could be applied to all the categories described in this chapter, where impairment is high, and where the withholding of a diagnosis on 'a technicality' would also withhold vital support for the child or young person.

Autism: definition

To be autistic in a world of non-autistic people has been described as being akin to visiting a strange country, where the language and rules are different to one's own. The things that are important to you seem to be much less so to everyone else, and vice versa.

Now accepted as a disorder that can occur at any intelligence level, autism or the autistic spectrum disorders have become a common consideration for CAMHS clinicians. They often, however, require a sophisticated approach to diagnosis.

As in some other areas, such as hearing impairment, an autism 'culture' has become established, where the assumption of the features of autism as being abnormal and 'a disorder' are questioned.

Autism: definition (ICD-10)

- The presence of abnormal or impaired development that is manifest before the age of 3 years
- The characteristic type of abnormal functioning in each of the following three areas of psychopathology, the so called *triad of impairment*.

Social deficits

Of the many facets of autism, difficulties with reciprocal social interaction and relationship-forming are perhaps both the most characteristic and the most disabling, manifesting in children in ways such as:

- An infant that does not enjoy being held, or fails to anticipate being lifted
- A lack of interaction such as pointing, imitating, offering comfort, sharing enjoyment, parallel play with other children
- Verbal/lingual signs of social difficulty: e.g. will rarely speak regarding concern for others, but will often make use of specific, direct—and often gauche—statements and questions
- Unusual eye contact and facial expressions.

The failure of those with autism to understand others' situations or feelings—a deficit in meta-representation—is often referred to as a lack of *theory of mind*.

Communication deficits

Deficits in communication are recognizable by an asocial quality, rather than reduced quantity.

- The normal flow of reciprocal conversation is often absent from the babbling stage onwards
- There is an unusual social quality and pitch/stress/rhythm/intonation of speech (referred to as odd *prosody*)
- Echolalia (repeating the words or phrases of others) and pronominal reversal (e.g. referring to themselves as 'she').

Restricted/repetitive interests and behaviours

These can be summarized as being; showing an interest things that others would regard as rather mundane or functional aspects of life; and behaviours that are repetitive and semi-purposeful (termed stereotypies). Such interests may begin as the enjoyment of a functional, rather than imaginative aspect of toys in early play, a commonly cited example being sorting toy cars according to shape rather than engaging in pretend drives.

In later childhood these restricted interests may become more sophisticated, an example being deriving fascination from particular types of stones, car hub-caps, or lamp-post serial numbers in place of the usual football, or boy bands.

Stereotypies can manifest as a part of an unusual interest either as an isolated occurrence, for example, the act of smelling part of an inanimate object, or as part of a repetitive ritualized system of actions. Stereotypes by definition also include acts occurring in response to an unpleasant situation or stimulus; for example, hand flapping in response to a disliked noise (📖 sensory defensiveness, below). These often predictable acts may help to ease the anxiety associated with the sufferer's unease at these situations.

Self-harming in autism (commonly hitting or biting) is most often a form of stereotypy and often a response to anxiety.

Associated features

Various other difficulties are commonly associated with autism. Of these the most common is:

Sensory defensiveness

- This may include an idiosyncratic dislike and extreme unease in response to otherwise innocent sensory stimuli. Commonly quoted examples include the sounds made by domestic appliances or the feeling of certain textures against the skin (types of fabric, bare feet on carpets, etc.)
- The intensity of response to these stimuli has been likened to the discomfort that many non- autistic spectrum disorder (ASD) individuals feel in response to sounds such as fingernails on a blackboard or wet woollen clothing.

ICD-10 atypical autism F84.1:

Differs from autism in terms of either age of onset or of failure to fulfil all three sets of diagnostic criteria. Atypical autism may present in severe learning disability, for example, where functioning is so limited that one or more the triad of impairments may be absent.

Autism: epidemiology

The concept of autism has changed over the past 4 decades, most notably in our understanding of its relationship to learning disability. Epidemiological research has allowed the expansion of the classical definition from Kanner's original description of autism as pertaining to a non-communicating, stereotypy-laden and severely learning disabled individual, to a disorder that includes individuals with a wide range of intellectual abilities, including the normal range, referred to as part of ASD.

The 'autistic spectrum' is bound together by the presence of qualitatively similar characteristics defined by the classic triad of impairments. However, the concept has been broadened considerably such that 'the spectrum' extends to the autism-like phenotypic traits seen in relatives of those diagnosed as autistic, and to other conditions where autistic traits are seen. This broader group will include the other PDDs and also non-PDDs such as extreme early deprivation or even congenital blindness.

The relationship between autism and Asperger's syndrome is described later in this chapter.

Epidemiology: incidence and increased rates of diagnosis

- In terms of the autistic spectrum disorders, including those of normal IQ, but excluding some of the more extended concepts, incidence is currently estimated at 0.3–0.6%
- Taking recent studies together an estimate for the incidence of autism is 7.5 per 10,000
- These figures represent around a 10-fold increase over estimates of incidence from the 1960s
- It is generally argued that the bulk of this increase is explainable by the expansion of diagnostic criteria and improved awareness of the disorder, rather than an increase in occurrence
- Boys are at greater risk of ASD, outnumbering girls by around 4:1
- The associations of increased rates of autism with certain social classes or ethnic origins await definitive research evidence.

Autism: aetiology

The most common over-riding and unequivocal results of research into the aetiology of autism are that:
- The causes of autism are *multifactorial*
- Autism is subject to a significant degree of *heritability* (90% heritability overall)
- The true mechanisms underlying the symptoms of autism remain unknown.

Genetic factors

Family and twin studies show:
- Increased risk of ASD in siblings of those with an ASD
- Greatly increased risk in monozygotic compared with dizygotic twins
- Increased risk of the broader phenotype in family members of those with autism.

Genetic linkage (family patterns) and association studies (disease patterns) show:
- There is no one 'gene for autism'; as with the vast majority of disorders (in any system), genetic susceptibility to autism is likely to arise from a combination of genes from a required array of gene variants, and that in most cases these are also likely to occur in combination with a range of non-genetic factors
- Several promising chromosomal locations for susceptibility genes have been identified, including locations on chromosomes 2 and 7
- ASD-like features found in the single gene disorder Tuberous Sclerosis have added to knowledge of likely susceptibility genes, whereas chromosomal disorders such as Fragile X syndrome, also which involves ASD features, are thought to be less important in the genetic aetiology of autism.

Prenatal factors

There are various associations between ASD and adverse factors during pregnancy; the most robust of these being with congenital rubella, which itself is now thankfully rare. Most associations are with first trimester effects, implying that an impact on early brain development is of particular importance. Obstetric complications are currently not thought to represent a causative factor.

Postnatal factors, including the mumps, measles and rubella (MMR) vaccine

Many postnatal factors have been linked with autism; however, few if any of these links are supported by robust evidence.

The postnatal links of most recent interest and subject to some disproportionate lay media interest, are the hypothesized links between ASD and the childhood vaccination programme, which arose largely in response to the findings of a single, methodologically flawed study. This link may have initially been made because the typical onset of ASD symptoms occurs in the 12–24-month period, coinciding with the MMR given at 12–15 months.

- Measles/mumps/rubella vaccination was hypothesized to be related to a regressive form of autism. Many studies that aimed to replicate these findings were unable to do so
- Thiomersal, a mercury-based preservative used in some vaccines, has also been implicated, but again no proven link exists.

Whilst the majority of the increase in diagnosis of ASD is attributed to increased recognition, rather than increased incidence, it is not possible to rule out the contribution by the environment as being contributory.

Autism: causal theories

Structural and imaging studies

Have not implicated any closely localized structures, which again may implicate a process occurring early in development.

In particular, these studies have found:

- Increased total brain volume and early acceleration in brain growth, with over-connectivity in some regions
- Disordered cortical functioning in which connectivity/synchronization of brain regions and cortical activity are abnormal.

Neuropsychological approaches

One potential approach to understanding the mechanisms that result in autism is to identify the neuropsychological dysfunctions that underpin the various ASD symptoms. These dysfunctions may in turn implicate brain structures responsible for that process, i.e. *neural substrates*. Examples include:

- Failure to recognize affective significance of stimuli, perception of emotion, orientating to social stimuli; all may map to dysfunction in the amygdala
- Motor planning/flexibility dysfunction—mapping to frontal lobe dysfunction
- Attention shifting problems—mapping to cerebellar dysfunction.

The next step will be to identify the *cognitive genomics* of these changes.

- Related are the 'deficient empathizing vs. drive towards systematizing' theories of autism include the 'extreme maleness' theory of the disorder. Males tend to empathize less well than females, but are more often driven to indulge in restricted and absorbing interests. This includes hypotheses about the effects of differential foetal androgen exposure, suggesting that the prenatal response to testosterone, which results in neural structure/function changes may be relevant in ASD.

Other research directions

- Immune system dysregulation has been found in some children with ASD and also a suggestion of aberrant immune activity during critical periods of development
- Neurotransmitter abnormalities have been associated with ASD, such as plasma and urine serotonin changes, as well as implication of the serotonin transporter gene as a susceptibility locus
- Failure of imitation and modelling of others' behaviours mediated via structural abnormalities in brain regions related to the so called mirror neuron system.

Autism: assessment 1

Screening

Screening programmes are often controversial, and this is certainly the case in autism. Although in the majority of cases unusual behaviours have been noticed by the age of 2, early intervention is accepted to be key to maximizing potential in ASD, and hence American Academy of Paediatrics guidelines currently recommend screening at 18 and 24 months. However, in the UK screening is not currently recommended for any developmental disorders. This is because the available tools are not considered sufficiently robust, particularly in terms of the rates of false positives and negatives identified, and therefore the benefits accrued are not great enough.

There are, however, several checklist tools available for children for whom concerns have been raised or for children at increased risk include the Checklist for Autism in Toddlers (CHAT) and M-CHAT (parental report)

Available UK guidelines include the 2003 National Autism Plan for Children and the 2007 Scottish Intercollegiate Guidelines Network (SIGN) guideline, with National Institute for Health and Clinical Excellence (NICE) due to publish guidelines in 2011.

Although screening is not generally recommended there are several warning signs that may suggest an increased risk of ASD.

Developmental warning signs of ASD in preschool children

- Delay or absence of spoken language
- Looks through people; not aware of others
- Not responsive to other people's facial expression/feelings
- Lack of pretend; little or no imagination
- Does not show typical interest in or play near peers purposefully
- Lack of turn-taking
- Unable to share pleasure
- Qualitative impairment on non-verbal communication
- Does not point at an object to direct another person to look at it
- Lack of gaze monitoring
- Lack of initiating of activity or social play
- Unusual or repetitive hand and finger mannerisms
- Unusual reactions, or lack of reaction, to sensory stimuli.

Warning signs of possible ASD in school age children

- Communication impairments
  - Abnormalities in language development including muteness
  - Odd or inappropriate prosody
  - Persistent echolalia
  - Reference to self as 'you', 'she', or 'he' beyond 3 years
  - Unusual vocabulary for child's age/social group
  - Limited use of language for communication and/or tendency to talk freely only about specific topics

- Social impairments
  - Inability to join in play of other children or inappropriate attempts at joint play (may manifest as aggressive or disruptive behaviour)
  - Lack of awareness of classroom 'norms' (criticizing teachers, overt unwillingness to co-operate in classroom activities, inability to appreciate or follow current trends)
  - Easily overwhelmed by social and other stimulation
  - Failure to relate normally to adults (too intense/no relationship)
  - Showing extreme reactions to invasion of personal space and resistance to being hurried
- Impairments of interests, activities and/or behaviours
  - Lack of flexible co-operative imaginative play/creativity
  - Difficulty in organizing self in relation to unstructured space (.g. hugging the perimeter of playgrounds, halls)
  - Inability to cope with change or unstructured situations, even ones that other children enjoy (school trips, teachers being away, etc.)
- Other factors
  - Unusual profile of skills/deficits
  - Any other evidence of odd behaviours including unusual responses to sensory stimuli.

Autism: assessment 2

Diagnosis

Timing

More severe forms of ASD can be diagnosed at an early age, but rarely earlier than 18 months, when language and rudimentary social skills are absent in most children. Less severe ASD may not be recognized until much later in childhood, perhaps only when social or educational demands increase. A small proportion of children appear to lose skills and develop an ASD later in life, this is sometimes referred to regressive autism.

Personnel

Whilst a wide range of people known to the child may raise concerns, current recommendations are that the diagnosis of ASD is made by a multidisciplinary team with experience of their own facet of the disorder. An example of core members of such a team could be psychologist, psychiatrist, speech therapist, paediatrician/neurologist.

Clinical diagnosis

Interviews with the child, and those who know them well, may be supplemented by the use of diagnostic tools such as the revised Autism Diagnostic Interview (ADI-R), which aims to make a categorical diagnosis, or the Diagnostic Interview for Social and Communication Disorders (DISCO) or Developmental, Dimensional and Diagnostic Interview (3Di). The Autism Diagnostic Observation Schedule (Generic) (ADOS-G) is a structured method of observing the child, which employs provision of specific scenarios and is associated with strong diagnostic validity.

Individual profiling

A facet of all mental health issues, but of particular importance in ASD, is the inter-individual difference in presentation, in terms of differing severities of problems, and areas of relative weakness and strength.

As a consequence the assessment of each individual's pattern of ASD is an important part of the assessment process. It is here in particular that the multidisciplinary team comes into its own. Assessment of speech and language abilities is, therefore, a standard part of any ASD assessment, and assessments for other specific domains, such as IQ and adaptive functioning should also be considered.

Assessment for co-existing or causal conditions

- **Co-morbidity:** there are several other conditions that occur more commonly in those with ASD compared with the general population and these should always be considered/excluded:
  - Epilepsy
  - Visual impairments
  - Speech impairments
  - Anxiety
  - Depression
  - ADHD
  - Behavioural disorders
  - Sleep disorders
  - Tic disorders
  - Dyspraxia
- **Causal conditions:** 1 in 10 cases of ASD currently have an identifiable medical cause. Hence, assessment should usually include:
  - General physical examination for neurological stigmata
  - Appropriate investigation to rule out specific disorders associated with ASD, e.g. tuberous sclerosis and associated epilepsy
  - Karyotyping for Fragile X syndrome
  - Detection of hearing and specific language disorders.

Autism: management

General principles of management

ASD can present substantial barriers to normal daily functioning, and the approach to its management is a combination of symptom modification together with the removal of these barriers wherever possible. It is often equally important to address co-morbid or co-existing difficulties and symptoms as it is to manage the core ASD symptoms.

Careful recording of pre-intervention status and a priori agreement of aims of intervention is useful.

Non-pharmacological management

These can be broadly separated in to parent-delivered and clinician-delivered interventions; the best combination will be dictated by the child's ASD profile, and the preferences of the child, the parents and the clinicians.

Management is based around several factors

Communication Interventions

These include a wide range of methods and techniques designed to improve communication, including social non-verbal communication, which itself has overlaps with development of joint attention and symbolic play skills. Often this work is conducted by speech and language therapists.

Social skills interventions

Designed to encourage more effective interpersonal interactions, such as social communication therapy, tactile prompting, and visual reinforcement.

Behavioural interventions

These include both entire behavioural programmes and specific interventions for problems ranging from self-harming behaviours to difficulties in shops.

- Intensive programmes using applied behavioural analysis are often used as an early intervention for preschool children, the best known being the Lovaas programme
- An example of a specific intervention is Auditory Integration Training for excess sensitivity to certain sounds.

The ideal setting for implementation of ASD management depends on severity of disorder and availability of provision. The move towards inclusion into mainstream schooling in the UK, with the placement of children with ASD in either a standard class or in a resource base, rather than in separate 'special schools' has largely been seen to be a success. Concerns remain, however, as to the level of expertise in autism within schools and bullying remains a problem for many children.

The alternative to mainstream school is full time special school attendance or dual placement, these being required for more severe disorders.

Pharmacological interventions

No medication has any direct effect on the triad of impairment, and the place of medication is therefore mainly in alleviating associated conditions and problems.

The most commonly used medications are the antipsychotics, stimulants, antidepressants, and melatonin.

Additional caution is advised when using any medication in autism because of the increased likelihood of unpredictable effects and adverse effects in this group.

- Antipsychotics
  - There is now reasonable evidence for the use of risperidone in the management of aggression, tantrums and self injury in ASD
  - UK guidelines recommend maximum daily doses of between 2 and 3.5 mg for children weighing under and over 45 kg, respectively. In practice many authorities recommend using very small doses, starting at 0.25 mg, and increasing very slowly if required
  - The usual caveats apply in terms of adverse effects. The major difficulty associated with risperidone, is its tendency to cause significant weight gain and it may also result in the metabolic syndrome developing
- Stimulants
  - Children with ASD and co-existing ADHD respond to stimulant medications in a similar way to those with ADHD alone
  - There is some evidence that the non-stimulant ADHD medication atomoxetine may also be effective
  - In both cases adverse events may be increased in this group requiring a slower titration and lower end doses
- Antidepressants: a small amount of evidence supports use for low mood, but also some utility in improving repetitive behaviours
- Melatonin
  - Available as a food supplement in the US, as a special order prescription in the UK. Whilst little 'official' information exists about its safety profile, dosing, etc., melatonin does appears to be both safe and effective in helping children with ASD who have sleep-wake cycle problems that fail to respond to behavioural intervention
  - Commonly used doses are 1–9 mg at night.

Autism: prognosis and outcome

A 2004 study reported the outcome of 68 individuals with ASD and an IQ over 50 who had been diagnosed as children and followed-up into adult life.

- 12% were rated as having a 'Very Good' outcome
- 10% as 'Good'
- 19% as 'Fair'
- 46% as 'Poor'
- 12% as 'Very Poor'.

The other main findings were:

- Most remained dependent on families or other services
- Only a small minority lived independently, had employment or close friends
- Communication, reading and spelling were impaired in most
- Stereotypies and restricted interests remained for most.

A similar study that included those with lower IQ's suggested that these children have worse outcomes.

Factors associated with good prognosis

- IQ over 50
- Language acquisition before the age of 6
- Having a skill that is consistent with securing employment.

Although those who did better generally had IQ over 70, the variability within this group was too great to consider this as a sensitive prognostic factor.

Special skills and high functioning autism

The vintage term idiot savant is a representation of the phenomenon by which an apparently very impaired autistic individual may have supra-normal abilities in one specific area. Beyond the effects of practice secondary to constantly attending to a restricted interest, these abilities are often considered, for example, as a natural genius at an art, such as painting or music, or an extraordinary memory. Whilst the overwhelming majority of the ASD population lacks such a talent, this and less spectacular, but no less positive attributes, such as an ability to systematize, may support a theory of localized brain over-connectivity.

Autism culture and neurodiversity

This represents a movement for a reduction in the perception of ASD as an illness that must be cured, and aims to re-frame many of the features of ASD as being a form of diversity, of which non ASD people ('neuro-typicals') should be more tolerant. Reinforcing to this movement are web based communities such as Wrong Planet, literature by ASD and Asperger's syndrome-diagnosed authors such as Temple Grandin and Mark Haddon, and artworks by artists such as Steven Wiltshire.

The opponents of the movement accuse those embracing autism cultures of being insensitive to the extreme and daily difficulties faced particularly by those at the severe or low functioning end of the spectrum.

A fitting summary is an extract from a New Statesman interview with Simon Baron-Cohen a leading autism researcher, in 2007:

Autism involves disability, but it also involves areas of strength—fantastic attention to detail and a good memory. There are aspects of autism to be proud of that can lead to gifts and talents.

Rett's syndrome

Rett's syndrome has been described as the least common, but most devastating of the pervasive developmental disorders. It is also the youngest, having been first described in only 1966.

Definition and presentation

ICD-10 F84.2 Rett's syndrome: a condition, so far found only in girls, in which apparently normal early development is followed by partial or complete loss of speech and of skills in locomotion and use of hands, together with deceleration in head growth, usually with an onset between 7 and 24 months of age. Loss of purposive hand movements, with hand-wringing, mouthing, and bruxism stereotypies, and unusual breathing patterns, such as hyperventilation, breath-holding, and sighing, amongst other behaviours, which are hallmarks of the condition. Social and play development are arrested, but social interest tends to be maintained. Trunk ataxia and apraxia start to develop by age 4 years and choreo-athetoid movements frequently follow. Severe mental retardation almost invariably results.

Rett's syndrome is clinically diagnosed.

Associated features

- **Epilepsy:** one of the most commonly associated problems is seizures originating in early childhood—co-morbid in around 80% of Rett's syndrome
- **Gastrointestinal problems:** in particular constipation, are common
- **Growth problems and scoliosis**
- **Motor problems:** including ataxia, chorea, dystonia, hypotonia
- **Cardiac conduction problems** (prolonged QT interval).

Epidemiology

- Prevalence 1 in 10–15,000
- Almost always occurs in females (the incidence in males is unknown). That this is secondary to lethality of the mutation (see aetiology) to males *in utero* has not been proven.

Differential diagnosis

- **Cerebral palsy:** differentiated by the pattern of onset of problems—in cerebral palsy there is rarely the regression seen in Rett's syndrome
- **ASD:** the high incidence of epilepsy and the characteristic stereotypies assist with the differentiation of Rett's syndrome from autism.

Aetiology

Rett's syndrome was recently discovered to be caused by a mutation of the gene encoding methyl-CpG binding protein 2 on the X chromosome. Most mutations are sporadic, but a small percentage may be inherited from a maternal germ line mutation.

A separate gene mutation results in a similar picture to Rett's syndrome, but also includes infantile spasms as the associated epilepsy.

Management

With gene therapy still at the animal-based hypothesis stage, management of Rett's syndrome is rooted in providing support and maximizing potential (for example, by facilitating communication) and treatment of associated problems, with common interventions including the use of atypical antipsychotics, such as risperidone for self-harming behaviours.

Prognosis

Life expectancy is reduced in Rett's, to middle age in females, and in rare surviving males, not beyond infancy. The exception to the latter is a co-existing condition, which adds a balancing extra X chromosome, such as Klinefelter's syndrome.

Childhood disintegrative disorder (CDD): Heller's disease

Definitions and presentation

ICD-10 F84.3—other childhood disintegrative disorder: a type of perva-sive developmental disorder that is defined by a period of entirely normal development before the onset of the disorder, followed by a definite loss of previously acquired skills in several areas of development over the course of a few months. Typically, this is accompanied by a general loss of interest in the environment, by stereotyped, repetitive motor mannerisms, and by autistic-like abnormalities in social interaction and communication. In some cases, the disorder can be shown to be due to some associated encephalopathy, but the diagnosis should be made on the behavioural fea-tures. Excludes Rett's syndrome

Alternative terminology
- Dementia infantilis
- (Progressive) Disintegrative psychosis
- Symbiotic psychosis.

The hallmark of childhood disintegrative disorder is the cruel and devas-tating loss of previously acquired developmental progress at a relatively late stage, from around 3 years to as late as 10 years old.

This loss of skills will usually include 2 out of the 3 of the autistic triad of impairments (see autism section), but can also include more wide ranging difficulties, such as enuresis/encopresis.

Epidemiology
Most data on childhood disintegrative disorder is derived from case series, and as such prevalence figures are approximate. Overall, there appears to be:
- A prevalence of around 1–6 per 100,000
- An excess of males affected.

Differential diagnosis
- **Autism:** particularly the regressive subtype, although the lateness and severity of the regression are characteristic of childhood disintegrative disorder
- **Landau–Kleffner syndrome** (acquired epileptic aphasia): a sudden loss of language at around 5–7 years old. However, the other 2 impairments in the triad remain intact, and EEG is abnormal
- **Other epilepsies** especially in the setting of persistent seizures. However, the loss of skills is usually thought to fluctuate in this situation.

Aetiology
The aetiology of childhood disintegrative disorder is unknown. Current research leads include the possibility of genetic risk, storage-like disease, and an immunopathological mechanism.

Management

The general encouragement of communication and support in behavioural management are the most appropriate supportive measures taken in management of childhood disintegrative disorder. Frequently co-existing epilepsy will require anti-epileptic pharmacotherapy.

Prognosis

- Outcome IQ's for childhood disintegrative disorder are usually in the severely learning disabled range. A minority display a slowly progressive ongoing regression
- Once regression is complete, the clinical picture of childhood disintegrative disorder is often similar to that of autism with a comparable IQ
- Overall, the course of childhood disintegrative disorder is poorer outcome than for ASD, with lower functioning and greater problems with co-existing epilepsy.

Asperger syndrome: definitions

Definition

ICD-10 describes Asperger syndrome (or Asperger's) as being of unknown nosological validity, and indeed, as with the PDDs in general, classification along either dimensional or categorical lines is still at times difficult to achieve.

However Asperger's current place among the PDDs is accurately summarized by ICD-10, describes the disorder as being characterized by:

The same type of qualitative abnormalities of reciprocal social interaction that typify autism, together with a restricted, stereotyped, repetitive repertoire of interests and activities. It differs from autism primarily in the fact that there is no general delay or retardation in language or in cognitive development. This disorder is often associated with marked clumsiness. There is a strong tendency for the abnormalities to persist into adolescence and adult life. Psychotic episodes occasionally occur in early adult life.

Presentation

Typical presentation features of Asperger's are:

Restricted interests

- A narrow focus on sometimes (but not always) unusual or left-field topics, with a variable understanding of the wider picture
  - The tendency of many small boys to be interested in dinosaurs or space travel may mask this issue until primary school age, where this interest reveals an unusual intensity or depth
  - Intense interests can be associated with ritualized and rigid behaviours or stereotypies such as the classic hand flapping and twirling.

Social awkwardness

- A failure to read others' feelings results in
  - A tendency to talk at length despite signals that the listener is disinterested
  - A tendency towards socially *gauche* comments in public or a precocious style of discourse
  - An odd style of social discourse resulting from a rigid attempt to simulate normal interactions (excessive eye contact, interrupting in conversation)
  - Social difficulties arising from rigid or *concrete* interpretation of situations, and so a failure to grasp humour, irony or teasing
  - Withdrawal from peer groups as a result of past social failures.

Unusual communication style

- May be excessively formal in younger children (when associated with intense interests leading to the 'little professor' label
- Unusual/inappropriate rate, rhythm, volume and prosody (the use of tonal variation and stresses in conversation)
- Use of unusual or novel words and idiosyncratic humour.

Gillberg's criteria for Asperger's syndrome

All six criteria must be met
- Severe impairment in reciprocal social interaction (at least two of the following)
  - Inability to interact with peers
  - Lack of desire to interact with peers
  - Lack of appreciation of social cues
  - Socially and emotionally inappropriate behaviour
- All-absorbing narrow interest (at least one of the following)
  - Exclusion of other activities
  - Repetitive adherence
  - More rote than meaning
  - Imposition of routines and interests (at least one of the following)
    —on self, in aspects of life
    —on others
- Imposition of routines and interests (at least one of the following)
  - On self, in aspects of life
  - On others
- Speech and language problems (at least three of the following)
  - Delayed development
  - Superficially perfect expressive language
  - Formal, pedantic language
  - Odd prosody, peculiar voice characteristics
  - Impairment of comprehension including misinterpretations of literal/implied meanings
- Non-verbal communication problems (at least one of the following)
  - Limited use of gestures
  - Clumsy/gauche body language
  - Limited facial expression
  - Inappropriate expression
  - Peculiar, stiff gaze
- Motor clumsiness: poor performance on neurodevelopmental examination.

Asperger's syndrome and normality

A not uncommon perception of Asperger's is as a problem that becomes less important or even an advantage under certain circumstances. For example, a surgeon may be very successful as a result of being quiet and determined, but paying extreme attention to detail in theatre, despite being a little odd on post-operative rounds (and hopeless at dinner parties).

There is an emphasis on Asperger's being a disorder, which allows a much higher level of or normal functioning in relation to other ASDs. There is, on the other hand, a risk that the disorder may remain unnoticed or be assumed to be a quirk of personality, whilst actually causing significant functional impairment.

It may be for this reason that Asperger's frequently presents late, if at all, by which time it is accompanied by a range of secondary problems, such as anger outbursts and frustration in younger children, or low mood and anxiety, and associated peer/social difficulties in adolescents.

Asperger syndrome: epidemiology, aetiology, diagnosis, management, prognosis

Epidemiology

Because of uncertain diagnostic boundaries, prevalence estimates vary widely: from 3 per 10,000 to 3%, with male diagnoses exceeding females by 2–10 fold.

Aetiology

Although many of the theories around the aetiology of autism are also considered as viable for Asperger's syndrome, it is not necessarily assumed that Asperger's and autism share the same aetiology. There is evidence for as strong if not stronger heritability as is seen in autism. Some environmental risk factors, particularly those impacting early in foetal brain development, have been suggested, but there is, as yet, no clear unifying causal theory.

Diagnosis

Diagnosis is usually made using either ICD-10 criteria, or commonly used alternatives, such as those proposed by Gillberg or the Szatmari criteria.

Gillberg's criteria are more inclusive than those in ICD-10, for example, as there is no requirement for 'normal' development of cognitive skills, language, curiosity and self-help skills in Gillberg's criteria. As such the ICD-10 most likely corresponds to a more strictly defined categorical diagnosis, whereas the Gillberg criteria encourage a more dimensional view of Asperger's within the broader ASD/PDD constructs.

Asperger's may often be diagnosed later in childhood than autism, although retrospectively traits may have been present at the ages of 2 or 3 years. Individuals in whom a suspicion of Asperger's or autism has been raised should be investigated a thorough multidisciplinary assessment which can be supplemented by the ADI or ADOS-G questionnaires, which also encompass the Asperger's diagnosis. There are also screening questionnaires which are more specific to Asperger's, such as the Gillberg or the Australian Scale for Asperger' syndrome.

Management

As with autism, management is dictated by specific aspects of the individual's difficulties; many of the approaches are similar to those employed in autism and include behavioural and/or cognitive strategies aimed at:

- Normalizing social discourse
- Normalizing language
- Minimizing difficulties associated with restricted interests, sensory defensiveness, etc.

Asperger's is frequently is associated with dyspraxia type difficulties, in which case occupational therapy assessments can be helpful.

Prognosis

Although there is a lack of reliable long-term data, the core elements of Asperger's course seem likely to remain relatively unchanged throughout life. Whilst difficulties from co-morbid anxiety and depression continue to be a risk, there does seem to be a tendency for many of those diagnosed with Asperger's to be less impaired by their difficulties as life progresses. It may be that as the all absorbing importance of peer relationships in adolescence and early adulthood fades, a more comfortable niche is found.

Recommended reading

Rutter M & Schopler E. (1992) Classification of pervasive developmental disorders: some concepts and practical considerations. *J Autism Dev Disord* **22:** 459–82.

Arndt TL, Stodgell CJ, Rodier PM (2005) The teratology of autism. *Int J Dev Neurosci* **23**(2–3): 189–99.

Newschaffer CJ, Croen LA, Daniels J, et al. (2007) The epidemiology of autism spectrum disorders. *Ann Rev Public Hlth* **28**: 235–58.

Rutter M. (2005) Aetiology of autism: findings and questions. *J Intellect Disabil Res* **49**(Pt 4): 231–8.

Scottish Intercollegiate Guideline Network Guideline 98. *Assessment, Diagnosis and Clinical Interventions for Children and Young People with Autism Spectrum Disorders.*

Time out with Nick Cohen (2007) *New Statesman*, 26 February.

Trevatham E, Naidu S. (1988) The clinical recognition and differential diagnosis of Rett syndrome. *J Child Neurol* **3**(Suppl.): S6–16.

Attention deficit hyperactivity disorder

Definitions

Attention deficit hyperactivity disorder (ADHD) is a complex neurodevelopmental disorder. The core symptoms are:
- Inattention
- Impulsivity
- Over-activity.

These symptoms are required to be:
- Present from an early age (before the age of 7 years)
- Pervasive across at least two situations (e.g. home, school, and social life)
- The cause of significant impairment to the child's functioning

The DSM-IV diagnostic criteria for ADHD are detailed in Table 11.1.

The ICD-10 criteria for hyperkinetic disorder are somewhat more restrictive in that they require:
- Hyperactivity, impulsivity, and inattention all to be present
- All symptoms to be impairing across two or more settings

For this reason hyperkinetic disorder defines the subgroup of those with combined type ADHD with the most severely impairing symptomatology.

Table 11.1 Diagnostic criteria for DSM-IV ADHD

Symptoms	Requirements
Inattention	*Subtypes:* Combined type: at least 6 inattentiveness items plus 6 hyperactivity/Impulsivity items
Fails to give close attention to details or, makes careless mistakes in, schoolwork, work, or other daily activities	Inattentive type: at least 6 inattentiveness items
Has difficulty sustaining attention on tasks or play activities	Hyperactive/impulsive type: at least 6 hyperactivity/impulsivity items
Does not seem to listen to when spoken to directly	*Onset:* symptoms that caused impairment must be present before the age of 7 years of age
Does not follow through on instructions and fails to finish schoolwork chores, or duties in the workplace	*Pervasiveness:* impairment must be present in two or more settings
Has difficulties organizing tasks and activities	*Impairment:* there must be clear evidence of clinically significant impairment of functioning
Avoids, dislikes, or is reluctant to engage In tasks that require sustained mental effort such as schoolwork or home work	*Co-existing disorders:* symptoms should not be better accounted for by another mental disorder
Looses things necessary for tasks or activities (e.g. toys, school assignments, pencils, books or tools)	
Is easily distracted by extraneous stimuli	
Is forgetful in daily activities	
Hyperactivity	
Fidgets with hands or feet or squirms in seat	
Leaves seat in classroom or in other situations in which remaining seated is expected	
Runs about or climbs excessively in situations in which it is inappropriate	
Has difficulty playing or engaging in leisure activities quietly	
Is 'on the go' or often acts as if 'driven by a motor'	
Impulsivity	
Difficulty waiing turn	
Interrupts often	
Blurts out answers	
Talks excessively	

Epidemiology

Initial epidemiological studies of ADHD resulted in widely varying estimations of prevalence with rates from as low as 0.9% to as high as 20% being reported.

A recent systematic review identified 102 studies, from across all world regions. The overall prevalence of ADHD based on all studies was 5.3%. The prevalence for children was 6.5% and for adolescents 2.7%.

Differences between studies were mainly accounted for by:

- The use of differing diagnostic criteria (DSM-III, DSM-III-R, DSM-IV, or ICD-10)
- The source of information used to elicit symptoms (best-estimate procedure, parents, teachers, or subjects)
- The requirement, or not, for impairment to be present in order for the diagnosis to be made.

After adjustments were made to account for these methodological issues, the estimates from North America and Europe were not significantly different from each other.

The prevalence of the more restrictive ICD-10 hyperkinetic disorder diagnosis has been estimated to be around 1.5%.

Studies in children consistently suggest that ADHD is more common in boys than in girls with a male:female ratio between 2:1 and 9:1 depending on how the sample is gathered. In epidemiological studies of non-referred children the pooled ADHD prevalence for boys is 2.45 times higher than that for girls. The increased prevalence among girls found in community samples compared with clinical samples, suggests that there are greater barriers to recognition, referral and diagnosis of ADHD in girls than in boys.

The impact of ethnic and socioeconomic issues on the prevalence rates of ADHD has been much less well investigated. However, in general, it appears that ADHD is a worldwide disorder and that, as long as similar methodologies are used, the prevalence rates are similar in most ethnic communities.

Aetiology

ADHD displays considerable heterogeneity at the genetic, pathophysiological, cognitive, and behavioural levels of analysis. Whilst the exact aetiology of ADHD is unknown considerable research supports a strong genetic component with non-shared environmental factors contributing most of the residual variance. Gene-environment interactions seem likely to be important, but have not yet been studied extensively.

Genetic factors

- ADHD aggregates within families with a 3–5 times increased risk in first degree relatives
- Behavioural genetic studies suggest a heritability of 0.6–0.9
- Molecular genetic studies have implicated a number of possible genes (📖 Table 11.2). However, each of these genes only increases the relative risk of ADHD slightly. This is consistent with the hypothesis that ADHD is a complex polygenic disorder with high levels of heterogeneity, influenced by the interaction of multiple aetiological factors
- Some rarer genes, including fragile X and resistance to thyroid hormone, may show larger effects, but only in a small number of cases

Table 11.2 Genes potentially involved in ADHD for which there are replicated findings

Dopamine receptor 4 (DRD4 7-repeat allele)
Dopamine receptor 5 (DRD5 148 bp-allele)
Dopamine transporter (DAT1 10-repeat allele)
Dopamine receptor gene (DRD1) and Serotonin receptor gene 5-HT(1B)
Dopamine beta hydroxylase gene (Taq 1 polymorphism)
SNAP-25 gene replicated findings

Environmental factors

Potentially important environmental factors include:
- Prenatal and perinatal obstetric complications
- Low birth weight
- Prenatal exposure to benzodiazepines, alcohol, and nicotine
- Brain diseases and injuries
- Severe early deprivation
- Institutional rearing
- Idiosyncratic reactions to food
- Exposure to toxic levels of lead

The quality of relationships within the family and at school can be considered as maintaining or protective factors.

Neurodevelopmental factors linking causes to behaviours

There are, however, many consistent findings that provide empirical evidence for the biological basis of ADHD. Several potential causal pathways have been described, however it is now recognized that each of these is probably too simplistic to explain all cases of ADHD and that there are almost certainly multiple causal pathways that interact with each other.

Structural and functional brain imaging studies

Studies have identified various structural and functional abnormalities in frontal, temporal, and parietal cortical regions, the basal ganglia, callosal areas, and cerebellum. These abnormalities appear to be evident early in development, are non-progressive, and are not a result of treatment with medications.

Pathophysiology

Evidence from molecular genetics, the effectiveness of stimulants, some animal models and functional imaging studies are all in keeping with the theory that catacholaminergic dysregulation (probably involving both dopamine and noradrenaline) is central to the aetiology of ADHD.

Neuropsychological and electrophysiological studies

Studies have found alterations in a range of higher-order 'executive' cognitive functions, motivational processes and more basic 'non-executive' stages of information processing.

Several potential cognitive endophenotypes have been described including:
- Working memory
- Non-executive short-term memory
- Timing regulation
- Inhibitory dysregulation
- Delay aversion

Assessment

At the level of primary care, the first responsibility is to recognize and detect the symptoms of ADHD. There is considerable evidence to suggest that, despite increasing recognition rates, most cases of ADHD still remain unrecognized in the United Kingdom and most European countries. Parental checklists and accounts from teachers are valuable in helping to make sure that ADHD symptoms are, indeed, the presenting problems, rather than the commoner difficulties of sleep or conduct disturbance. Physical examination can ensure that there is no evident underlying physical illness, hearing should be checked, and any history of epilepsy sought. If the symptoms of ADHD are causing social impairment, then the next step should be referral to a community child mental health service or to developmental paediatrics.

A full assessment should be multidisciplinary, and will almost always require more than one visit. ADHD symptoms must be evaluated carefully against what is expected at that developmental level. The assessment needs to be full enough to find any alternative explanation of the symptoms, and any significant co-morbidity. A full assessment should include the following

Clinical interview with the parents, including:
- A general mental health evaluation as described in Chapter 9.
- Specific questioning should include:
  - The behaviours that comprise the ADHD diagnosis, any situational variation in these, their times of onset and development, and their presence in other family members
  - Symptoms of co-morbid and differential diagnoses should be enquired about (in addition to those listed below borderline personality disorder, substance abuse, and schizophrenic disorders should also be considered in adolescents).

A separate interview with the child
- This should be considered standard practice
- The purpose is to address general adjustment and co-morbidity and should focus on:
  - General functioning in the family, the school and the peer group
  - The presence of emotional problems and low self-esteem
  - The child's attitudes to and coping with their ADHD

Information from preschool and school

This is essential, as long as parents agree to it being obtained, and it should focus on information from the teacher about:

- Behaviour and behaviour problems
- Developmental and social functioning
- Situational variations in behaviour, and symptoms indicating potential co-morbid or differential diagnoses
- Written or telephoned reports can help provide a full view of the child at school, and to assess the coping style of the teacher and the teacher-child relationship.

Psychometric tests

- These are not routinely required and do not generally help with the diagnostic process; however, they may be helpful when there are problems related to classroom adjustment or academic progress
- When time is scarce, a short Wechsler Intelligence Scale for Children (WISC) or equivalent is better than no assessment
- Speech and language tests are needed when there is evidence of difficulty in communication
- Tests of attention and impulsivity are still essentially research tools, and have not been standardized for individual diagnosis.

General physical evaluation

This is always required, and should include:

- Assessment of physical health, any evidence of breakdown of care, and signs of congenital disorders (e.g. foetal alcohol syndrome, Williams' syndrome, neurofibromatosis)
- A check on vision and hearing
- Neurodevelopmental assessment is important and should include assessment for evidence of immaturity in gross and fine motor functions, and for motor and vocal tics
- Height, weight, and head circumference should always be recorded.

Differential diagnosis

In most cases differential diagnoses can be addressed by a careful initial assessment, although in some situations observation over time is required. Potential differential diagnoses include:

- Pervasive developmental disorders
- Anxiety and mood disorders
- Acute adjustment disorders (readily distinguished by their time course)
- Attachment disorders
- Chronic brain syndromes may present with hyperactive behaviour and are therefore not a differential diagnosis, but a possible cause
- Mental retardation can co-exist with ADHD and does not exclude the diagnosis of ADHD
- Conduct disorders may sometimes give difficulty in the differential. It may be difficult to tell whether an apparently inattentive pattern of failing to do activities is, in fact, due to defying adult expectations to conform.

Co-morbid disorders

The co-existence of several other types of psychopathology along with ADHD is very common; indeed in clinical samples it is relatively rare to see a case of 'simple' ADHD with no other co-morbid problems.

Conduct disorder

Oppositional defiant and conduct disorders are very common in ADHD they should most often be seen as a complication, rather than a co-morbidity or differential diagnosis. Hyperactive behaviour is a risk factor for developing conduct disorder, even in children who showed a pure pattern of hyperactivity without conduct disorder at the beginning of their problems. Conduct disorder does not give rise to ADHD in the same way.

Emotional disorders

The reasons for the frequent co-existence of hyperactivity, and problems of anxiety and depression are not well understood. Some children may develop low self-esteem and insecurity as a result of failures at school and interpersonal relationships.

Specific learning disorders

Children with ADHD disorders are more likely to show other neurodevelopmental delays of various types. Language milestones are achieved later than normal, expressive language is unduly simple, sensory motor co-ordination is often impaired, handwriting is poor and reading ability is behind that expected for chronological age. Some children may enter school with their cognitive function compromised by neuropsychological deviations. The subsequent stress in adjusting to classroom demands leads to disturbances in the control of activity and attention. For other children, a primary disturbance of attention and impulse may give rise to secondary academic problems, either through inability to cope with the work or an aversion to it.

Pervasive developmental disorders

Children with autism often show hyperactive behaviour and autistic symptoms are sometimes seen in the hyperactive. Clinically, children with ADHD and an autistic type of social impairment will sometimes show a partial response to stimulants (although caution is needed in view of possible adverse effects). It is therefore desirable to recognize both disorders when they are present.

Tic disorders

A number of children with ADHD develop co-morbid tic disorders during their early school years. In these cases, the degree of psychosocial impairment is usually determined by ADHD and it will often be the target for therapy.

Developmental co-ordination disorder

ADHD is often accompanied by problems in sensory motor coordination, especially seen as poor handwriting, clumsiness, poor performance in sports and marked delays in achieving motor milestones. If significant interference with academic achievements or activities of daily living is observed, further assesment by occupational or physiotherapists may be helpful. Treatment with stimulants could be indicated: it may improve motor co-ordination and increase the motivation of the child for further sensorimotor training.

Bipolar disorder

There is still some controversy about the existence and definition of pre-adolescent mania (□ Chapter 16 for a fuller discussion). More work is needed on the phenomenology and diagnosis of mania in children, on its natural history, and on its familial correlates. Nevertheless, some studies which describe high rates of overlap between ADHD and mania exist. This might have implications for treatment approaches in such cases, but consensus is not reached yet.

Substance abuse

The relationship between ADHD and substance abuse is complex and relatively understudied. Elevated rates of ADHD are reported among adults seeking treatment for substance use disorders. Those with ADHD present younger and report earlier onset of drug abuse, more frequent and intense drug use, higher rates of alcoholism, and higher rates of previous treatment. Prospective studies of referred and non-referred children with ADHD followed up into adolescence and early adulthood also report increased rates of drug use and abuse, including smoking. Whilst controlling for co-morbid disorders (particularly conduct disorder) substantially weakens this association there is some evidence that non-co-morbid ADHD in adults does act as an independent risk factor for substance misuse.

Management: general issues and decision making

Psychoeducational, behavioural, and medication treatments all have a place in the treatment of those with ADHD. Treatments should be planned on an individual basis taking into account the severity and pervasiveness of the core ADHD symptoms and impairments, the presence of co-morbidity, and the individual's circumstances and preferences. Most cases seen by clinicians will have problems in several functional domains and will therefore require some form of multimodal intervention.

Psychoeducation

Psychoeducation will form the cornerstone of any treatment package and should be offered to every individual diagnosed with ADHD, their families, teachers, and others in regular contact with the child. Psychoeducation should include an assessment of the child and parents' beliefs and understanding about ADHD, its causes and consequences, followed by an informed discussion of the current scientific and clinical knowledge about ADHD, its co-morbidities and treatment including acknowledgement of both what is and is not known. Even if formal parent management training is not being offered, it is almost always appropriate to help parents and teachers to identify specific problem situations and find behaviour management techniques for them. If medication is being considered, a full and frank discussion about the various drug treatments, addressing potential benefits and risks should be implemented. Discussing patient and parental beliefs and fears about medication to treat ADHD is likely to improve adherence with treatment.

Which treatments for which patients?

With several effective treatments approaches available, an important decision concerns the order in which these treatments are offered. Many of these decisions are currently based on the various results of the influential Multimodal treatment of ADHD (MTA) study. The primary findings of this 14-month randomized trial were that:
- The children in all four treatment arms (community 'as usual' treatment, intensive behavioural treatment, intensively monitored medication treatment, and a combination of the behavioural and medication arms) improved considerably
- The medication and combined arms were significantly better on most measures than the other two arms
- The addition of the behavioural package to the medication arm produced few benefits.

As a consequence it has been suggested by some authorities that medication treatments should be considered as 'first line' for cases of combined subtype ADHD. This position is challenged by a reanalysis of the MTA dataset which suggests that whilst the superiority of medication was clear for children meeting criteria for ICD-10 defined hyperkinetic disorder, the situation was less clear for those children with the broader DSM-IV combined type ADHD, with the behavioural and medication treatment arms having equal effectiveness. The European Guidelines Group have therefore suggested that medication should be the first treatment for those with hyperkinetic disorder, whilst those with combined subtype ADHD, but not hyperkinetic disorder should be first offered a trial of behavioural treatment with medication reserved for those whose symptoms persist.

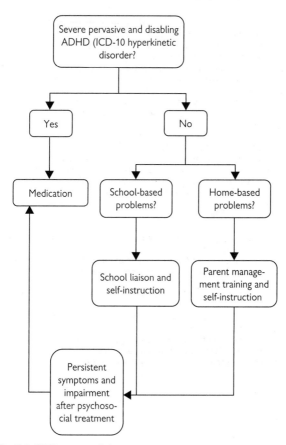

Fig. 11.1 ADHD treatment choices.

Management: psychosocial treatments

Psychosocial treatments, in particular family-based behavioural interventions, reduce ADHD symptom, and are well supported by randomized trials.

Parental training and behavioural interventions in the family

There are many approaches, including (but are not limited to):

- The identification of specific problem situations and the immediate precipitants of disruptive behaviour
- Encouraging continual monitoring of the child's progress
- Analysis of the positive and negative consequences and contingencies of appropriate and problem behaviours along with the parents
- Identification of marked inconsistencies in applying negative consequences to problem behaviour and positive consequences to appropriate behaviours
- Reduction of coercive and unpleasant parent–child interactions, while increasing positive parent-child interactions
- Enhancing parental attending skills during supervised playtime sessions
- Teaching parents effective methods of communicating commands and setting rules (e. g. making eye contact with the child; not giving too many commands at once; framing commands positively) and of paying positive attention to child compliance
- The use of specific problem situations (e. g. mealtimes) in order to train these skills
- The use of token systems in order to reinforce appropriate behaviour in specific situations
- Encouraging the use of preferred activities should be used as back-up reinforcers, rather than material rewards, such as sweets
- The development, together with the parents, of appropriate negative consequences for problem behaviour, which should be closely and consistently linked to the problem behaviour
- The use of response cost systems to reduce very frequent problem behaviours
- The use of time-out from reinforcement as a punishment procedure for more serious forms of child non-compliance and where negative consequences to problem behaviour are not effective

Behavioural interventions in the preschool or the school

School-based approaches can include:

- Discussion of classroom structure and task demands with the teacher, e.g.
  - Having the child sit close to the teacher
  - Brief academic assignments
  - Interspersing classroom lectures with brief periods of physical exercise
- The identification of specific problem situations and the immediate precipitants of disruptive behaviour
- Frequent monitoring of the child's progress with a rating scale
- Analysis of the positive and negative consequences and contingencies used by the teacher to manage behaviour
- If coercive and unpleasant teacher–child interactions occur very often while positive teacher–child interactions rarely occur, then it may be possible to enhance the differential attending skills of the teacher
- Discussion of effective methods of communicating positive commands, setting rules, paying positive attention to child compliance
- The use of token systems in order to reinforce appropriate behaviour in specific situations with potential reinforcements at home
- Response cost systems are useful to reduce very frequent problem behaviours
- The use of brief time-out from reinforcement as a punishment procedure for more serious forms of child non-compliance.

Work with the child

The child needs to be integrated as an active member into this therapeutic process. The use of self-management procedures in school-aged children may enhance both home- and school-based interventions. Self-monitoring of problem behaviours can be taught and used in specific situations (e.g. leaving seat during meals, school work, or homework). Children can also be taught to evaluate their own behaviour and to reinforce themselves. In adolescence, use contingency contracting, rather than token systems or response cost systems and stress self-management procedures. Problem solving and communication training, as well as cognitive restructuring can be used to reduce parent-adolescent conflicts.

Management: pharmacological 1

Pharmacological treatments for ADHD are supported by a strong evidence base. The most commonly used medications in the UK and Europe are the psychostimulants methylphenidate and dexamfetamine. The non-stimulant drug atomoxetine is also licensed for treating ADHD and is widely used.

Methylphenidate and dexamfetamine

These drugs block monoamine transporters, thus inhibiting the re-uptake of dopamine and noradrenalin from the synapse.

Effects

The literature supporting their use includes numerous placebo-controlled randomized control trials that confirm substantial short-term benefits with a pooled effect size of around 0.9. The psycho-stimulants markedly and rapidly reduce the core ADHD symptoms, decrease aggression, improve the quality of social interactions, and increase compliance. Both methylphenidate and amphetamines are each effective in around 70% of children with ADHD, and between 90 and 95% of those treated respond to one or both medication.

Adverse effects

Although relatively few subjects drop out of clinical trials due to problems with tolerability, a significant minority (around 20–25%) of clinic treated patients do not wish to remain on stimulants due to adverse effects. The main adverse effects of both medications are interference with sleep and loss of appetite.

The 36-month results of the MTA study suggest that stimulant medications can result in the initial slowing in growth rates and that whilst the rate of growth was normalized by 36 months, there was no rebound growth during this time and children were on average 1 inch shorter than expected. It is therefore recommended that both height and weight should be routinely monitored.

A recent Food and Drug Agency (FDA) review identified 25 deaths and 54 serious cardiac complications in patients taking stimulant medications, in the USA between 1999 and 2003. It should be noted that these adverse reports equated to less than 2 non-fatal cardiovascular events per million prescriptions, and less than 1 death per million, which is unlikely to be greater than the rate in the untreated population. The main practical implications of these findings are:

- To include physical examination before prescribing stimulants
- To seek cardiovascular abnormalities, such as raised blood pressure or heart murmurs [electrocardiogram (ECG) is optional]
- To enquire about symptoms such as syncope on exercise, with a cardiology evaluation being recommended if any warning signs are found.

Pulse and blood pressure should continue to be routinely monitored during treatment.

Motor tics may emerge or worsen during treatment in a proportion of cases, although recent evidence suggests this is less of an issue than previously thought.

Whilst stimulants probably lower the convulsive threshold, experience suggests that they can be used safely and effectively in children with co-existing seizure disorders, as long as seizures are well controlled.

A meta-analysis of the available literature reported that stimulant treatment reduced, rather than increased the risk of substance misuse problems.

Extended release preparations

Recently several long-acting oral stimulant preparations, which are a mixture of immediate- and extended-release medications, have been developed and licensed. These preparations differ with respect their duration of action (Equasym XL®/Metadate CD®, Ritalin LA®, Medikinet Retard® = 8 h duration; Adderrall XR® = 8–10 h; Concerta® = 12 h) and the proportion of immediate-release to extended-release (Concerta® 22:78; Equasym XL®/Metadate CD® 30:70; Ritalin LA®, Medikinet Retard®, Focalin XR®, Adderrall XR® 50:50). As a consequence, each preparation has a different profile over time, a factor that can be useful when matching a particular patient to a particular drug. Although still to be fully demonstrated empirically, these preparations have several potential advantages over their immediate-release predecessors including:

- A reduction in stigma at school
- Improved compliance
- A reduced risk of misuse.

In view of these potential benefits, most commentators have agreed that, whilst they should not replace short-acting drugs, extended-release preparations should be available and should be used.

Other long-acting stimulant preparations licensed in the USA, but not yet available in the UK or Europe include a methylphenidate transdermal patch system (Daytrana®) and lisdexamfetamine (Vyvanse®), an amphetamine pro-drug.

Management: pharmacological 2

Atomoxetine

Is a selective noradrenalin transporter blocker and the first non-stimulant drug licensed for the treatment of ADHD.

Effects

Its efficacy in reducing ADHD symptoms and increasing quality of life is supported by several randomized clinical trials. Although it may have some immediate effects, full clinical effects take around 6–8 weeks to appear. Whilst the half-life is relatively short (around 5 h), the clinical effects appear to last longer and, once established, daily dosage is sufficient for most patients and may last across the whole 24-h period.

A systematic review of published and unpublished data estimated the effect size of atomoxetine to be 0.7.

Adverse effects

Common adverse effects include nausea, sedation and appetite loss. Most adverse effects appear to diminish over the first months of treatment. As with stimulants, pulse and blood pressure may increase, and should be monitored. Although atomoxetine is metabolized by the cytochrome P450 2D6 enzyme, there does not appear to be a significant increase in adverse events in poor metabolizers. The most common serious events reported with atomoxetine have been seizures, although in many cases those affected were already prone to seizures or were taking other drugs that can cause them. Thus, it is not clear whether atomoxetine can cause seizures. The warnings given for serious idiosyncratic hepatic events are similar to those for stimulants and medication should be discontinued in patients who present with signs or symptoms of liver injury. Routine monitoring of hepatic function is, however, not recommended. Preliminary data on atomoxetine do not show any potential for abuse or long-term effects on growth.

Other non-stimulants

Since the licensing of atomoxetine and the extended-release stimulants, other unlicensed non-stimulant drugs known to have some efficacy in treating ADHD are currently used much less frequently. These include the tricyclic antidepressants, clonidine, guanfacine, and bupropion.

Management: pharmacological 3

Which medication should be used in which circumstances?

This will depend on a range of patient and practical considerations, and individual choices need to be made for each patient. However, general recommendations can be made.

- Methylphenidate will usually be the first choice medication
- Both release modified and immediate release methylphenidate preparations should be used
  - Modified release preparations can be considered when it is important to maximize convenience, improve adherence, reduce stigma, avoid taking medication in school, and when a smoother pharmacokinetic profile is required
  - Immediate-release preparations should be considered when a more flexible dosing regimen is required
- If starting a patient on an extended-release stimulant preparation, the choice of preparation will depend upon the profile of action required over time and availability
- Atomoxetine may be preferred in some cases particularly where
  - There is a history of substance abuse
  - There is a co-morbid tics disorder
  - There is a strong family preference for a non-stimulant
  - A 24-h action is particularly strongly required
  - There is co-morbid anxiety
- Where a child has suffered adverse effects on methylphenidate, then the next step will often be to proceed to atomoxetine
- If a child has failed to respond to methylphenidate, because of lack of efficacy, rather than adverse effect, then the next option is to try dexamfetamine or atomoxetine depending on the relative balance of advantages.

Monitoring ongoing treatment

The superiority of the medication arm of the MTA study over the community treatment arm, in which a substantial proportion also received medication, suggests that the effectiveness of medication treatment depends on more than just selecting the right drug and gives some pointers to several of the other potentially important treatment factors.

The children in the medication arm were managed much more intensively and were more closely monitored than those in the community treatment arm. Differences included:

- Starting treatment with an intensive 28-day double-blind titration trial
- They were treated with higher doses (10 mg/day greater)
- They received their stimulant medication 3 times daily dosing as opposed to twice daily dosing in the community group
- They received supportive counselling and reading materials at the beginning of and during treatment
- They had their dose adjustments informed by monthly teacher consultation with the pharmacotherapist.

It is therefore recommended that clinicians try to arrange continuing care for their ADHD patients in an organized manner that can capitalize on these benefits as much as is possible.

Prognosis, course, and outcome

Whilst ADHD was originally conceptualized as a disorder restricted to childhood and adolescence longitudinal studies have shown that, whilst symptoms decline with age, they persist in a variable proportion of people. A meta-analysis of longitudinal studies of ADHD found a 15% persistence rate when full diagnostic criteria were required and one of between 40 and 60%, when cases of ADHD in partial remission were included. These findings have led to a debate as to whether the symptom threshold should be lower in adults. Recent evidence has suggested that the age-dependent decline in symptoms observed in referred ADHD samples is true only for males, i.e. there is greater persistence of symptoms in females.

The risk factors determining the persistence of ADHD diagnosis in adults remain unclear. However, some studies suggested that higher persistence is associated with:

- Increased severity of ADHD symptoms
- The presence of co-morbidities
- Adversities during childhood
- Family history of ADHD.

There is a large amount of data that documents a worse outcome in subjects affected by ADHD compared with non-ADHD controls right across the life span. Thus, a diagnosis of ADHD is associated with a higher rate of:

- Several psychiatric co-morbidities, such as disruptive behaviour disorders, anxiety, mood disorders, and substance use disorders
- School problems, such as having to repeat a year, suspensions, lower than predicted academic performance, and school dropout
- Accidents and driving impairments
- Unemployment and sub-employment
- Family dysfunction, such as divorce and poor quality of family relations
- Social and legal problems
- Risk-taking behaviours
- Increased medical care costs.

There is a paucity of good quality long-term out-come studies. The MTA group has published their 36-month data (14-month clinical trial and 22 months observational follow-up). This data is consistent with the findings from the 14-month study, which suggested that good quality medication treatment seems likely to deliver the most favourable outcome. They found that the earlier advantage of having had 14 months of the intensive medication algorithm over the behavioural and community treatment arms was no longer apparent at 36 months. The overall message is that to achieve maximal effectiveness requires careful titration at the beginning of treatment, and well-designed and executed continuing care protocols constructed to ensure that treatment continues to be effective. Whilst such practices are possible in routine clinical care, they require thoughtful planning and careful execution.

Clinical example

Jake was a much wanted first child for his parents. However, from a very early age they found him more difficult to manage than they had expected. He was restless as a baby, taking a long time to settle after feeds and once he started walking he was noted to be very active. As a toddler he was a 'nightmare' to take anywhere. In the supermarket he would not settle in the trolley, always trying to climb out and on the few occasions that he was allowed to walk he would hurtle down the aisles and on several occasions knocked down food displays by fiddling with them. His mother would get exasperated with him and their relationship deteriorated into frequent arguments. The parental relationship was also very strained. Jake became very oppositional at home and this continued when he went into nursery school. His mother took him to the health visitor and the GP on several occasions, but felt that they were blaming her for being a bad parent and stopped asking for help.

At the end of his first year at primary school Jakes parents were called into the school to discuss Jake's 'bad' behaviour. He would not sit in his seat, was always 'attention seeking' by shouting out at the teacher and butting into the other children's games, he never finished his work and was dropping behind. Jakes parents were asked to be stricter with him. Jake stopped being invited to play with the other children and was not often invited to their birthday parties. Things continued to go poorly at home and at school for the next 2 years. Jake's mother then read an article about ADHD and felt that she recognized several of the symptoms in Jake. She discussed Jake with someone from one of the ADHD support groups who gave her more information and supported her going back to the GP to ask for a referral. Although the GP was initially reluctant to make the referral as child psychiatry waiting lists were very long, in the end it was agreed and the referral made.

Jake was finally seen at the local CAMHS service. A full history was taken, and Jake and his parents were seen on two occasions. Jake spent some time with the doctor alone during which he described how difficult he found being in class at school and how lonely he felt. As it was during the summer holidays it was not possible to get information from school straight away. The doctor informed Jake's parents that it was not possible to give a diagnosis before speaking to school as, whilst the symptoms they described were consistent with ADHD, there were too few to confirm the diagnosis. After obtaining written school reports and speaking to the teacher the clinicians reviewed all the information and agreed that Jake met the criteria for ADHD combined type as defined by DSM-IV, but that he did not meet the criteria for ICD-10 hyperkinetic disorder.

The consultant met with Jake and his parents, and spent time discussing the diagnosis with them, during which they talked about the causes of ADHD, its course, and the types of treatment available. Following the clinic's protocol the consultant suggested a course of parental training and liaison with school. Initially, Jake's parents were reluctant as the felt the doctor was blaming them for Jake's problems, but after some discussion they agreed, realizing that, whilst they had not caused Jake's problems, they could help manage them and reduce his impairment. The family was seen 4 months later following the parental management course. Although they had found the course useful in reducing Jake's oppositional behaviour, he still had considerable problems with over-active and impulsive behaviours at home. Staff in school had also worked hard to manage Jake's ADHD there, but he remained symptomatic and impaired in class and at break-times would intrude into other children's games. Indeed, his inattentiveness in the classroom setting seemed to have become more apparent as the school year progressed.

After discussion it was agreed to titrate Jake onto a trial of immediate-release methylphenidate. The titration was carried out over a 4-week period starting at 5 mg tds, increasing to 20 mg tds. Jake and his parents attended the clinic weekly where Jakes ADHD symptoms were rated, adverse events enquired about using a structured and standardized protocol, and pulse and blood pressure were recorded. At the end of the titration it was clear that Jake had not responded to the methylphenidate. As he had not suffered from any adverse effects either, it was agreed to titrate him on to dexamfetamine, again over a 4-week period using the same structured protocol starting at 2.5 mg/kg tds increasing to 10 mg tds. At the end of the first week there was no reduction in symptoms, but as Jake had some insomnia and loss of appetite, the dose frequency was reduced to 5 mg bd. At the end of the second week Jake had a complete loss of appetite that continued throughout the day and he was not sleeping well at all. His ADHD symptoms, however, were much improved and school were very pleased with him.

He remained on the dexamfetamine at 5 mg bd for several months with support from the nursing staff regarding sleep hygiene and the dietician for his eating. Whilst his ADHD symptoms remained well treated, he continued to have problems with sleep and had lost a significant amount of weight. It was therefore agreed to try him on a course of atomoxetine. This was started in the standardized way at 0.5 mg/kg for 1 week then increased to 1.2 mg/kg. His dexamfetamine was tapered off and stopped after 6 weeks. When the dexamfetamine was stopped Jake's ADHD symptoms returned somewhat, but they were never as bad as they had been before he was treated. He had some nausea in the first 2 weeks of the atomoxetine, but this resolved, and when the dexamfetamine was stopped his sleep and appetite improved greatly. Over the next few weeks Jake's symptoms started to improve again and by 12 weeks his ADHD, whilst not as well controlled as it was on the dexamfetamine was rated as only mildly impairing.

Jake remained on the atomoxetine and continued to be reviewed at the continuing care clinics at least once every 6 months, where the staff continued to rate symptoms and adverse effects using the same standardized protocol that had been used during titration.

Three years later Jake remains well and is progressing well at school, although he has a scribe in some lessons as he was found to be dyslexic. He has many friends, and has joined the scouts and a local football club. His mother runs a local ADHD support group and is working with professionals to improve the recognition of ADHD in the community.

Recommended reading

Banaschewski T, Coghill D, Santosh P, et al. (2006) Long-acting medications for the hyperkinetic disorders. A systematic review and European treatment guideline. *Eur Child Adolesc Psychiat* **15**: 476-95.

Jensen PS, Arnold LE, Swanson JM, et al. (2007) 3-year follow-up of the NIMH MTA study. *J Am Acad Child Adolesc Psychiat* **46**: 989–1002.

MTA Cooperative Group (1999a) A 14-month randomized clinical trial of treatment strategies for attention-deficit/hyperactivity disorder. The MTA Cooperative Group. Multimodal Treatment Study of Children with ADHD. *Arch Gen Psychiat* **56**: 1073–86.

MTA Cooperative Group (1999b) Moderators and mediators of treatment response for children with attention-deficit/hyperactivity disorder: the Multimodal Treatment Study of children with attention-deficit/hyperactivity disorder. *Arch Gen Psychiat* **56**: 1088–96.

Swanson JM, Elliott GR, Greenhill LL, et al. (2007) Effects of stimulant medication on growth rates across 3 years in the MTA follow-up. *J Am Acad Child Adolesc Psychiat* **46**: 1015–27.

Taylor E, Dopfner M, Sergeant J, et al. (2004) European clinical guidelines for hyperkinetic disorder—first upgrade. *Eur Child Adolesc Psychiat* **13(Suppl 1)**: 17–30.

Chapter 12

175

Oppositional defiant disorder and conduct disorder

Definitions and epidemiology

Definitions

Oppositional behaviour and conduct problems continue to be the most common reasons for referral to child and adolescent mental health services. The essential features of oppositional defiant disorder (ODD) are a recurrent pattern of negativistic, defiant, hostile, and disobedient behaviour towards authority figures that leads to impairment. Conduct disorder (CD) describes more serious aggressive and antisocial behaviour.

There has been considerable research regarding the degree to which ODD and CD are related to each other (📖 Box 12.1). The majority of the research to date supports them continuing to be seen as distinct disorders.

Box 12.1 DSM-IV diagnostic criteria

ODD	CD
Often loses temper	Often tells serious lies e.g. 'cons' others
Often argues with adults	Has bullied threatened or intimidated others on several occasions
Often actively defies or refuses to comply	Has stolen items without confronting the victim (usually less than £20) in value
Often deliberately annoys people	Destruction of the property of other, such as vandalism, breaking into houses, buildings, or cars
Often blames others	Forces others into sexual activity
Often touchy or easily annoyed	Has run away from home overnight at least twice
Often angry or resentful	Often initiates physical fights
	Has used or threatened to use a weapon
Often spiteful or vindictive	Has been physically cruel to animals or killed an animal
	Aggressive Stealing
	Playing with fire or settings fires with intent to damage
	Has trusted from school
	Physical cruelty to persons

In addition these behaviours must have been present for at least 6 months and be evident at a level that:
- Is developmentally inappropriate (there is sub-classification according to age of onset)
- Caused functional difficulties in a least one domain, there is no requirement that the individual has been charged by the police.

Within ICD-10 the symptoms are the same, but the ODD symptoms are described as a subcategory of the CD symptoms. ICD-10 also uses similar criteria to DSM-IV, but places greater emphasis on the social network surrounding the young person and includes a classification of 'socialized' or 'non-socialized', which is a reflection on whether or not the young person is integrated within a deviant peer group. An additional difference is that the ICD-10 system recognizes the possibility that conduct problems arise as part of another disorder (e.g. hyperkinetic CD), whereas DSM-IV would give multiple diagnoses where the criteria for each individual disorder is met.

The potential to include age of onset and the quality of the young persons' social relationship into the diagnosis is helpful as both are important predictors of prognosis.

Epidemiology

Prevalence rates vary between 1 and 16% depending on the age of the sample and diagnostic criteria used. However, in general:

5–10-year-olds	ODD	Conduct disorder
Boys	4.8%	1.7%
Girls	2.1%	0.6%

- Prevalence is higher in lower socioeconomic groups
- There is no clear difference between urban and rural rates of ODD/ CD once the degree of poverty has been taken into account

Aetiology

Much of the data concerning aetiology comes from research on CD as there have been few studies investigating the causal factors for ODD.

Current research would suggest that none of the factors below can be considered as causal, but should be viewed as risk factors.

Biological factors

- Studies suggest a familial clustering of ODD, CD, attention deficit hyperactivity disorder (ADHD), and substance use disorders
- Temperament: 'callous-unemotional'
- Autonomic under-arousal, with lower electrodermal activity, and lower mean resting heart rate
- Prenatal or early developmental exposure to toxins, e.g. lead
- Exposure to nicotine *in utero*
- Deficient nutrition and vitamins
- Abnormalities in the pre-frontal cortex
- Altered neurotransmitter function in the serotonergic, noradrenergic, and dopaminergic systems
- Low cortisol and elevated testosterone
- Physical illness especially those affecting the central nervous system

Psychological factors

- **Attachment difficulties:** similarities have been noted between the behavioural manifestations of insecure attachment and disruptive behavioural disorders, but research findings have been inconsistent
- Deficient social learning and information processing
- Reading problems

Social factors

- Low socioeconomic status
- Peer relationship difficulties
- Parental mental illness
- Parental substance abuse and criminality
- Parental disharmony, family dysfunction including domestic violence
- Poor supervision by parents
- Erratic harsh discipline and hostile critical parenting
- Rejection of the child
- Low parental involvement in the child's activities
- Child maltreatment, neglect and abuse

The most likely situation is that is that ODD and CD arise out of a complex mix of risk and protective factors. There is much debate about which factors provide protection and how they might interact with risk factors.

- Are protective factors simply the opposite of identified risk factors, e.g. high intelligence is protective as low intelligence increases risk?
- Do protective factors buffer the impact of risk factors?
- Does the presence of protective factors, in the absence of risk factors, result in a positive outcome?
- Do multiple risk factors interact with each other in an additive or multiplicative ways?

With respect to the relationship between ADHD, ODD, and CD, longitudinal data suggests that ADHD in early life is a predictor of ODD and CD later in life, and that this association is frequently mediated by hostile and critical parenting styles. On the other hand, early ODD and CD (in the absence of ADHD) do not predict later ADHD.

Assessment

Should be comprehensive and involve the collection of information from different informants, about behaviour in different settings.

Clinical interview with the parents

Including:
- **Description of current problems:** onset, duration, frequency, and location
- **Developmental history:** child's temperament, periods of separation and peer relationships
- Medical history paying particular attention to review of head injuries, seizures, or central nervous system (CNS) infections
- Physical examination including neurological if indicated
- **Parenting behaviour:** behavioural strategies that have been tried or are currently being tried
- Family history of medical or mental health problems
- **Social history:** parental employment, accommodation, current stressors, and support.

Assessment should also consider ethnic and cultural issues with regard to different ideas about obedience and parenting in ethnic subgroups.

Clinical interview with the child or adolescent

The nature of oppositional behavioural problems is such that they may not be perceived as a problem by the young person who may rationalize or attempt to justify their oppositional or aggressive behaviour. It is important to try and build a working relationship with the young person, but without condoning or being perceived to judge their behaviour. An empathic, listening stance may enable the young person to engage with the assessment process allowing their views to be elicited.

Collateral information

From teachers, or others who are in regular contact with the child.

Note: there is generally a low rate of agreement between multiple informants, but teachers and parents' ratings tend to agree more on externalizing behaviour than child ratings.

Psychological assessment

- Intellectual capacity
- Language development
- Reading and arithmetic skills
- In circumstances where a full cognitive assessment may not be possible detailed evaluation of the school reports may be helpful in identifying areas of weakness or underachievement. The British Picture Vocabulary Scale (BPVS) is easy to administer and can provide a useful assessment of verbal ability.

Neuropsychological assessment

Although impaired executive control functions, (e.g. difficulties in planning, changing responses to inhibit or initiate action, and self-monitoring of behaviour) have been found individuals with ODD and CD, none of these deficits are either unique to these disorders or universally present, and therefore do not assist the diagnostic process.

Specific questionnaires and rating scales

- Child Behavioural Checklist (Achenbach and Edelbrock, 1991)
- Conner's Parent and Teacher Rating Scales (Conners 1989, 1998)
- Eyberg Child Behaviour Inventory (Eyeberg, 1992).

Note: there are a number of other rating scales available, but not all are suitable for younger children.

In summary

Assessment should be:

- Comprehensive and include information from different informants
- Take into account the child's behaviour in different settings
- Examine the function of the behaviour and the parents/adults response.

In addition, there may also be a need to consider a more structured risk assessment for significant aggressive and/or sexualized behaviour.

Differential diagnosis and co-morbidity

Differential diagnosis

- Attention deficit hyperactivity disorder
- Mental retardation
- Substance abuse
- Specific developmental disorders
- Post-traumatic stress disorder
- Adjustment disorder
- Anxiety disorder
- Seizure disorders
- Major depressive disorder
- Psychoses.

Careful evaluation of the history of symptom development and information from multiple informants is essential in delineating ODD and CD from other disorders.

Co-morbidity

Assessment of co-morbidity is an important part of any evaluation because ODD and CD have high levels of co-morbidity with a very wide range of conditions. In the past it was common for ADHD in children co-morbid ODD or CD to be missed, and therefore remain untreated. Whilst it is likely that this occurs less often now it is important to keep an open mind regarding the presence of co-morbid disorders as if they are appropriately treated this may lessen the oppositionality and conduct problems.

All of the disorders listed above as differentials may also present co-morbidly with ODD or CD.

Management: psychological interventions

An individualized treatment plan should be developed in accordance with the biopsychosocial formulation of the case and taking into account any identified co-morbidity. Parental and family psychopathology also commonly co-exists with ODD and CD and this needs to be considered when planning treatment packages.

Psychological interventions

A wide range of behaviourally-orientated treatment programmes have been developed, which attempt to address the multiple risk and perpetuating factors associated with ODD and CD. The National Institute for Health and Clinical Excellence (NICE) recommends that group-based parent training/education programmes should be the mainstay of treatment for children of 12 years and under with ODD and CD. They also suggest that individual-based programmes should only be recommended where the family's needs are too complex for a group-based programme.

Parent management training

Evidence from randomized trials suggests that parent management training strategies based on the principles of social learning theory (an approach to learning that includes learning from observing other people) are effective in the treatment of oppositional behaviours. This is particularly true if these programmes:

- Include ways of improving family relationships
- Reduce the positive reinforcement of disruptive behaviour
- Increase the reinforcement of pro-social behaviour and compliant behaviour. The type of positive reinforcement varies depending on the programme, but parental attention is important
- Use punishment selectively. This usually consists of a form of time-out, loss of tokens, and/or loss of privileges
- Make parental response predictable, contingent, and immediate
- Help parents to identify their own parenting goals
- Include role play during sessions and homework between sessions so that parents can apply what they have learnt to their own family's situation
- Are given by trained staff that follow an evidence-based programme manual and use whatever resources are needed to ensure that this programme is followed consistently.

Whilst individual treatment may be appropriate in some cases, group parent training has a number of benefits:

Advantages of group parent training

- Helps socially isolated families meet each other
- Builds a sense of cohesiveness
- Provides opportunities to share views and learn from others
- Provides appropriate role models
- Provides support
- Groups can be powerful in developing confidence and self-esteem
- Are likely to be more cost-effective.

Most current parent training programmes are 10–20 weeks in duration, which may be too short when there are severe problems.

Other psychological Interventions

- **Individual or group behavioural training** for the child focusing on emotional recognition and problem solving. These are most effective when run in conjunction with parent management training
- **Trials of school based interventions** have led to inconsistent results and require further investigation
- **Family therapy:** limited evidence of effectiveness, but there have been very few studies.

In general, many of these programmes lack empirical evidence that improvements in behaviour are maintained in the long term. Unsurprisingly, early intervention with younger children is associated with better outcomes.

Most of the evidence discussed above is from studies in ODD. Unfortunately, psychological interventions for established CD appear show little effectiveness. There is, however, some evidence that multimodal interventions, such as 'Fast Track' or 'Multisystemic Therapy', are of modest benefit

These benefits may be linked to these approaches by being:

- Intensive
- Proactive
- Addressing therapeutic barriers
- Involving all domains of a young person's life.

Dramatic treatments, such as boot camps or exposure to frightening situations meant to induce young people to desist from aggressive behaviours, are not effective and may only worsen symptom.

Management: pharmacological interventions

Medication should not be the first or only intervention for ODD or CD and should not be started until psychological interventions have been attempted. Psychopharmacological treatments for oppositional or aggressive behaviour have not been well studied. There have been few double-blind placebo controlled trials with most studies being small scale or open label. Polypharmacy should be avoided and careful monitoring of compliance and side-effects is required. Evidence to date would suggest:

- In ADHD with co-morbid ODD and CD, stimulants and atomoxetine may help reduce oppositionality
- Typical and atypical antipsychotics may help in aggression in the context of mental retardation and pervasive developmental disorders
- Very limited evidence that SSRIs may be helpful for ODD in the context of a mood disorder
- Lithium carbonate has been shown to reduce aggression and temper outbursts, but studies were all conducted in in-patient settings and, therefore, may have limited applicability in out-patient settings
- Carbamazepine has been used in aggressive, explosive behaviour, but double-blind studies show lack of superiority to placebo.

Prognosis

Oppositional defiant disorder
The developmental trends are shown in Fig. 12.1.

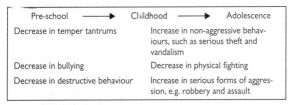

Pre-school ⟶	Childhood ⟶ Adolescence
Decrease in temper tantrums	Increase in non-aggressive behaviours, such as serious theft and vandalism
Decrease in bullying	Decrease in physical fighting
Decrease in destructive behaviour	Increase in serious forms of aggression, e.g. robbery and assault

Fig. 12.1 Developmental trends.

Poor prognosis is associated with
- Early onset of symptoms
- Longer duration of symptoms
- Co-morbid mood, anxiety, impulse control, and substance use disorders
- Development of CD.

Remission from ODD symptoms most often occurs before age 18. Approximately 30% with early onset ODD will progress to develop CD.

Conduct disorder
Research has shown that compared with the late onset form early onset CD has a particularly poor prognosis. This is also the case for CD, which is co-morbid with ADHD

Almost 50% of all youths that initiated serious violent acts before the age of 11 continued this type of offending beyond the age of 20—twice the rate of those who started in adolescence.

Approximately 40% of prepubertal children with CD may develop antisocial personality disorder (Zoccolillo *et al.* 1992) and most antisocial adult report a history consistent with CDs as a child.

Conduct disorder has also been linked to:
- Failure to complete schooling
- Joblessness and consequent financial dependency
- Poor interpersonal relationships
- Family break-up and divorce
- Higher rates of unemployment and state benefits.

The estimated annual cost per child if CD is left untreated is around £15,000, and a recent study suggested that by age 28, costs for individuals with CD were around 10 times higher than for those with no problems, with a mean cost of £70,000. Criminality incurs the greatest cost, followed by educational provision, foster and residential care, and state benefits. Only a small proportion of these costs fall on health services.

The cost of CDs in terms of the reduced quality of life of those affected, those around them, and society in general, is extremely high. Parent training/education programmes appear to be an effective and potentially cost-effective therapy for children with CD. However, the relative effectiveness and cost-effectiveness of different treatment models require further investigation.

Clinical example

Michael was first referred to the Child and Adolescent Mental Health Services by his GP when he was 3 years old.

His mum reported that he would have frequent temper tantrums and did not seem to listen to her. She had thought that this was just and extension of the 'terrible twos', but his behaviour was making it difficult for him to make friends at his play group and she was worried how he would get on at nursery.

Initial assessment established that Michael lived with his mum and 2 older siblings in a local council housing estate. The family were hoping to move house as his mum felt the local area was very rough and was reluctant to let any of the children out to play as there were lots of fights between the neighbourhood children. His parents were separated, but his dad lived nearby and maintained regular contact with the children. Both parents generally tried to be consistent in their management of the children, but his dad agreed that he tended to let the kids away with some behaviour because he felt guilty about leaving their mum.

At this time the recommendation was parenting work with the local Child and Family Centre, and Michael was discharged from CAMHS.

Michael was referred back to the CAHMS service when he was 8 Years old. He was now in a local primary school and was having significant problems with his peers, and had problems at home—fights with his siblings, ongoing temper tantrums, defiance of mum and dad. He had been cautioned by the police for vandalism on several occasions. Someone at school had mentioned that Michael might have Attention Deficit Hyperactivity Disorder. A further assessment identified that the inconsistency in the rules between mum and dad had increased. Mum, but not dad had attended the parenting classes recommended previously. Dad felt that some of Michael's behaviour was just being a typical boy and was reluctant to impose the same consequences as mum. Conner's Rating Scales from home and school were inconsistent, and full clinical assessment ruled out a diagnosis of ADHD, but identified sub-clinical symptoms of a generalized anxiety disorder.

On the basis of the assessment a diagnosis of ODD was made with emerging conduct problems. Specific behavioural recommendations were made and psychoeducation information was provided to school about anxiety. It was suggested that both parents attend a group-based parenting training programme, whilst Michael attended a social skills training group. The family attended a follow-up appointment once the group work was complete and they reported that, although Michael continued to test the boundaries at home they were now able to be consistent in their approaches. Michael's end of term report was the best he had received since starting primary school; he had been invited to a classmate's party for the first time a few months ago and his mum said home was no longer like a 'warzone'. Michael himself reported that he was happier than he had ever been at school, and that he now had 3 good friends who he plays with both in and out of school.

Recommended reading

National Institute for Health and Clinical Excellence (NICE) (2006) *Technology Appraisal—Conduct disorder in children—parent-training/education programmes.* Available at: http://www.nice.org.uk/TA102 (accessed 12 April 2008).

Steiner H, Remsing L. (2007) Practice parameter for the assessment and treatment of children and adolescents with oppositional defiant disorder *J Am Acad Child Adolesc Psychiat* **46**: 126–41.

Zoccolillo M. *et al.* (1992) The outcome of conduct disorder. *Psychological Medicine* **22**: 971–986.

Tics and Tourette's

Definitions and typical presentation

Definitions

Tics are involuntary stereotypic or patterned (but non-rhythmic), non-purposeful motor movements, or vocalizations of sudden onset.

Tic disorders can be categorized as:
- Transient or chronic
- Simple or complex
- Motor or vocal.

Typical clinical presentations

- Simple motor tics commonly occur in the upper body especially face, neck, shoulders, including blinking, eye rolling, head jerking, sniffing
- Simple phonic tics can include grunting, barking, hissing, screeching, shouting specific words
- Complex motor tics can include self-harming or hopping
- Complex vocal tics include the shouting or repetition of phrases
- A minority of those with tics exhibit the infamous trait of profane verbal tics (coprolalia) or repetitive obscene gestures (copropraxia); however, repeating actions/sounds of others (echopraxia/echolalia) or repeating one's own sounds (palilalia) are somewhat more common
- Other types of complex tics can include unacceptable or dangerous actions, such as touching a hot iron
- Sensory tics can occur, especially around the glottis, leading to the common throat clearing or coughing tics, or even a sensation of a hard to define pain.

ICD-10 definitions

- **F95.0 Transient tic disorder:** tics of duration between 4 weeks and 12 months
- **F95.1 Chronic motor or vocal tic disorder:** tics of duration longer than 12 months, either motor or vocal, but not both. Usually multiple, but may be single
- **F95.2 Combined vocal and multiple motor tic disorder (Gilles de la Tourette)—Tourette's syndrome:**
  - Multiple tics, both motor and vocal, are present and have persisted for over 1 year. Vocal tics often multiple with explosive repetitive vocalizations
  - Onset is in childhood, usually worsening in adolescence
  - Tic free periods last no longer than 3 months
  - Tourette's syndrome is often qualified by an additional requirement for functional impairment, but this is no longer an official diagnostic requirement.
- **F95.8 Other tic disorders** and **F95.9 Tic disorder, unspecified.**

Aetiology

The cause of tics is not known, however:

- Twin and family studies suggest a strong heritable component, with rates of 10–15% in first degree relatives. They also suggest that these genetic effects show incomplete penetrance with variable expression, and that tic disorders are likely to be polygenic
- There appears to be an aetiological overlap between Tourette's syndrome and obsessive compulsive disorder (OCD). Relatives of patients with Tourette's patients have increased rates of OCD, and possibly also of attention deficit hyperactivity disorder (ADHD)
- The frequent clinical response of tics to antipsychotic medications and data from neuroimaging studies have supported the hypothesis that tics arise due to a dopamine mediated effect. This may be related to a dysfunction in the basal ganglia 'brake' that is normally applied to damp down unwanted motor activity
- There is also evidence supporting the involvement of several environmental factors, including perinatal complications and psychosocial factors, such as stressful life events. Non-heritable tics do occur and are reported to occur differentially in monozygotic twins
- Potential autoimmune triggers, such as those implicated following streptococcal infection in paediatric autoimmune neuropsychiatric disorders associated with streptococcal infections (PANDAS) are a focus of current research interest.

PANDAS: paediatric autoimmune neuropsychiatric disorders associated with streptococcal infections

- OCD and or tic disorder arising following Group A beta-haemolytic streptococcal infection
- Possible mechanism is via autoimmune sequelae of infection in the basal ganglia, in a process analogous to the post infective movement disorder Sydenham's chorea
- Characteristically a child will acutely develop a combination of OCD symptoms, tics, and emotional and mood disorders following a streptococcal throat infection. Some authorities also require a prepubertal onset, relapsing/remitting course and other motor abnormalities
- Treatments are still experimental. As the process is a post-infective, processes such as plasma exchange and immunoglobulin have been used.

Epidemiology

The variability of what is often described as a tic disorder (and an almost certain tendency towards under-recognition and under diagnosis) means that exact incidence is hard to ascertain and, as a consequence, studies report very different rates.

However it would appear that overall, tics of any type may be present in as many as about 1–2% of children. Milder tics are more common than more severe ones, and tics are more common in males than females (on average around 5:1).

Until recently, the best study of the prevalence of Tourette's syndrome came from a study where more than 28,000 adolescents entering military service in Israel were screened, revealing a prevalence of about 0.05%. However, more recent studies such as a review of 4500 Swedish school-children suggest that definite Tourette's syndrome occurs much more commonly—in about 0.5% of school-age children.

Onset is in childhood, by definition, and usually between the ages of 5 and 15 years. Simple tics are seen at earlier ages, whereas vocal tics, complex tics, and compulsions are seen later.

A predominance of Caucasian children in studies is thought to reflect a referral bias, rather than a true ethnic variation.

Assessment

Tics can present in many ways, but there are several unifying features that often allow a diagnosis to be made from a careful history and observation, and without the need to instigate specific neurological investigations. There are, however, times when tics are not observed in the clinic and sometimes the use of a home video can help in assessment.

Important aspects to bear in mind when making an assessment of tics include:

- Whilst tics appear to be involuntary, they are probably better described as a *voluntary response to an irresistible urge*
- Tics are often postponable, especially during voluntary movement (in contrast to dystonias, choreaform movements, etc., which cannot be postponed). Tics may, indeed, be postponable for an entire clinic visit and, therefore, not seeing the tics does not mean that they are not occurring
- Tics are often associated with a sensory urge or premonition immediately prior to their occurrence and a sense of tension when suppressed
- Tics naturally wax and wane, occur in groups, and can migrate from site to site, e.g. a shoulder shrug tic can become a mouth stretch tic over a short period of time
- Tics are often triggered by stressful situations (or specific triggers such as the word 'relax!') and are rarely experienced during sleep. They may reduce during an interesting or enjoyable activity

The functional impact of tics remains a crucial part of the history in particular:

- **Social impairments:** very noticeable tics can often result in extreme stigmatization and prejudice, with subsequent social withdrawal
- **Interference with daily thoughts and tasks** as a consequence of the interrupting and time-consuming nature of the tics
- **Self injury:** this can occur as a direct consequence of a self-injurious tic (e.g. hitting self, especially if around the eyes and face); indirectly as result of a tic-mediated accidental injury, or secondary to a co-morbid or reactive mood disorder.

Other important factors in the history include:

- The presence of a positive family history of tics, Tourette's syndrome, or OCD
- Timing of onset
- It is essential that assessment is comprehensive enough to identify or rule out co-morbid disorders and, in particular, ADHD and OCD. Some specific symptoms may prove difficult to label as either a tic or a compulsion satisfactorily
- It is also essential that any mood and anxiety disorders are identified.

Physical examination is primarily for the exclusion of potential differential diagnoses. In particular neurological examination including eye examination for Kayser–Fleischer rings (indicative of Wilsons disease), and for abnormal movements, tone, and gait, which may be suggestive of choreas or dystonias.

Differential diagnosis

- A differential diagnosis should always be considered, but particularly so in the absence of a family history of tic disorder
- Tics in the absence of tic disorder as a primary cause are sometimes referred to as *tourettism*
- Whilst ADHD often co-exists with tics and Tourette's, it should also be considered as a potential differential diagnosis to ensure that movements being described as tics are not due to a failure of impulse control, rather than true tics. However, the line between the two disorders may not always be clear
- There are also overlaps between OCD and Tourette's syndrome and the two disorders frequently occur together. However, they may also sometimes be confused with each other. OCD will usually involve more preoccupation about carrying out actions or thoughts, and evoke an associated guilt or anxiety. Obsessions and compulsions will often be associated with symmetry or contamination, whilst tics are generally more random and less purposeful in nature. However, complex and seemingly purposeful tics do occur, and may be very difficult to distinguish from compulsions
- There are several other conditions that include tics as part of the overall disease presentation. In these cases, tics may present a relatively unimportant facet in relation to more severe impairments. In particular, this is the case for general learning disabilities, developmental disorders such as autism, movement disorders (e.g. chorea seen in ataxia-telangiectasia) and some chromosomal disorders (e.g. tuberous sclerosis).

Co-morbidity

There is an important and common co-occurrence with ADHD (see Chapter 11) and OCD (📖 see Chapter 20). These may represent a common genetically transmissible aetiology, rather than a simple co-morbidity.

Additionally, co-morbidity in Tourette's syndrome also comes from:

- Increased incidence of co-occurring, but genetically independent conditions
- The psychological sequelae of the impact of the syndrome itself. Examples include depression, anxiety, substance abuse, and behavioural disorders.

Management

The successful management of tic disorders and Tourette's typically involves a combination of:

- Education
- Psychological counselling and therapies
- Tic reduction using medication
- Specific management of co-morbid conditions.

The order in which these treatment approaches are considered will depend on severity and which symptoms/problems are the most impairing. Often the tics alone will not require medication, and mild cases can be managed by education and reassurance for both the sufferer and those around them. Assesment of treatment response shoud take into account the tendency of tics to wax and wane.

Psychological Therapies for tics and Tourette's

Both tics and obsessive compulsive symptoms may improve with CBT, if successful exposure–response prevention can be achieved.

Techniques include:

- Relaxation
- Exposure-response prevention
- Massed practice (forced repetition of the tic)
- Habit reversal (movements incompatible with the tic)

Medication used for tics and Tourette's

Medication may be indicated when:

- Tics are severe and significantly interfering with daily functioning
- Tics are placing the sufferer or others at risk
- There are cognitive impairments that prevent satisfactory psychoeducation, counselling, or psychotherapy
- Tics and ADHD or OCD co-exist

Once the decision to use medication has been made, the choice of drug is a risk-benefit-based decision to be made with the child and their family.

The algorithm in Fig. 13.1 is based on one used by a specialist Tourette's treatment centre in the USA, and is helpful particularly when considering co-occurring OCD and ADHD.

- Dopamine receptor antagonist antipsychotics have the best trial evidence for efficacy, but are marred by greater incidence of adverse effects. Atypical antipsychotics, such as risperidone, and typical antipsychotics, such as haloperidol are often used
- Alpha-2 agonists: most commonly used are clonidine and guanfacine—have less robust trial evidence of efficacy, but are more acceptable in terms of adverse effects
- Whilst tics co-morbid with ADHD stimulants have frequently been associated with tics, reviews of the literature suggest that the bulk of this observation is probably down to co-morbidity, rather than cause. Under most circumstances children with ADHD and tics should not be refused the option of stimulant medication.

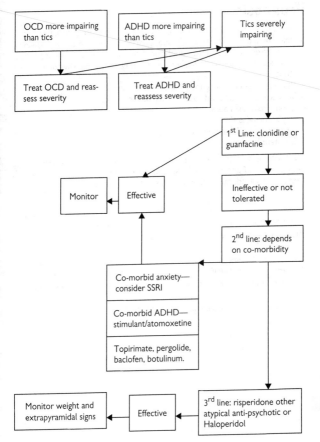

Fig. 13.1 Algorithm for treatment of tics including ADHD and OCD. Modified version of algorithm from Gilbert D. (2006) Treatment of children and adolescents with tics and Tourette's syndrome. *J Child Neurol* **21**: 690–9.

Prognosis

Overall, tic disorders in childhood have a favourable prognosis, peaking in middle childhood and frequently disappearing by the late teens. However, a minority do continue into adulthood, both in severe and milder forms. In this case, symptoms are likely to be lifelong, following a waxing-waning pattern.

Poorer long-term prognosis is associated with:
- Tourette's (as opposed to the other tic disorders)
- Co-morbid disorders
- Physical illness
- Unsupportive home environments
- Substance abuse.

Much of the morbidity from tics is derived from secondary or co-existing conditions, and prognosis will depend very much on the skill with which these are treated, rather than treatment of the tics alone.

Recommended reading

Black K, Webb H. (2007) *Tourette syndrome and other tic disorders.* Emedicine.com 2007. Available at: www.emedicine.com/neuro/TOPIC664.HTM (accessed 1 April 2008).

Gilbert D. (2006) Treatment of children and adolescents with tics and Tourette syndrome. *J Child Neurol* **21**: 690–9

Robertson M. (2006) Attention deficit hyperactivity disorder, tics and Tourette's syndrome: the relationship and treatment implications. A commentary. *Eur Child Adolesc Psychiat* **15**: 1–11 .

Snider L, Swedo S. (2004) PANDAS: current status and directions for research. *Molec Psychiat* **9**: 900–7.

Special issue on Tics and Tourette's Syndrome. (2006) *J Child Neurol* **21** Issue 8.

Psychiatric complications of epilepsy in childhood

Background

Around 5% of children have seizures, with 0.5–1% being diagnosed as having epilepsy. Psychiatric problems are common in those with epilepsy because:

- There can be a shared aetiology between psychiatric illness and epilepsy
- Seizures may have psychiatric content
- The presence of psychiatric co-morbidity in those with epilepsy
- The behavioural consequences associated with having seizures
- There may be cognitive consequences of severe or prolonged seizures in a small proportion of individuals
- There are psychiatric adverse effects associated with several epilepsy treatments.

Assistance with managing the psychiatric aspects of epilepsy is one of the most common requests made of child psychiatry/paediatric liaison teams. Child psychiatrists are also frequently asked to assist with the assessment of suspected pseudoseizures (non-epileptic seizures).

Seizures with psychiatric content

Several types of seizure can present with psychiatric content.

Frontal lobe epilepsy

- Paroxysms of complex or bizarre emotional-type behaviours with sudden onset and conclusion. There is frequently no apparent prodrome or post-ictal period
- Seizures can include kicking or laughing, with a preservation of normal responsiveness to external stimuli
- Inter-ictal electroencephalogram (EEG) may be normal
- Average age of onset is around 10 years
- Need to exclude *space occupying lesions* and *head trauma*.

Temporal lobe epilepsy (TLE)

- Auditory hallucinations, visual distortions, and odd sensations, such as fear during the aura may mimic psychotic phenomena
- Anxiety and depersonalization in TLE may mimic anxiety states
- The onset of the post-aura part of the seizure may include a period of staring, similar to absence seizures.

Absence seizures

- May mimic inattention and TLE
- Are common in children
- Can be distinguished from inattention by EEG. Hyperventilation during the recording of the EEG is often used to encourage the occurrence of an absence seizure
- May be distinguished from TLE by the absence of a post-ictal confusion period.

Assessment

In each case, a careful history/examination (including assessment of dysmorphism and cutaneous signs) *and* a discussion with a paediatric neurologist should occur *before* referral for EEG or magnetic resonance imaging (MRI).

Differential diagnosis

This includes:

- Breath holding attacks
- Sleep problems
- Syncope
- Benign paroxysmal vertigo
- Inattention.

Behavioural problems associated with epilepsy

There are several potential reasons for the higher incidence of behavioural problems in children with epilepsy. These include:

- The increased likelihood of global cerebral insult
- Academic and social limitations secondary to the epilepsy and its treatment
- The stigma and uncertainty associated with epilepsy
- Secondary gain related to seizure activity.

As is the case generally the risk of behavioural problems are further increased by:

- Being male
- Young age
- Low socioeconomic status
- Stress at home.

The incidence of behavioural problems is greater in epilepsy than that it is in other chronic physical childhood illnesses, such as diabetes.

Psychiatric disorders co-morbid with epilepsy

One-third to one-half of children and young people with epilepsy will be co-morbid for at least one psychiatric disorder, much of which is not identified. Important conditions to consider (in order of decreasing likelihood) include:
- Attention deficit hyperactivity disorder (ADHD) and the other disruptive behaviour disorders
- Affective or anxiety disorders
- Psychotic disorders.

The increased risk of psychiatric disorder in this group may occur as a consequence of common aetiological factors, which increase risk for both epilepsy and psychiatric illness, or secondary to the impact of epilepsy on development. Most often it will be a combination of the two together.

Risk of co-morbid psychiatric disorder appears to be increased by:
- A clear neurological cause for the epilepsy
- Increased seizure frequency
- The presence of cognitive impairments
- The presence of family difficulties.

Pseudoseizures

30% of reported childhood 'seizures' are thought to be non-epileptic in origin. Psychiatrists are often asked to differentiate between these and true epileptiform seizures.

The differentiation between true and pseudoseizures is difficult because:
- Pseudoseizures are common in children with true epilepsy
- Both true and pseudoseizures can be triggered by stress
- True frontal lobe seizures can be very atypical in appearance and be misinterpreted as pseudoseizures.

Factors suggestive of pseudo, rather than epileptiform seizures

Pseudoseizures
- Usually occur in the presence of an observer and rarely when the individual is alone
- Often have a gradual, rather than sudden, onset
- Present with quivering or random movements, rather than rhythmic/clonic ones
- Are often accompanied by shouting or screaming
- The individual avoids painful stimuli and falls, and as result is rarely injured
- Are associated with a rapid recovery back to complete normality with no post-ictal period.

The best approach to assessing problematic pseudoseizures is to be *non-accusatory in manner* and to carefully explore possible underlying stressors, including a history of trauma or abuse. Some case reports suggest a high incidence of unspeakable dilemmas lying at the root of pseudoseizures.

Psychiatric adverse effects of antiepileptic drugs

Whilst most of the drugs used to treat epilepsy are associated with a range of potential psychiatric adverse effects the risk profile for each drug is summarized in Table 14.1.

Table 14.1 Risk profiles of psychiatric problems from studies of antiepileptic drugs

Drug	Behavioural problems	Depression	Psychosis
Phenobarbital	+++	+++	−
Gabapentin	+	−	−
Valproic acid	+	−	−
Carbamazepine	+	+	−
Lamotrigine	+		+
Phenytoin	+	−	−
Oxcarbazepine	+	−	−
Zonisamide	+	−	++
Levetiracetam	+	−	+
Topiramate	+	−	+

From Glauser (2004) *J Ch Neurol* **19**: S28–38. Reproduced with permission.

The risk of psychiatric adverse effects should also be considered with newer drugs. They are also more likely to occur in the presence of:
- Polypharmacy
- Pre-existing behavioural problems
- Developmental delays
- A family history of psychiatric disorder.

Approach to assessment

Assessment of children with epilepsy and psychiatric problems can be complex, and it is easy for a psychiatrist to suddenly feel deskilled when attending a 16-year -old with complex seizures on the neurology ward.

The aims of assessment may not always be to make an immediate diagnosis, but rather look at relative contributions made by various factors or to direct further investigations.

With pseudoseizures in particular, one of the necessary aims of assessment may be the protection of the child.

Neuropsychiatric assessment

It is often helpful to begin the assessment by taking accurate and fairly detailed history of epileptic episode. Whilst there may be a history documented in the notes already, this will usually bear repeating in the search for clues.

Good histories of a possible seizure are similar to a detailed behavioural 'ABC' analysis:

A What was happening before the first signs of the seizure? Who was there? What time of day? Where did it occur?

B What was the first sign of the seizure occurring? Actions/movements/ speech? Responsiveness? Course of the seizure. Timescale? First signs of recovery?

C How did the person behave afterwards? What did they do/say? How did they feel? Did anything else happen between the episode and normality returning? How long did it take?

Once the seizure history is assessed, salient parts of the examination and investigations should be gathered. Of particular importance are EEG (ideally video-EEG combining video of episodes with EEG recording) and imaging, and resultant diagnostic impressions, although both remain only a guide to formulation in many cases.

Psychosocial assessment

Once a clear picture of the presentation and neurological opinion is achieved, the psychiatric history should be obtained with a focus on psychosocial factors, usually involving the family, but also allowing the patient to speak in confidence. A comprehensive assessment may also require information from third parties, such as teachers and social workers, if appropriate permissions are granted by the patient and their family.

Important aspects in the history may include:

• The nature of any behavioural problems, especially the timing of these in relationship to onset of seizures. Chronological relationship may clarify the direction of causality

• A careful assessment of the possibility of child protection and risk issues

• Systemic family issues

• School and wider social issues.

Some of the possible outcomes of assessment with examples

- **Primary seizures mimicking psychiatric problem:** frontal lobe epilepsy and odd outbursts of behaviour with typical ictal findings on EEG report
- **Primary seizures with psychiatric problem secondary to seizure:** depression resulting from life-long self-consciousness
- **Primary seizure with psychiatric problem secondary to treatment:** psychosis coinciding with initiation of topirimate
- **Primary psychiatric problem mimicking epilepsy:** inattentive sub-type ADHD
- **Primary psychiatric problem co-morbid with epilepsy:** conduct disorder
- **Primary psychological problem resulting in epilepsy-like picture:** pseudoseizures in a girl who witnesses sexual abuse of a sibling by a family member
- A combination of two of the above
- Problem remains idiopathic despite assessment and basic investigations.

Approach to management

Overarching principles

- It can be helpful for psychiatrists and neurologists to jointly manage complicated cases of childhood epilepsy, (each having expertise on different aspects of the same system—the brain/mind)
- Psychoeducational work should be offered for all children and young people with epilepsy, and their families. This should aim to provide clear explanations about epilepsy and the potential behavioural consequences and family burdens associated both with the epilepsy and its treatment
- Clinicians should always bear in mind the potential for neuropsychological and cognitive deficits that may be longstanding and that can be related to the causes of the epilepsy or to the seizures themselves. These cognitive difficulties may interfere with a person's ability to make use of psychotherapy.

Specific outcomes

Primary seizures mimicking psychiatric problem

The management of seizures that result in odd behaviours will often involve both pharmacological and non-pharmacological approaches. These epilepsies usually respond to antiepileptic drugs, with carbamazepine being the first line for partial seizures. Ideally, medication would be instituted following a careful recording of baseline seizure activity to allow assessment of benefit. The patient and their families will also benefit from psychoeducation and practical advice in managing the day-to-day problems associated with the seizures.

Primary seizures with psychiatric problem secondary to seizures

In this situation, the patient and family psychoeducational inputs become first line; the type and source of the problem will require careful deconstruction before a practical approach can be taken. This will vary from a course of parental management techniques to psychotherapy or pharmacotherapy.

Cognitive behavioural therapy plays a key role in the treatment of mood and anxiety disorders in childhood. In children with epilepsy cognitive behavioural therapy (CBT) can be helpful in assisting the child to examine the role that epilepsy may have played in the formation of cognitive distortions.

Several of the drugs used to treat depression and psychosis have the potential to lower seizure threshold; however, this is likely to present a low risk in practice, especially with newer compounds and *careful monitoring*.

Primary seizures with psychiatric problem arising secondary to treatment

Management should be as with any psychiatric problem in epilepsy. However, a discussion with the patient, family, and their neurologist about the risk/benefit balance of changing epilepsy treatment is also required.

Primary psychiatric problem mimicking epilepsy

Treatment as usual, although an increased level of vigilance is required to ensure that the original formulation is correct and that new features more suggestive of true epilepsy do not develop.

Primary psychiatric problem co-morbid with epilepsy

Part of the routine follow-up of a child diagnosed with epilepsy should be monitoring of mental health, ideally in liaison with a Child and Adolescent Mental Health Services (CAMHS) professional. Treatment of co-morbid or emerging psychiatric conditions should be timely, but a degree of caution should also be maintained.

Although there is some evidence to suggest that the stimulant drugs used to treat ADHD may reduce the seizure threshold, the available clinical evidence suggests that it is safe and appropriate to treat ADHD in the presence of epilepsy using stimulant drugs as long as seizures are well controlled using antiepileptic medications. There is less evidence to support the use of the non-stimulant ADHD drugs, such as atomoxetine in children with ADHD and epilepsy.

Many antiepileptic medications will interact with antidepressant or neuropleptic drugs. Whilst this is less of an issue with some of the newer antiepileptic drugs, such as gabapentin, it is always advisable to make checks before prescribing.

A lack of sleep, which is a common problem for children with ADHD and mood disorders, can also lower the seizure threshold. Therefore, sleep problems should be actively managed in this group. Sleep hygiene is vital and melatonin may have a role in some cases.

Primary psychological problem resulting in epilepsy-like picture

The approach to pseudoseizures should recognize the possibility of a somatoform /conversion /dissociative aetiology (📖 Chapter 21).

It may take time for a patient to build up a degree of trust with the clinician before they can divulge information regarding specific stressors. It is therefore important that the clinician attempts to build up a good therapeutic alliance when such concerns are around to maximize the chances of accessing this information.

Some drugs implicated in lowering seizure threshold*

- High dose (usually intravenous) antibiotics
- Antidepressants—serotonin reuptake inhibitors (SSRIs) and TCA
- Antipsychotics, especially clozapine
- ADHD treatments, including the stimulants methylphenidate and dexamfetamine, and the non-stimulant atomoxetine
- Aminophylline
- Cyclosporin
- Pethidine.

* Good unconfounded data is difficult to find; therefore, this table is not comprehensive.

Recommended reading

Buchanan, N. (2001) Medications which may lower seizure threshold. *Australian Prescriber* **24:** 8–9.

Glauser A. (2004) Behavioural and psychiatric adverse events associated with antiepileptic drugs commonly used in paediatric patients. *J Child Neurol* **19:** S25–38.

Haut S. (2008) Frontal lobe epilepsy. Available at: www.emedicine.com/NEURO/topic141.htm (accessed 1 April 2008).

Rutter M. (2005) *Child and Adolescent Psychiatry*, 4th edn. Blackwell, Oxford.

Schizophrenia and psychotic disorders

Concepts and definitions

Schizophrenia is a neurodevelopmental disorder, and is extremely rare in children and adolescents. However, psychotic symptoms in themselves are not uncommon in children and adolescents (4 and 8%, respectively).

Historical perspective

The term 'dementia praecox' invoked by Kraepelin (1919) distinguished patients with psychosis that typically began in early adult life and ran a progressive and deteriorating course from those with manic depressive illness, which was thought to be more episodic and benign nature. Kraepelin described that 3.5% of cases of dementia praecox began before age 10 and a further 2.7% between ages 10 and 15. The patterns of symptoms described in these younger patients were similar to those seen in the adult form, and were distinct from symptoms of autism and pervasive developmental disorders. However, from the early 1930s until the early 1970 the term childhood schizophrenia was widened to include autism, and other developmental disorders that were seen as childhood manifestations of adult symptoms. This grouping together of different disorders under the category of childhood schizophrenia has made the research from this period very difficult to interpret.

The work of Kolvin (1971) and Rutter (1972) demonstrated the similarities and continuity between schizophrenia in childhood and adolescence with the adult form of the disorder. From ICD-10 (1979) and DSM-III (1980) onwards the same diagnostic criteria have been used for schizophrenia regardless of the age of onset.

Symptom dimensions

The concept of positive and negative symptoms was first developed by the nineteenth century neurologist Hughlings Jackson, but it was not applied to the symptoms of schizophrenia until the 1970s. Factor analysis and correlational studies have confirmed that schizophrenia symptoms consist of at least 3 dimensions recent work has linked these symptoms dimensions with dysfunction in specific brain regions.

Table 15.1 Symptom dimensions and Putative Neurological associations

Positive symptoms	Hallucinations and delusions	Temporal lobe dysfunction
Negative symptoms	Affective blunting	Poor performance on frontal lobe tasks and hypo-function of the dorsolateral prefrontal cortex (DLPFC)
	Avolition	
	Alogia	
Disorganization	Formal thought disorder	Functional abnormalities of the ventral prefrontal cortex(predominantly on the right) and anterior cingulate
	Bizarre behaviour	

'Positive symptoms' in children and adolescents with early onset psychosis cannot, however, be considered pathognomic of schizophrenia, and have no clear prognostic value.

Negative symptoms have been associated with pre-morbid developmental impairments and an increased familial risk of schizophrenia.

Age of onset
- Early onset schizophrenia (EOS) onset before age 18
- Very early onset schizophrenia (VEOS) onset before 13.

Diagnostic criteria
The ICD-10 and DSM-IV diagnostic criteria for schizophrenia in children and adolescents are the same as the adult criteria.

Psychotic symptoms
- At least 2 of the following symptoms present for 1 month, which may include delusions, hallucination, disorganized speech or catatonic behaviour, and/or negative symptoms
- Only 1 symptom is required if delusions are bizarre or hallucination are 3rd person or in the form of a running commentary on thinking or behaviour.

Social/occupation dysfunction
For children this may include the failure to achieve age-appropriate levels of interpersonal, academic, or occupational development.

Duration
DSM-IV states that duration is at least 6 months of disturbance including at least 1 month of active symptoms.

ICD-10 states that symptom should be present most of the time for a 1-month period.

Exclusion of schizoaffective and mood disorders, and medical conditions/drug abuse
DSM-IV uses the category of schizophreniform disorder where there are psychotic symptoms, but the overall duration of illness is less than 6 months. These differences between the two systems result in the ICD-10 definition of schizophrenia having greater sensitivity, but lower specificity in first-episode psychosis and unsurprising given the longer duration of illness requires cases of schizophrenia defined by DSM-IV have a worse prognosis.

Developmental issues
There is some concern about applying unmodified adult criteria for childhood onset schizophrenia, but studies have indicated that schizophrenia can be reliably identified in children as young as 7 using these unmodified criteria. Long-term follow-up studies showed a high level of diagnostic stability with 80% having the same diagnosis recorded at adult follow-up. Early onset schizophrenia is characterized by greater disorganization both of thought and sense of self, and more negative symptoms, whereas later onset cases have a higher frequency of systematized and paranoid delusions.

Epidemiology

Very few studies have adequately examined the prevalence of early onset psychosis (EOS). Those that have along with clinical experience would suggest that onset prior to the age of 13 years of age is rare.

The rate of onset increases through adolescence with the peak age of onset between 15 and 30 years of age.

A Swedish study using case-register data found the prevalence for all psychoses (including schizophrenia, schiziophreniform, affective psychosis, atypical psychosis and drug psychoses) at age 13 was 0.9 in 10,000, reaching 17.6 in 10,000 at age 18.

There does not appear to be a clear relationship between onset of puberty and onset of psychosis.

In very early onset schizophrenia (VEOS, onset before age 13), the sex ratio is approximately 2:1 with males predominating. The sex ratio tends to even out in adolescence.

Aetiology and risk factors

Genetics

- Heritability estimates are as high as 82%
- Likely that mode of inheritance multiple genes of small effect (polygenic)
- The parents of children with childhood onset schizophrenia are themselves at 10 times increased risk for developing schizophrenia
- Several chromosomal deletions have been associated with psychosis including:
  - 22q11 deletion syndrome [velocardiofacial (VCFS) syndrome] 30% developed psychosis, most commonly schizophrenia (24%)
  - 8q21 deletion association with psychosis and mental retardation.

Pre- and perinatal factors

- Maternal infections, e.g. rubella
- Obstetric complications e.g. foetal hypoxia
- Stressful events during pregnancy are thought to affect foetal neurodevelopment and disrupt subsequent functioning of hypothalamic-pituitary-adrenal (HPA) axis
- Higher childhood rates of neurodevelopmental disturbance, e.g. motor impairments, abnormal growth, sensory sensitivity, and attentional problems.

Neurobiology

Neuropathology

In post-mortem examination of brains of those who have suffered from schizophrenia there is often an absence of gliosis, the hallmark of neurodegeneration, this is due to loss or reduction in dendritic spines, and synapses, vital elements in neuronal connectivity.

Neuroimaging

This is difficult in children and many of the findings are inconsistent. Much of the evidence comes from the US National Institute for Mental Health (NIMH) Childhood Schizophrenia Project.

- Decreased cerebral volume approx 10%, primarily a reduction in grey matter
- Progressive decrease in cortical volume through adolescence, prefrontal cortex (11%) and temporal lobe (7%) are disproportionately affected. The rate of reduction declines into adult life
- Larger lateral ventricles with progressive increases in size
- Hyper-intensities in white matter
- Basal ganglia and cerebellum changes, but findings inconsistent
- Functional studies [cerebral blood flow (CBF) and glucose metabolism] have demonstrated hypofrontality
- Cerebellar hypermetabolism, which is consistent with a pre-frontal thalamic-cerebellar network dysfunction, has been found in adults with schizophrenia

- Positron emission tomography (PET) studies show reduced activation in the mid- and superior frontal gyrus, and increased activation in the inferior frontal, supramarginal gyrus and insula.

In summary the neuropathological and neuroimaging findings in childhood onset schizophrenia are consistent with those found in adults.

It is not clear if the progressive brain changes including excessive synaptic elimination resulting in aberrant neural connections are a consequence of neurotoxic effects of the developing psychosis or precede the psychosis. These findings suggest a model of schizophrenia that focuses less on the concept of 'hypofrontality', and more on 'disconnectivity' in neural systems or networks.

Electrophysiology
- Lower prepulse inhibition
- Reduction in P300 amplitude.

Neurotransmitters
The 'dopamine hypothesis' remains predominant, but there is increasing evidence of a number of interacting models with other neurotransmitters including, glutamate, acetylcholine, and noradrenaline being involved.

Biomarkers
A number of studies have followed young people at high risk of developing schizophrenia and have identified a number of factors that were predicted a later schizophrenia related illness:
- Early attentional deficits
- Deficits in social functioning
- Deficits in organisational ability
- Intellectual ability at age 16 and 17.

Puberty
Although the temporal association between onset of puberty, and a marked increase in the incidence of schizophrenia suggests that events around puberty perhaps biological or social may be related to the expression of psychotic symptoms this has not been supported by research studies.

Psychological and social factors
Expressed emotion
There is little evidence to suggest a causal link between high parental expressed emotion and childhood onset schizophrenia (although it may moderate response to treatment).

Socioeconomic status
The results from studies are contradictory and at this time it is not possible to say if there is any relationship with socioeconomic status.

Environmental factors, whilst not established as causative agents, may interact with biological risk factors to mediate the timing of onset, course and severity of the disorder.

Assessment

Many clinicians are, understandably, reluctant to make a diagnosis of schizophrenia in children and adolescents, even if the diagnostic criteria are met because of the implied poor prognosis and potential social stigma it may bring. However, a failure to accurately diagnose, and early or very early onset psychosis denies these children and their families prompt access to adequate and appropriate treatment and support. The principles of a comprehensive psychiatric assessment should be followed and where possible include interviews with both the child or adolescent and their family.

Psychiatric assessment

- Symptom presentation
- **Course of illness:** VEOS generally has an insidious course
- **Developmental history:** high rates of fine and gross motor problems
- **Pre-morbid functioning:** high rates of pre-morbid difficulties especially in VEOS, particularly, social withdrawal and isolation, disruptive behaviour, academic difficulties
- Presence or absence of mood symptoms
- Family psychiatric history, particularly history of psychosis
- **Mental state examination, including details of psychotic symptoms and thought disorder:** hallucination, thought disorder, and flattened affect commonly found, systematic delusions and catatonic symptoms are much less frequent in EOS
- History of substance misuse
- Risk to self and others, particularly if over-involvement in fantasy, or with aggressive or violent behaviour
- Comprehensive semi-structured diagnostic interview protocols, such as the Schedule for Affective Disorders and Schizophrenia (K-SADS), are time consuming and requiring training to administer but have explicit definitions of disorders and samples of probe questions that can be a helpful guide to interviewing
- Assessment of family functioning.

Physical assessment

Particular attention should be paid to excluding potential medical causes of psychotic symptoms.

- Physical history and examination, particular attention should be given to detecting dysmorphic features, which may indicate an underlying genetic syndrome
- Neurological examination, particularly abnormal involuntary movements and other signs of extrapyramidal dysfunction. Spontaneous abnormal involuntary movements have been detected in a proportion of drug-naïve first episode schizophrenic or schizophreniform patients, and well as in those receiving antipsychotic medication.

Further investigations as indicated based on history and examination

- Neuroimaging, MRI
  - Ventricular enlargement
  - Structural brain abnormalities
  - Demyelination (metachromatic leukodystrophy)
  - Hypodense basal ganglia (Wilson disease)

- Karyotpe/cytogenetics
  - Sex chromosome aneuplodies
  - Velocardiofacial syndrome (22q11 microdeletions)
  - 8q21 micro deletions
- Electroencephalogram (EEG)
- U&E
- LFTs
- FBCs including arylsulphate A (metachromatic leukodystophy)
- Serum cooper and caeruloplasmin
- Urinalysis, including urinary copper and drug screen
- Electrocardiogram (ECG).

Potential organic causes for psychosis
- Acute intoxication
- Delirium
- Central nervous system (CNS) lesions
- Tumours
- Infections
- Metabolic disorders
- Seizure disorders.

Psychological assessment
10–20% of children with EOS have IQs in the borderline to mild learning disability range.

Cognitive testing may be useful where there is evidence of developmental delay since these deficits may influence the presentations of symptoms. It can also guide treatment planning, particularly education and rehabilitation.

Psychological testing, including personality and projective testing is not indicated as a method of diagnosing schizophrenia.

Neuropsychological assessment
A range of deficits have been identified including:
- Working memory
- Sustained attention
- Verbal memory deficits.

These deficits are not specific to psychosis and such testing remains a research tool at present.

Other assessments
- **Speech and language therapy:** higher rates of deficits in those with EOS and, language disorders can create diagnostic difficulties
- **Occupational therapy:** gross and fine motor problems together with co-ordination problems.

Differential diagnosis and co-morbidity

- The cognitive level of the child will influence his or her ability to express and understand complex psychotic symptoms
- Younger children may have greater difficulty differentiating between true hallucinations and dreams
- Internal localization of hallucinations is commoner in younger children, which may make it more difficult to differentiate them from internal thoughts or speech
- Children with immature language development may have patterns of illogical thinking that appear similar to formal though disorder
- Psychotic symptoms in children and adolescents are diagnostically non-specific, occurring in a wide range of functional psychiatric and organic brain disorders.

Table 15.2 Differential diagnosis of schizophrenia on childhood and adolescence

Organic conditions	Drug-related psychosis (amphetamines, 'ecstasy', LSD, PCP)
	Complex partial seizures (temporal lobe epilepsy)
	Wilson disease
	Regressive psychotic disorders, e.g. Rett's Disorder
Developmental disorders	Autistic spectrum disorder (Asperger syndrome)
	Developmental language disorder
	'Multidimensional impaired' disorder
Other psychotic disorders	Affective disorder (bipolar/major depressive disorder)
	Schizoaffective disorder
	Atypical psychosis
	Benign psychosis, e.g. hypnagogic and hypnapompic hallucinations
Other psychiatric disorders	Attention deficit hyperactivity disorder (ADHD)
	Conduct disorder
	Personality disorder, e.g. schizotypal personality disorder
	Reactive attachment disorder
	PTSD-related psychosis
	Dissociative identity disorder

LSD, lysergic acid diethylamide; PCP, phencyclidine. Reproduced from Rutter, M and Taylor, E, *Child and Adolescent Psychiatry*, Blackwell publishing, 4th Edition, with permission.

Co-morbidity

In general co-morbidity is the rule, rather than the exception in VEOS and EOS.

Co-morbidity in VEOS tends to include high rates of speech and language problems, developmental delay, ODD, and ADHD, mood and anxiety problems.

With the older age of onset of EOS, the range of co-morbidities as expected is similar, but includes higher rates of substance abuse, conduct problems, and personality disorders.

Management

General

Treatment recommendations for children and adolescents with schizophrenia will vary depending on the phase of the illness:

- Prodromal
- Acute phase
- Recuperative phase
- Recovery/residual phase.

Children and adolescents will require both:

- Specific therapies, aimed at the core symptomatology
- General therapies, relating to the psychological, social, and educational needs of the child and their family.

The aim of most CAHMS services will be to deliver treatment on an out-patient basis, but it may occasionally be necessary to consider day or in-patient treatment, in consultation with the young person and their family.

Early intervention

There has been considerable research and a number of early intervention programmes have been developed targeting 'high-risk' children and adolescents with a strong family history and/or suggestive prodromal symptoms, which attempt to ensure prompt early treatment (including medication) aimed at preventing the development of the active phase of schizophrenia. Unfortunately, the predictive validity is low (only about one-fifth of these high risk cases go on to develop frank psychosis) and there are ethical concerns about giving antipsychotic medication to essentially non-psychotic individuals.

Pharmacological treatments

There have been few RCTs of antipsychotics in children and adolescents, and many of the trials have been open label and have only included small sample sizes. Therefore, therapeutic recommendations are still primarily based on adult literature. There are no licensed antipsychotic medication approved for use in psychosis with children and adolescents, and medication use tends to be off licence. Current recommendations suggest using atypical antipsychotics as first line treatment in the acute phase (📖 Fig. 15.1, p. 225).

Duration of treatment

When initial treatment results in improvements in symptoms, it is suggested that medication be continued for a further 6–12 months after remission. Adult studies have shown 65% of patients relapse within 1 year and 80% relapse at least once in 5 years. In newly diagnosed patients who have been symptom-free for at least 6–12 months, a medication-free trial may be considered.

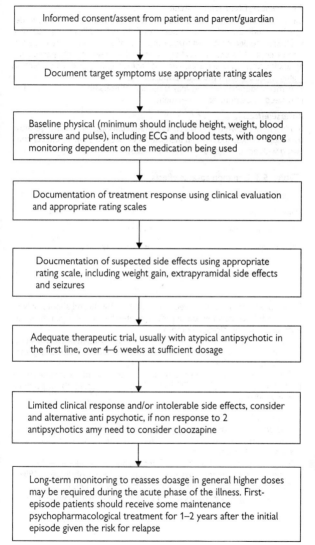

Informed consent/assent from patient and parent/guardian

↓

Document target symptoms use appropriate rating scales

↓

Baseline physical (minimum should include height, weight, blood pressure and pulse), including ECG and blood tests, with ongong monitoring dependent on the medication being used

↓

Documentation of treatment response using clinical evaluation and appropriate rating scales

↓

Doucmentation of suspected side effects using appropriate rating scale, including weight gain, extrapyramidal side effects and seizures

↓

Adequate therapeutic trial, usually with atypical antipsychotic in the first line, over 4–6 weeks at sufficient dosage

↓

Limited clinical response and/or intolerable side effects, consider and alternative anti psychotic, if non response to 2 antipsychotics amy need to consider cloozapine

↓

Long-term monitoring to reasses doasge in general higher doses may be required during the acute phase of the illness. First-episode patients should receive some maintenance psychopharmacological treatment for 1–2 years after the initial episode given the risk for relapse

Fig. 15.1 Flowchart for initiation of antipsychotics.

Treatment resistant schizophrenia

Only clozapine is currently licensed in these circumstances and only under specific conditions. There have been several small studies using clozapine in EOS; these demonstrated that clozapine is of benefit in symptom reduction or control. Its use, however, is associated with side effects, particularly agranulocytosis and seizures, and the incidence of these side effects is higher in EOS than in the adult population.

A medication-free period may be useful to reassess the diagnosis. This may need to be done as an in-patient

Adverse effects

Studies have shown that children and adolescents are particularly sensitive to antipsychotics, and have an increased incidence of adverse effects compared with adult subjects (📖 see Table 15.3).

Table 15.3 Common adverse effects

Extrapyramidal side effects	Seizures
Tardive dyskinesia	Sedation
Hyperprolactinaemia	Hypotension
Weight gain	Hepatotoxicity
Tachycardia	Hypersalivaltion

Depot preparations are not recommended for VEOS and should only be used in adolescents when there is documented history of psychotic symptoms and poor medication compliance.

Other medications including lithium and anticonvulsants have been used in adults with schizophrenia, but there is little evidence supporting their use in VEOS and EOS.

There is insufficient evidence to support the use of electroconvulsive therapy (ECT) in VEOS and EOS, and there are concerns about potential cognitive effects.

Rating scales

Rating scales give quantitative measures and psychopathology and functional impairment and can be useful to record the longitudinal course of the illness and treatment response.

- Scale for Assessment of Positive Symptoms (SAPS; Andreason, 1984)
- Scale for Assessment of Negative Symptoms (SANS; Andreason, 1984)
- Abnormal Movement Scale (AIMS; Rapoport *et al.*, 1985)
- Simpson-Angus Neurological Rating Scale (Simpson and Angus, 1970).

Psychological treatments

Traditional psychodynamic psychotherapeutic approaches have been shown to have little effect, but learning-based therapies, incorporating cognitive, behavioural, and social skills training can improve functioning and decrease relapse rates a range of interventions include:

- Psychoeducation
- Family interventions aimed at:
  - Reducing expressed emotion
  - Building supportive relationships and Limit setting
  - Addressing feelings of guilt for child' illness
- Parental support groups
- Individual therapy
  - Social skills training
  - Emotion recognition and management
  - Problem solving and communication skills
  - Cognitive behaviour therapy
- Group therapy.

Course and outcome

Schizophrenia is a phasic disorder and this has implications for assessment and treatment. The phases include:

- **Prodrome:** may last from days to months
- **Acute phase:** generally lasts 1–6 months depending on treatment response
- **Recuperative/recovery phase:** usually lasts several months, with significant impairment and some patients may develop significant depressive symptoms
- **Residual phase:** there may be months or years between acute episodes with few residual positive, but more negative symptoms
- **Chronically ill:** there may be some individuals who remain chronically symptomatic and impaired to a varying extent by their symptoms

There is limited data on recovery rates from childhood onset schizophrenia, (and disputes over what constitutes 'recovery'), but given that the emergence of the disorder disrupts psychosocial development, and schooling it is unsurprising the VEOS and EOS often has a relatively poor prognosis even with psychopharmacological treatment (📖 Table 15.4).

- 12.5–15% of VEOS/EOS obtain full recovery (5-year follow-up)
- 80–90% will have 2 or more episode in a 5-year period
- 20–25% recovery from affective psychosis
- 30–40% recovery from psychosis NOS.

Table 15.4 Predictors of outcome

Poorer outcome	Better outcome
Onset before age 10	Shorter duration of psychosis
More negative symptoms at baseline	Cerebral asymmetry
Lower premorbid functioning	Presence of affective symptoms

Mortality

There a few studies, but the risk of suicide or accidental death as a result of psychotic symptoms appears to be about 5% (suicide rate for adults with schizophrenia approx 10%).

Case example

David a 15-year-old schoolboy was referred to the local CAHMS service by his GP. He had been taken to the GP by his mum who wondered if David might be depressed about his forthcoming exams and a recent break-up with his girlfriend. David spoke to the GP with his mum present and confirmed that he had lost interest in schoolwork and friends; he denied thoughts of self-harm. He was agreeable to a referral to CAHMS.

At his initial CAHMS appointment David asked to see the psychiatrist without his mum. He agreed he had been worried about his exams, but there were a number of things that had been happening in his life that puzzled him and he was trying to work out the meaning of them. He said that although his girlfriend had broken up with him he felt sure that she was trying to communicate with him in different ways to say that she was sorry. He had heard a song on the radio and just knew that this was a message from his girlfriend. He also said that he was building up evidence of a plot at school to smuggle diamonds into the country, but he thought that the plotters might have realized that he was 'on to them' as he had begun to notice that people were following him. He had been staying up through the night watching the cars passing his house and recording the number plates. He was writing everything down in case anything should happen to him. He was not sure if he was in danger and during the interview appeared perplexed about what was going on around him. He said that he was having difficulty concentrating in class, but attributed that to trying to collect further 'evidence' as he believed that coded conversations about the plot were taking place in classes.

History from mum was that David had always done well at primary school; there had been no concerns about his behaviour until about 6 months ago. David had become more withdrawn at home, spending increasing amounts of time on his own. He had been a very sporty boy, but this again has slipped lately and David was less interested in meeting friends. Mum reported that she had often heard David wandering about at night in his room and she had heard him talking, but had assumed he was speaking to friends.

David lived at home with his mum and dad, and older sister. There was no family medical or psychiatric history. David said that he had smoked cannabis with friends occasionally, but denied any use over the past 3 months. There was no history of alcohol misuse.

At the end of the initial appointment a possible diagnosis of a psychotic episode was raised with David and his mum. They were advised that David should take some time off school and further physical investigations, including a urine drug screen and MRI, were arranged (no abnormalities were detected).

At subsequent out-patient appointments David began to discuss more openly his feeling that his room has been bugged as he had begun hearing voices inside his head commenting on what he was doing. He was becoming more concerned about his safety and had started sleeping with a knife under his pillow.

Following further discussion with David and his family he was admitted to the day service, and attended 3 days a week, receiving regular individual and family psychotherapy sessions. After 3 months there had been no improvement in David's psychotic symptoms. Further treatment options were discussed with David and the family, and a trial of risperidone in addition to ongoing psychotherapy suggested. Gradually, David reported that the diamond plot must have been abandoned as he was no longer under surveillance. He returned to school part-time and began to play rugby again. The CAHMS team discussed with David and his family that, although his symptoms appeared to be improving and he no longer required the intensive support of the day programme, it would be advisable to continue with treatment for the next 6–12 months on an out-patient basis.

References and recommended reading

Cepeda C. (2006) *Psychotic Symptoms in Children and Adolescents: Assessment, Differential Diagnosis, and Treatment.* Routledge, New York.

Kolvina I. (1971) Studies in the Childhood Psychoses. *British Journal of Psychiatry* **6**:209–234.

McClellan J, Werry J. (2001) Practice parameters for the assessment and treatment of children and adolescents with schizophrenia. *J Am Acad Child Adolesc Psychiatry* **40**: 4S–23S.

Rutter M. (1972) Childhood Schizophrenia Reansidered. *Journal of Autism and Childhood Schizophrenia* **2**: 315–337.

Bipolar disorder

Definitions

The diagnosis of bipolar disorder (BPD) in children and adolescents remains controversial, not least due to concern about how best to apply the diagnostic criteria to children and young people, particularly prepubertal children, and how best to operationalize symptoms such as grandiosity in these populations.

Both the DSM-IV and ICD-10 diagnostic criteria define and recognize episodes of hypomania and mania, but use different terms to describe these episodes. Although there are differences, both systems require that episodes must represent a significant departure from baseline functioning and that the mood disturbance be sufficiently severe to cause marked impairment in functioning.

Table 16.1 outlines the different terms used by both systems.

Table 16.1 The different terms used by both systems

DSM-IV	ICD-10
Bipolar I disorder: requires only a single manic or mixed episode. The manic symptoms must be present for at least 7 days (or any duration if hospitalization is necessary) Episodes of depression are not required for a diagnosis although often individuals' minor or major episodes of depression during their life span.	**Bipolar affective disorder:** at least 2 episodes required one of which must be mania or hypomania. The episode can be further classified according to the current mood present. The duration criteria for a manic or hypomanic episode are the same in DSM-IV
Bipolar II disorder: periods of depression and hypomania (episodes lasting least 4 days), but not a full manic or mixed episode	**Manic episode:** including hypomania, and mania with or without psychotic symptoms
Mixed episode: a period lasting 7 days or more in which both symptoms of a manic and depressive episode are met	**Bipolar affective disorder, current episode mixed:** both mania and depressive symptoms present for at least 2 weeks
BPD not otherwise specified	**Bipolar affective disorder, unspecified**
Rapid cycling: when there are at least 4 mood episodes a year (the episode still meets the duration criteria)	

Several other definitions have been used in childhood onset BPD, but have not as yet been adopted as part of any diagnostic system.
- **Ultrarapid cycling:** brief frequent manic episodes lasting hours to days, but less than the 4-day criteria for hypomania
- **Ultradian cycling:** repeated brief (minutes to hours) cycles that occur daily.

Recent National Institute for Health and Clinical Excellence (NICE) guidelines also make the following recommendations:

- In prepubertal children irritability should not be considered a core diagnostic criterion
- Bipolar II disorder should not be diagnosed in children and adolescents due to a lack of consensus regarding diagnostic criteria.

Diagnostic concerns

There is no doubt that there are many children and adolescents who present to Child and Adolescent Mental Health Services (CAHMS) service with mood disturbance, irritability, and outbursts of aggression and particularly in the USA, the diagnosis of early onset (pre-pubertal) BPDs is increasing. The debate surrounding early onset BPD centres on a number of issues:

- Are these symptoms best characterized as BPD?
- Is early onset BPD the same illness as adult BPD? A number of studies have shown that those diagnosed with symptoms of early onset BPD do not show increased rates BPD over time, which is surprising as adult BPD is generally considered a lifelong condition
- How specific are symptoms, such as irritability and over-activity, to BPD in children and young people given the overlap between the criteria for mania and those for attention deficit hyperactivity disorder (ADHD) and the other disruptive behavioural disorders? Are clinicians identifying true pre-pubertal BPD or severe cases of disruptive behaviour disorders such as ADHD, conduct disorder (CD), and oppositional defiant disorder (ODD)?
- What are the risks of labelling children and young people with a major psychiatric disorder, particularly one that has treatment with psychotropic medication as an option?
- The diagnostic criteria have been interpreted and used in very different ways by different investigators. This has caused further confusion about the diagnostic specificity of symptoms
- Although the early descriptions of BPD such as those used by groups from St Louis (Geller) and Boston (Biederman) were very broad and generally considered over inclusive by clinicians in Europe, more recent studies have utilized a much narrower phenotype and have identified groups of children whose symptoms and presentation are much closer to those recognized as being consistent with descriptions of adults with BPD (e.g. Youngstrom, Leibenluft).

Epidemiology and aetiology

Epidemiology

There have been few epidemiological studies addressing this issue (📖 AACAP parameters for more information); the main findings are summarized below:

- All epidemiological studies have reported mania as being very rare or non-existent in prepubertal children, in a study of rural youths aged 13 or younger no cases of mania were found
- A number of epidemiological surveys of 9–18-year-olds found estimated prevalence of mania was 0–0.6%. If sub-threshold symptoms or symptoms of hypothymia or cyclothymia were included prevalence rates rose to 5.7–13.3%
- Large retrospective surveys of adults with BPD noted that onset before age 10 occurred in 0.3–0.5% of patients, although many described mood symptoms (commonly depression) beginning in childhood.

There is some evidence that adolescent onset BPD may be on the increase reasons for this may include:

- Genetic process of anticipation
- More sensitive diagnostic methods
- Increasing alcohol and substance abuse.

Aetiology

Given the sparse literature on early onset BPD and the variability in diagnostic criteria used in different studies, relatively little is known about the aetiology of early onset BPD.

Genetics

- There have been no large scale genetic studies of pre-pubertal or adolescent onset BPD
- Adult twin, family, and adoption studies of the broad phenotype support a genetic component with a 4–6-fold increase risk in first degree relatives of affected individuals
- In early onset and highly co-morbid cases the degree of familiarity appears higher
- Molecular genetic studies to date have not identified any candidate genes.

Imaging

Studies have identified white matter hyperintensities in both cortical and subcortical regions of the brain in early onset BPD. Functional neuroimaging studies have shown variable results and have been limited by small sample size.

Neuropsychology

Children and adolescents with early onset BPD have been demonstrated to have significant cognitive deficits that impact on academic functioning. Studies have identified a range of deficits, including attentional set shifting and interpretation of facial expression, which may be impaired in early onset BPD, but it is not clear that these deficits are specific for early onset BPD.

Psychosocial risk factors

Many of the children and adolescents diagnosed with BPD have poor social skills, conflictual relationships with peers, siblings, and parents, together with poor problem solving skills. High levels of hostility and low warmth in maternal relationships, and elevated rates of novelty seeking have also been noted. These deficits are non-specific to BPD and further studies are required to identify if they are related to the BPD, co-morbidity, or family psychopathology.

A number of other factors have been identified as being more common in early onset BPD:

- Mood lability with irritability, anxiety, attention problems, depression, somatic complaints, and school problems is more common in offspring of bipolar parents and may precede the development of BPD
- Pre-morbid psychiatric problems are common in early onset BPD especially disruptive behavioural disorders (ADHD and ODD/CD), irritability and behavioural dyscontrol
- The rates of premorbid disruptive behaviour disorder are higher in childhood onset than adolescent onset BPD.

Assessment

- The diagnosis of BPD should only be made by a clinician with specialist training in child and adolescent mental health.
  Any assessment should include:
- A detailed account of the presenting problems from the child, parents, or carers, and other significant adults such as teachers. The purpose is to:
  - Confirm that the symptoms described represent a marked change from baseline and are impairing in a range of situations, e.g. home and school
  - Ascertain the duration of symptoms and any association with psychomotor and sleep changes (although studies of early onset BPD found sleep disturbance in ≤50% of cases)
- A description of current and past functioning:
  - Consider using a life chart to capture the patterns of episodes, severity, and association with significant life events and previous treatment response if appropriate. Using a longitudinal perspective may help with diagnosis as the presentation in the acute phase can often be confused with other disorders
  - Early onset mania especially in young children more often presents with ultrarapid or ultradian cycling (10 and 77%, respectively, in one study) than the more protracted cyclical course typically found in adults
- A full developmental and neurodevelopmental history including:
  - Birth history
  - Family history of mental illness
  - Speech and language development
  - *Behavioural problems:* early onset BPD may be associated with greater risk of behavioural problems in childhood. Serious childhood behavioural problems are more common in those with early-onset (60%) than adult-onset (10%) BPD
  - Attachment behaviour
  - Parent–child relationship conflicts
  - Temperamental difficulties (higher rates of irritability and mood lability)
  - History of abuse
- Mental state examination based on an individual interview with the child or young person:
  - Adolescent onset BPD is associated with high rates of psychotic symptoms, labile moods, and mixed maniac and depressive features
  - Children with early onset BPD more commonly present with irritability, change in energy level, and mixed episodes
  - There are high rates of co-morbid disorders particularly anxiety, ADHD, disruptive behaviours, and substance abuse
  - In addition, adolescents with BPD are reported to have higher rates of suicide attempts
  - It is also important to assess risk taking behaviour particularly where there is co-morbidity with ADHD and substance abuse

- Physical and neurological examination as appropriate consider:
  - Urine drug screen
  - Pregnancy test (vital if considering medication)
  - There are no biological tests, neuroimaging or genetic tests that are helpful in making the diagnosis of BPD
- Neuropsychological assessment: there are no specific tools or tests, but a cognitive assessment may be helpful in planning treatment.
- Cross cultural issues may influence the expression or interpretation of symptom and therefore must be considered.

Rating scales

- A specialist structured diagnostic interview such as the Washington University Kiddie Schedule of Affective Disorders and Schizophrenia (WASH-U-KSADS) may be helpful. This is completed by an clinician and makes diagnoses based on DSM-IV criteria
- Various reliable and validated rating scales that are completed by parents are available. These can be helpful in guiding the assessment, but are NOT diagnostic instruments and should not replace a full clinical interview. They include:
  - Child behaviour checklist
  - Conners' Abbreviated Rating Scale
  - Parents Young Mania Rating Scale.

The symptoms with the best specificity are:
- Elevated mood
- Grandiosity/inflated self-esteem
- Pressured speech
- Racing thoughts
- Decreased *need* for sleep
- Hypersexuality.

Special considerations in the assessment of BPD

In prepubertal children, symptoms must be assessed in the context of the developmental period, e.g. wearing a superhero costume as part of a role play game can be mistaken for grandiosity. Additionally, children and adolescents with learning disabilities may have difficulties describing their emotions and feelings.

Differential diagnosis and co-morbidity

Differential diagnosis

Symptoms of irritability and emotional reactivity are not diagnostically specific to BPD. The chronic and very rapid cycling of symptoms typical of early onset BPD presents considerable diagnostic challenges to clinicians. Differential diagnoses include:

- **Schizophrenia:** mania in adolescence frequently presents with psychotic symptoms
- **Schizoaffective disorder:** mixed presentation of depressive and manic symptoms is common in early onset BPD
- **ADHD:** ADHD and BPD share several common symptoms:

Symptom	Bipolar	ADHD
Irritability	Yes	Yes
Grandiosity	Yes	No
Elevated mood	Yes	No
Over-activity	Yes	Yes
Sleep problems	Yes	Yes
Distractibility	Yes	Yes
Impulsivity	Yes	Yes
Over-talkative	Yes	Yes
Episodic	Yes	No

- **Conduct disorder:** common symptoms in both this and BPD include:
  - Irritability
  - Hostility and violence
  - Impulsivity
  - Inappropriate sexual behaviours
- **Substance abuse** may mimic symptoms during acute intoxication and withdrawal (and can also arise as a consequence of BPD)
- **Pervasive developmental disorder (PDD):** the irritability, mood lability and aggression sometimes seen in PDD can be mistaken for mania
- **Personality disorder:** sub-syndromal cases of adolescent BPD have increased rates of antisocial and borderline personality disorder symptoms as young adults, but no increased risk of BPD
- **Organic causes**, e.g. acute confusional states, epilepsy (pre- or post-ictal confusional states) and medication side effects, e.g. akathisia due to neuroleptics
- Sexual, emotional, and physical abuse may present with hypervigilance, disinhibition and hypersexuality.

Co-morbidity

High rates of co-morbidity are seen in early onset BPD:
- ADHD 11–75% (depending on criteria used to define BPD)
- ODD 46–75%
- CD 6–37%
- Anxiety disorders 13–56%
- Substance abuse 0–40%
- Pervasive developmental disorder 11%.

Co-morbidity varies with age; children with paediatric BPD have higher co-morbidity with ADHD than adolescents, whereas adolescents have higher rates of substance abuse.

Treatment

The current evidence for both drug and psychological treatments of BPD in children and adolescents is extremely limited.

As would be expected treatment requires a comprehensive treatment plan that may include medication in addition to psychotherapeutic interventions. The goals of therapy will include:

• Reduction in core symptoms
• Psychoeducation
• Relapse prevention
• Facilitating normal growth and development.

Pharmacotherapy (📖 Fig. 16.1, p. 246)

Most of the recommendations for the pharmacotherapy of BPD in children and adolescents are based on findings in adults, the effectiveness and safety of anti-manic (this term is used as there is no agreed definition of mood stabilizer), antipsychotic, and anticonvulsant medications in early and adolescent onset BPD is not yet established. The type of medication used will depend on:

• The phase of the illness (acute mania, acute depression, mixed episode, maintenance)
• Presence of additional symptoms or co-morbidity
• Patient history of medication response
• Patient and family preference.

To date, only lithium in licensed in the UK for treatment of BPD in those 12 years and older. However, anticonvulsants and antipsychotics are also used, although evidence for use of these and Lithium in the young population remains scarce.

Prior to using medication the following baseline measures should be considered:

• Weight, height, and Body Mass Index (BMI)
• Electrocardiogram (ECG), blood pressure, and pulse
• Blood tests including full blood count (FBC), U&Es, LFTs, TFTs (esp. prior to lithium) prolactin, and blood glucose (neuroleptics)
• Urinalysis including pregnancy test.

These measures should also be checked on a regular basis (every 3–6 months) together with plasma levels of lithium, valproate, and carbamazepine during maintenance treatment.

Dose considerations

In general, the recommendations are to 'start low and go slow' compared to adult doses.

Co-morbidity

There is no evidence that stimulant treatment exacerbates mood symptoms in patients with co-morbid ADHD.

Duration of treatment

There have been few prospective studies, but one study found over 18 months that >90% of adolescents who were non-compliant with treatment relapsed. Current evidence therefore suggests that treatment should be continued for 12–24 months following the stabilization of the acute mania episode. Some young people may need lifelong treatment, but this should be discussed with the young person with consideration of the risks and benefits of continued treatment.

Electroconvulsive treatment

The evidence base for use in adolescents is mainly from case reports, but ECT is used in adults who have not responded to standard treatment.

ECT should only be considered for well documented bipolar I disorder with severe episodes of mania or depression, who are non-responsive to standard treatment. Side effects include short-term cognitive impairment, anxiety symptoms, disinhibition, and lowered seizure threshold.

Managing rapid cycling

- Treatment should focus on optimizing the long-term functioning, rather than treating the acute episode
- Review previous treatment to ensure that there was adequate durations of treatment and adherence.

Psychotherapeutic interventions

The development of BPD during childhood and adolescence disrupts academic, social, and family functioning. Although medication may help with the core symptoms the associated functional and developmental impairments, including pre-existing behavioural problems and co-morbidity mean than additional psychotherapeutic interventions are almost always necessary. The following treatment recommendations come from adult literature and preliminary studies of early onset BPD:

- Psychoeducational therapy including information regarding symptoms, course, impact on functioning and heritability
- Relapse prevention focusing on recognition of relapse symptoms, importance of compliance with treatment and general stress reduction, strengthening the therapeutic relationship
- Individual therapy. Consider cognitive behavioural therapy (CBT) for adolescents. Supporting skill building, and exploring impact of illness
- Social and family interventions, family focused therapy to address treatment compliance, positive family relationships, problems solving and communication
- Academic and occupational interventions to address education needs both in the short and long term, older adolescents may need support with higher education placements and vocational training.

Combining individual and family interventions appears to help decrease relapse and lessen depressive symptoms.

Treatment location

The majority of children and adolescents with a diagnosis of BPD will receive out-patient treatment by specialist CAHMS teams but intensive community treatment, specialist inpatient or day patient treatment in specialist CAHMS services (Tier 3–4) may be required for patients at risk of suicide or other serious self-harm.

Course and prognosis

Longitudinal studies show:
- Very low rates of conversion of depression to mania among prepubertal children
- Some studies suggest than approximately 20% of adolescents who have an episode of major depression experience a subsequent manic episode by adulthood. The following features have been found to predict subsequent development of mania in depressed children and adolescents:
  - Depressive episode of rapid onset with psychomotor retardation and psychotic features
  - Family history of affective disorder, especially mania
  - History of mania or hypomania following antidepressant treatment
- Adolescents presenting with an initial manic episode show higher relapse rates (approximately 50% during 5-year follow-up)
- The early course of adolescent onset BPD appears more chronic and refractory to treatment than adult onset. Long-term prognosis is similar or worse than that of adults
- Co-morbidity predicts functional impairment
- Age of onset predicts duration of episodes
- Studies have found that early onset BPD have high rates of relapse (approx 60% in 18 months) despite treatment
- Low rates of maternal warmth predict shorter duration to relapse
- Presence of psychosis is associated with chronicity
- Children with ADHD do not have an increased risk of BPD in later life
- No studies have demonstrated that prepubertal mania progresses to the classic adult disorder
- Later adolescent onset BPD tend to have a more similar relapsing and remitting course to the adult presentations.

Table 16.2 Summary characteristic of child and adult BPD

	Prepubertal and young adolescent	Older adolescent and adult
Initial episode	Major depressive disorder	Mania
Episode type	Rapid, ultra-rapid, or ultradian cycling	Discrete with sudden onsets and clear offsets
Duration	Chronic, continuous cycling	Weeks
Inter episode functioning	Non-episodic	Improved functioning

Clinical examples

Case 1

A 7-year-old boy was referred to local CAMHS services because of hyperactivity and oppositional behaviour. A full assessment including school reports suggested a cyclical pattern of mood disturbance with episodes consisting of 4–5 days of low mood with psychomotor retardation, reduced appetite, increased anxiety and self-doubt, followed by episodes lasting 2–7 days of increased activity, oppositionality, risk-taking behaviour (e.g. jumping off roofs, fighting with older children), elevated mood, and reduced need for sleep. There were brief periods between these episodes where baseline function appeared to be of mild hyperactivity and oppositionality. A diagnosis of ADHD with sub threshold bipolar symptoms was made. Following some psychoeducational work with the patient, family and school the patient and family felt that no further active treatment was required and out-patient follow-up was offered.

Case 2

A 13-year-old girl presented to CAMHS service via GP referral with a 6-month history of mood swings. There was a strong family history of affective disorder and her mother had a chronic BPD. When seen initially there were no significant mood symptoms but a clear history of a recent hypomanic episode with disturbed sleep, appetite, and school functioning. The girl was followed up in out-patients and developed a depressive episode which responded well to CBT. Over the next 12 months she was reviewed regularly in clinic and appeared to be doing well and was medication free. She was then referred as an emergency to the on call CAMHS service with a 4 days history of sleep disturbance, agitation, grandiose ideas (that she was a singer in a well known pop group), irritability, and increased sexual activity. She was clear that she had not used illicit substances. At interview there was marked pressure of speech, flight of ideas, and a clear elevation of mood. It was felt that she was not at risk and her mother was able to increase her supervision of her daughter by taking time off work, and she was commenced on lithium following discussion with the family. Over the next 4 weeks she was regularly reviewed in clinic and her mood stabilized. She regained insight and was able to recognize that prior to the episode she had been worried about her forthcoming exams and had frequently been staying up late studying. She had also been worried about her mum's physical health as she was due to go into hospital soon for a hip replacement. Both the patient and the mum attended several family sessions, and were able to discuss openly their concerns about each other, as well as some work on relapse prevention. The patient decided to continue on treatment throughout her exam period.

Treatment algorithms

Stop antidepressant medication (if taking) abruptly or gradually depending on clinical need and risk of withdrawal/discontinuation symptoms
Is the patient already taking an antimanic agent?

No

Consider:
- An antipsychotic
  - Aripipazole
  - Risperidone
  - Olanzapine
  - Quetiapine
- Valproate: avoid in girls and young women (risk of polycystic ovarian syndrome)
- Lithium: if responded previously and not severe symptoms

If already taking an antipsychotic with an inadequate response consider adding lithium or valproate

Carbamazepine, gabapentin, lamotrigine, and topiramate should not be use in acute mania

Avoid use of benzodiazepines if possible due to risk of disinhibition. Avoid use of haloperidol due to risk of extra pyramidal side effects

Yes

If taking an antipsychotic:
- Check dose
- If inadequate consider adding lithium or anticonvulsant

If taking lithium:
- Check plasma level (if <0.8 mmol/L increase dose to maximum blood level 1.0 mmol/L)
- If response inadequate consider adding an antipsychotic

If taking valproate consider:
- Increase dose but monitor carefully if dose >45 mg/kg
- Adding an antipsychotic

If taking carbamazepine:
- Do not increase dose
- Consider and antipsychotic
- Caution required as drug interactions common with carbamazepine

In general follow treatment recommendations as for adults BUT:
- Start medication at a lower dose
- Check weight and height regularly
- Measure prolactin level
- If considering an antipsychotic remember risk of increase prolactin with risperidone and weight gain with olanzapine
- Increased risk of extrapyramidal side effects with antipsychotics
- Advise patient and family to avoid excessive stimulation
- May need time off school
- Need to monitor closely as out-patient but may need to consider in-patient treatment

Fig. 16.1 Acute mania and hypomania. Adapted from NICE guidelines.

Monitor weekly; if symptoms mild and do not need immediate treatment and offer additional support at home and school

↓

If treatment required this should be undertaken within specialist CAHMS services

For moderate to severe depression treat as for adults BUT fluoxetine is the only licensed antidepressant for under 18s

Further considerations:

- Initially offer structured psychological therapy (☐ see Chapter 17, p.249) in addition to any prophylactic medication that may be being taken
- if no response after 4 weeks consider adding fluoxetine starting at 10 mg
- When starting an antidepressant need to explain to patient and family the risks of switching to mania
- If taking an antidepressant may also need to be taking an antimanic medication

↓

Avoid antidepressants for patients who have

- Rapid cycling bipolar disorder
- A recent hypomanic episode
- Recent functionally impairing mood fluctuations
- Instead consider increasing dose of antimanic medication

↓

If no response to fluoxetine consider using different SSRI (sertraline or citalopram)

↓

If symptoms remit or have reduced considerably for 8 weeks consider gradual discontinuation of antidepressant

If incomplete response consider:
- Re-assess for comorbidity
- Addition of lithium
- Addition of antipsychotic
- Follow adult guidelines

If concurrent depressive and psychotic symptoms augment treatment with antipsychotic or consider ECT

Fig. 16.2 Treatment of depression in the context of BPD. Adapted from NICE guidelines.

Recommended reading

AACAP Official Action (1997) Practice parameters for the assessment and treatment of children and adolescents with bipolar disorder. *J Am Acad Child Adolesc Psychiatry* **36**: 138–57.

Faraone SV, Glatt SJ, Tsuang MT. (2003) The genetics of pediatric-onset bipolar disorder. *Biol Psychiatry* **53**: 970–7.

Kowatch RA, DelBello MP. (2005) Pharmacotherapy of children and adolescents with bipolar disorder. *Psychiatr Clin N Am* **28**: 385–97.

NICE (2006) *Bipolar Disorder: NICE Guideline 38*. National Institute for Health and Clinical Excellence, London. Available at: http://www.nice.org.uk/guidance/index.jsp?action=byID&o=10990 (accessed 7 May 2008).

Depression

Definitions and epidemiology

Definition

Depression is an emotional disorder that can occur in childhood and adolescence. ICD-10 and DSM-IV classification of depression for adults apply to children and adolescents. Both classifications require that:
- Symptoms are present for more than 2 weeks
- Symptoms have a significant effect on functioning.

ICD-10 criteria

Depressive episode

Core symptoms for a 'depressive episode':
- Depressed mood
- Loss of interest and enjoyment
- Increased fatigability.

Diagnosis requires the presence of two out of the above three symptoms for diagnosis of mild to moderate depressive episode, and all three for severe depressive episode.

ICD-10 additional symptoms
- Reduced concentration and attention
- Reduced self-esteem and self-confidence
- Ideas of guilt and unworthiness
- Bleak and pessimistic views of the future
- Ideas or acts of self-harm
- Diminished appetite
- Disturbed sleep.

Mild depressive episode requires 2 additional symptoms.
   Moderate depressive episode requires 3–4 additional symptoms
   Severe depressive episode requires 4 or more additional symptoms, or for psychotic symptoms to be present.
   In ICD-10, severity is further determined by the effect the depressive episode has on daily functioning.
- **Mild depressive disorder:** continues to function with difficulty in some areas of life
- **Moderate depressive disorder:** experiences considerable difficulty in functioning at school, home, and with peers
- **Severe depressive episode:** functioning is significantly affected in all areas of life.

Dysthymia

Dysthymia is classified as chronic sub-clinical version of depression that has persisted for over a year.

DSM-IV

Major depressive disorder

The DSM-IV diagnostic criteria for Major Depressive Disorder require presence of depressed mood, irritable mood, or anhedonia plus five additional symptoms from the list below, and for these to have a significant effect on functioning.

DSM-IV symptoms

- Low or irritable mood with lack of reactivity
- Dysphoric mood
- Diurnal variation in mood
- Sleep disturbances
- Fatigue, loss of energy, and tiredness
- Change in appetite or body weight
- Motor agitation or retardation
- Worthlessness and negative self-perception
- Hopelessness, discouragement, and pessimism
- Rejection sensitivity.

Epidemiology

Rates of depressive disorder vary across studies depending on diagnostic classification, and whether studies include or exclude children and adolescents with co-morbid diagnoses.

Childhood prevalence of depression is reported between 0.5 and 2.5%, with girls and boys being equally likely to experience depression.

Prevalence of depression in adolescence is between 2 and 8%. In this age group girls are twice as likely as boys to experience an episode of depression, mirroring the gender bias seen in adulthood.

Aetiology

There are a number of predisposing, precipitating, and protective factors that contribute to the likelihood of a child or adolescent becoming depressed.

Genetic factors

- Genetic studies have demonstrated a significant heritability for depression that is estimated as accounting for approximately 40% of the risk for developing depression
- Lifetime prevalence of depression in parents of depressed children is double that of parents of a non-depressed children
- The genetic risk appears to have two components, an increased risk of developing a depressive disorder, and an increased risk of experiencing negative life events.

Pathophysiology

- The exact role of neurotransmitters in the aetiology of depression in children and adolescents is unclear
- In adolescents, response to treatment of depression with SSRI's may suggest that low levels of serotonin may contribute to the development of a depressive disorder in this age range.

Gender

- Post-pubertal females are twice as likely as males to become depressed. There are a number of theories regarding this, but little clear evidence. Possible links to oestrogen levels, either *in utero* or post-puberty, have been suggested
- Females may be more influenced by lack of positive relationships, close friendships, or a supportive peer network. These are particularly important in adolescence.

Environmental factors

- Early adversity and attachment difficulties
- Negative life events
- Death of a parent
- Traumatic life events
- Experience of abuse and neglect
- Drug and alcohol abuse
- Bullying.

Psychosocial factors

- Social isolation and negative interpersonal relationships
- Good academic achievement
- Unstable family environment
- Parental drug and alcohol abuse.

Assessment, differential diagnosis, and co-morbidity

Initial assessment needs to recognize the symptoms of depression and their impact on the child or adolescent.

Clinical presentation in childhood and adolescence depends on the young person's cognitive development, and their ability to recognize and identify their emotions. Prior to the development of these skills, depression is likely to be associated with increased irritability and challenging behaviour.

Anxiety, somatic complaints, and social withdrawal are also more common in children and adolescents than in adults.

Clinical interview with the parents

Should include:
- A general mental health evaluation as described in Chapter 9
- Specific questioning should cover:
  - The symptoms of depression
  - The effects of any mood disorder on functioning within the family, school and with peers
  - Behavioural changes associated with altered mood
  - The presence of symptoms suggestive of a manic episode
  - Psychotic symptoms
  - Risk of self-harm or suicide
  - Current level of self-care
  - Somatic symptoms
  - Anxiety symptoms
  - Short- and long-term predisposing, precipitating, and perpetuating factors
  - Previous history of depressive episodes and previous treatment
  - Past or present history of co-morbid psychiatric disorder
  - Premorbid functioning
  - History of abuse or neglect
  - Family functioning
  - Family history of psychiatric disorder, including bipolar disorder (BPD), and drug and alcohol abuse.

Mental state assessment should be completed.

A separate interview with the child or adolescent

This is essential to:
- Confirm the information obtained in the interview with parents present
- Elicit any information that the child or young person may not wish to discuss in the presence of their parents.

Particular attention should be paid to:
- Risk of self-harm or suicide
- Alcohol and drug use
- History of abuse or neglect
- Consent and capacity to consent to treatment.

Information from school
- Past and current social functioning, and quality of interpersonal relationships
- Educational abilities and academic attainments
- The impact of current mood disorder on levels of functioning.

General physical examination
This is required:
- In any child or young person with symptoms suggestive of a physical illness
- To exclude a physical cause for moderate to severe depression
- To exclude a physical cause for depressive symptoms that do not respond to the initial management plan.

Rating scales
These may be used to supplement the assessment, but should not be used on their own to make a 'diagnosis'.
    The following scales are often considered:
- Mood and feelings questionnaire
- Beck Youth Depression Scale
- Strengths and difficulties questionnaire.

Differential diagnosis
- BPD
- Anxiety disorder
- Obsessive Compulsive Disorder (OCD)
- Post-traumatic stress disorder (PTSD)
- Psychosis
- Physical health problems, neurological, metabolic, or endocrine illnesses
- ODD and conduct disorders (CDs).

Co-morbidity
Anxiety disorders are present prior to the onset of a depressive disorder in 50% of adolescents. In particular, separation anxiety disorder and social phobia.
    Rates of symptoms of depression and depressive disorders are increased in children and adolescents diagnosed with:
- OCD
- Psychosis
- Drug and alcohol abuse
- Oppositional defiant disorder (ODD) and CDs
- ADHD
- Pervasive developmental disorders (PDD)
- Learning difficulties
- Acute and chronic physical illness.

Management 1: general principles and psychological treatments

Initial assessment should identify:

- Symptoms of manic episode or psychotic disorder
- Significant risk of self-harm or suicide
- Significant lack of self care or neglect
- Co-morbid psychiatric disorder
- Previous history of moderate or severe depressive episodes.

When any are present, referral to Tier 2/3 Child and Adolescent Mental Health Services (CAMHS) service is appropriate.

First line treatment for mild depressive disorder with symptom duration less than 4 weeks

Supportive therapy and psychoeducation about depressive disorders are effective first line interventions in 30% of children and adolescents with recent onset of mild to moderate depressive symptoms.

Advice should be given on sleep hygiene, nutrition, activity, and exercise.

After 2–3 months if there is no response to supportive management, young people should be referred to Tier 2/3 CAMHS services for more intensive psychological therapy as described for moderate to severe depressive disorders.

Treatment for moderate to severe depressive disorders

The psychological therapies recommended for treating child and adolescent depressive disorders are:
- Cognitive behavioural therapy (CBT)
- Interpersonal therapy.

Families should be involved in a young person's care and treatment unless specifically excluded by the child or young person. Brief family therapy may be effective in some cases.

Recommended practice is that a block of psychological therapy should be undertaken prior to consideration of antidepressant medication.

Response to treatment should be reviewed after 12 weeks

Good response to treatment
- The course of treatment should be completed
- Follow-up should be provided for 12 months after remission of symptoms. If the patient has had one or more previous episode of depression follow up for 2 years is recommended.

Poor or no response to treatment after 12 weeks
- Review assessment, formulation and treatment plan
- Consider co morbid diagnoses
- Review any significant environmental factors
- If a diagnosis of depression remains, consider alternative psychological therapy and or antidepressant medication (📖 p. 258).

Treatment of dysthymia

Children and young people with a chronic sub-clinical version of depression that has persisted for over a year merit a diagnosis of dysthymia, and would also benefit from treatment for depression.

Inpatient care

Admission may be required for:
- Assessment and management of suicide risk
- Assessment and treatment of psychosis
- Physical care when severe depressive disorder is associated with significant self-neglect.

Inpatient care should be provided in an age appropriate setting.

Electroconvulsive therapy (ECT)

ECT is only recommended in life-threatening situations and it is used rarely in this age range. When used, ECT should be administered by a clinician experienced in its administration.

Management 2: pharmacological treatments

Antidepressant medication

Antidepressant medication should be used alongside psychological therapy. It is recommended that antidepressant medication is prescribed by a clinician with significant experience in the treatment of depression in children and adolescents.

Reasons for prescribing:
- If the young person is unable or unwilling to engage in psychological therapy
- If, following a 12-week block of psychological therapy, there is either no response or only a poor response to treatment, then an antidepressant medication is recommended for treatment of depressive disorders in adolescents, and should be considered as a treatment option for children.

If psychological therapy is initially refused, it should continue to be considered as a treatment option. Children and young people will often be more motivated and able to participate in therapy following response to medication.

Prior to prescribing

Elicit symptoms that may later be attributed to side effects including:
- Physical symptoms, such as nausea, vomiting, abdominal pain, sweating, headache, insomnia, tremor, and sexual dysfunction
- Suicidal behaviour and self-harm
- Anxiety or agitation
- Hostility
- Elevated mood, particularly if there is a family history of BPD.

If there is a family history of BPD, patients should be monitored closely for symptoms of elevated mood.

Fluoxetine

Fluoxetine is the drug of choice for treatment of depression in children and adolescents.

Prescribing guidance for fluoxetine
- Starting dose should be 10 mg daily
- Children may respond to 10 mg
- The dose should be increased to 20 mg daily after 1 week if clinically necessary
- There is little evidence regarding the effectiveness of doses higher than 20-mg daily in this age range.

NICE guidelines recommend further increases in older children of higher body weight with severe illness up to adult doses of 60 mg.

If there is no response to treatment with fluoxetine, or it is not tolerated, sertraline or citalopram may be prescribed. There is no evidence that tricyclic antidepressants are of benefit for treatment of depression in this age range.

In psychotic depression consideration should be given to augmenting antidepressant treatment with an atypical antipsychotic.

Monitoring of side effects and response to treatment

Patients should be seen weekly when medication is commenced, and when the dose of medication is changed.

Potential side effects of serotonin reuptake inhibitors (SSRIs) to check for are:

- Suicidal behaviour, self-harm, anxiety, or hostility, and agitation
- Physical side effects, nausea, vomiting, abdominal pain, sweating, headache, insomnia, tremor, and sexual dysfunction
- Rarer side effects include hyponatraemia and bleeding disorders.

Treatment duration

Treatment should be continued for 6 months after symptoms have remitted and normal level of functioning has been achieved. Patients should be followed up for a further 6 months after medication has been discontinued. If the patient has had one or more previous episode of depression, follow up for 2 years is recommended.

Medication should be decreased gradually over a 6-week period to avoid discontinuation syndrome, which presents with flu-like symptoms, insomnia, dizziness, vivid dreams, and irritability.

Legal status of use of antidepressant medication in children and adolescents

There are no antidepressant drugs with a current UK Marketing Authorisation for depression in children and young people (under 18 years). However, both the Committee on Safety of Medicine and NICE guidelines have made specific recommendations on use of antidepressant medication in the under 18 age range.

Committee on Safety of Medicines recommendations

- Fluoxetine in the treatment of major depressive disorder
- Alternative selective serotonin reuptake inhibitors (SSRIs) where drug treatment is indicated, but a patient is intolerant of or has not responded to fluoxetine.

NICE guidelines recommendations

- First line treatment fluoxetine
- Second line treatment sertraline or citalopram.

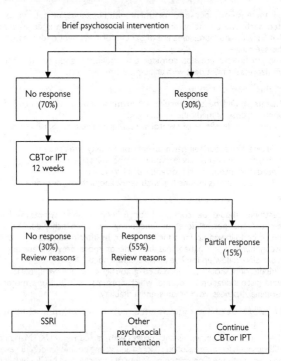

Fig. 17.1 Depression treatment algorithm.

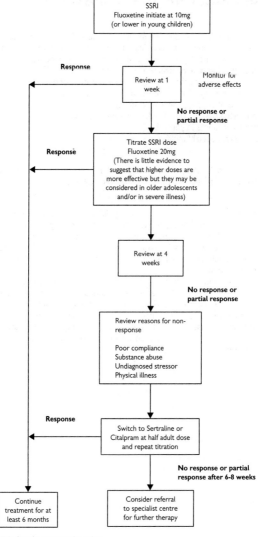

Fig. 17.2 Antidepressant algorithm.

Prognosis, course, and outcomes

Episode duration

In clinically referred samples the median duration of a depressive episode is 7–9 months; in community samples it is about 1–2 months. Approximately 90% of adolescent depressive disorders remit 1–2 years after onset and about 6–10% become protracted.

Maintaining factors that predict a longer duration of episode include:

- Greater severity of initial depression
- Presence of ongoing chronic adversity
- Co-morbid psychiatric disorders, personality disorder
- Psychiatric illness in parents
- Poor psychosocial functioning.

Relapse

Approximately 40–60% of young people with depression experience a relapse after successful acute therapy, either psychological or pharmacological.

Recurrence

Adolescent depression carries a strong risk of recurrence. In both community and clinical samples the recurrence rates for depressive disorders in teenage girls are between 20 and 60% by 1–2 years after remission from the index episode, increasing to 70% after 5 years. Between 40 and 70% of depressed adolescents will experience a recurrence of major depressive disorder in adulthood.

Compared with non-depressed adolescents, depressed adolescents are 2–7 times more likely to be depressed as adults even when controlled for adverse life events, intellectual achievement, and co-morbidity.

Currently, there is no evidence to suggest that childhood depression is linked to an increased risk of depressive disorder in adolescence and adulthood. Further research is required into the long-term prognosis of childhood depression.

One in five people experience depression at some time in their life.

Clinical example

David, a 15-year-old boy, was referred to CAMHS team for assessment by his GP. The referral letter stated that David had a 2-month history of low mood. The GP was concerned about David's suicide risk, as he described intermittent thoughts of self-harm and described not caring if he woke up in the morning.

At assessment, David's main mood symptoms were of low mood with no diurnal variation; he rated his mood as between 3–4/10 currently, with 8/10 being his best level in the previous year and 2/10 being the lowest. He also described poor concentration, difficulty in getting over to sleep with no early morning wakening problems, difficulty in making decisions about simple things, for example, what to wear.

He described himself as being more irritable and argumentative, and described falling out with family members and peers over small things that would not normally bother him. He was falling behind in his school work as he could not concentrate on his work and was not as motivated as previously to complete assignments. He had lost interest in hobbies, in particular sport, and had stopped attending training for his local team.

David described feeling guilty about his lack of effort in school and felt he was letting his parents down.

On reflection David thought things had actually become more difficult for him for 6 months. He described being anxious about his school exams and future career choices. In retrospect, he felt that his anxiety had affected his grades, which made him more concerned about his ability to get the required grades to go to university. He was the youngest of three children, and his parents and siblings had all gone to university.

David described intermittent thoughts that he would be better off dead. He had never made any plans to harm himself. He did sometimes wish he would not wake up in the morning. He felt guilty about these thoughts as he knew that his family and friends would be really upset. He did not like thinking about the future as he became anxious about career choices.

On mental state assessment David presented as being low in mood and anxious. He had no psychotic features, no active suicidal ideation, and good insight into his difficulties.

David's parents were concerned about his mood. They described David as previously being a confident, popular, and academically able boy who had increasingly been withdrawn from all activities that he had previously enjoyed. They were concerned that David was feeling pressured to attend university and wanted him to have a future that would be fulfilling for him. David was surprised by this.

Contact with school confirmed that David was an able pupil who had not been coping with the academic work. They did not feel that David's peer relationships were affected.

David and his parents spent time with the clinical team discussing symptoms of depression and how it affects young people. They were given reading material. David had a course of CBT treatment. This initially focused on helping David to gradually re-engage in pleasurable activities. David and his parents negotiated with school to ensure an achievable academic work load. It was agreed that he would drop two subjects.

In therapy David was able to explore his fears of letting his parents down and his preconceived ideas of what they expected from him. David's mood improved significantly over the 12-week treatment block.

The therapist contracted with David for another four sessions of therapy to address relapse prevention and anxiety management regarding David's forthcoming exams.

David's mood was kept under review by the therapist for a further 6 months. At this point he was discharged as he remained symptom-free during this period.

Recommended reading

Goldberg D. (2006) The aetiology of depression. *Psycholog Med* **36**: 1341–7.

National Institute for Health and Clinical Excellence (2005) Depression in children and young people: identification and management in primary, community and secondary care. Available at: http://www.nice.org.uk/guidance/CG28 (accessed 10 March 2008).

Suicide and deliberate self-harm

Suicide: definition and epidemiology

Definition
- Suicide is the intentional taking of one's own life
- A suicide attempt is an act focused on taking one's own life that is unsuccessful in causing death
- Suicidal thoughts are common; they become abnormal when there is intent and/or plan or when suicide is considered the only option.

Epidemiology
The World Health Organization found that suicide is among the top five causes of mortality in the 15–19-year age range across the world. In many countries it ranks first or second as a cause of death among boys and girls.

Incidence
Completed suicide is uncommon in childhood and early adolescence. The incidence rises in mid to late adolescence, peaking in the mid-twenties age range. While the incidence of completed suicides in males and females in the general population has fallen over the past 30 years, there is evidence that rates of completed suicides have increased in males aged 15–19 years.

Rates for males and females of completed suicide in adolescence have reported at:
- 1–2 per 100,000 age range 10–14 years
- 4–8 per 100,000 age range 15–19 years
- Male:female 3–4:1.

Some fatalities currently attributed to car crash, falling from heights, drowning, or overdose of illegal drugs may actually represent suicides, and the actual figure is likely to be higher.

Gender differences
Suicide is more common in males than in females. This may be related to gender bias in choice of method. Males are more likely to use more potentially lethal methods, hanging, or firearms (particularly in the USA); females are more likely to self-poison.

The availability of certain potentially lethal substances is controlled in many countries. Examples are limiting the number of paracetamol which can be bought at one time, and regulations for sale and storage of pesticides such as paraquat. Countries without such legislation have an increased mortality rate from overdose.

Family history
People who commit suicide are 2–4 times more likely to have had a first degree relative who committed suicide.

Co-morbidity

Mental illnesses are common in completed suicide. These include:

- Mood disorder
- Alcohol and substance abuse
- Anxiety disorder
- Conduct disorder (CD) or oppositional defiant disorder (ODD)
- Chronic physical illness.

The prevalence of psychiatric illness in people who commit suicide is estimated by the World Health Organization as between 80–100% across age range.

Youth suicide is a major global public health issue. While suicide rates are higher among 20–24-year-olds, the suicidal behaviours that precede the suicide are often established earlier in life. Suicide consistently ranks as one of the leading causes of death for adolescents between 15 and 19 years of age. Suicide accounts for 30% of deaths in the 15–24-year age group. There has been an increase in suicide mortality and morbidity over most of the 20th century among white adolescents in the USA and Europe.

Deliberate self-harm

Definitions and epidemiology

Definition

An act with a non-fatal outcome in which an individual deliberately does one or more of the following:

- Initiates a behaviour (e.g. self-cutting, jumping from a height), which they intended to cause harm to the self
- Ingests a substance in excess of the prescribed or generally recognized therapeutic dose
- Ingests a recreational or illicit drug (which they intended to cause harm to the self)
- Ingests a non-ingestible substance or object (e.g. batteries, razor blades).

Epidemiology

Suicidal thoughts and behaviours peak between the ages of 14 and 18 years.

Rates of deliberate self-harm have been difficult to assess accurately, and it is estimated that only 50% of adolescents present to hospital after taking an overdose. Significantly fewer young people who self-harm in other ways present to hospital.

A school survey by Hawton et al. (2002) found that:

- 6.9% of a school population aged 15–16 years had engaged in an act of deliberate self-harm in the previous year
- 10.3% had engaged in an act of deliberate self-harm in their lifetime
- 10% repeat the act of self-harm within a 1-year period
- Actual self-harm was more common in females with a female to male ratio of reported self-harm in previous year of 4:1 (11.2% girls 3.2% boy)
- Thoughts of self-harm were also more common in females, with a female to male ratio of 2.6:1 (22.4% girls 8.5% boys).

The World Health Organization estimates that as many as 50% of adolescents experience suicidal ideation at some point in adolescence.

Aetiology

Family history

The incidence of deliberate self-harm in adolescence is increased when there is a family history of deliberate self-harm. This is likely to be due to a combination of environmental and genetic factors.

Influence of others

Self-harm in friends and witnessing episodes of self-harm through the media increase risk of self-harm behaviour, suggesting that there may be an element of learned behaviour.

Biological

Trauma has been shown to cause damage to neurological pathways in the brain that are responsible for release of endorphins in response to stress and emotional arousal. It is known that self-harm by cutting causes release of endorphins. This may, in turn, play a compensatory role in regulating emotional responses to stress in individuals where these pathways have been damaged by previous traumatic experiences.

Abnormalities of serotonin level in the central nervous system (CNS) have also been recorded in adults who self-harm. The findings were present when the likely effects of co-morbid psychiatric disorder were controlled for. The functional significance of these findings is not clear.

Psychosocial factors

Several environmental factors have been demonstrated to increase the risk of deliberate self-harm. These include:

Early adversity
- Poor care and/or neglect
- Physical, emotional and sexual abuse
- Parental separation, divorce or family discord.

Individual factors
- Low self-esteem
- Lack of emotional support
- Poor social and inter personal skills
- Conflicting peer relationships
- Bullying
- Identity problems
- Confusion related to sexual orientation
- Females, poor body image
- Lack of academic performance
- Antisocial behaviour, in particular aggressive impulsive behaviour
- Alcohol and substance abuse.

Family factors
- Family inadequate or excessive authority
- High or low family expectation
- Parental mental health problems and alcohol or substance misuse.

Socioeconomic factors

Deliberate self-harm is reported to occur equally frequently across all socioeconomic groups in adolescence. This is in contrast to the adult population where higher rates occur in lower socioeconomic groups.

Assessment, differential diagnosis, and co-morbidity

Assessment

In addition to those cases where a disclosure of self-harm has been made, the possibility that a child or adolescent has self-harmed should be considered when they present with:
- Unexplained medical symptoms
- Acute confusional state
- Acute onset of hallucinations, particularly visual hallucinations
- Injuries that could have been the result of self-harm.

Physical assessment

Initial assessment of a child or adolescent who has, or is thought to have, self-harmed should identify:
- Injuries from self-harm
- Likely/potential effects of ingestion of substance
- The child/young person's capacity to consent to or refuse treatment
- Presence or absence of mental illness
- Risk of further episode of self-harm.
- Appropriate medical treatment should be provided.

Psychiatric assessment

A separate interview should be conducted with the child or adolescent. Issues addressed will include:

History of act of self-harm
- Circumstances leading up to self-harming behaviour
- Degree of suicidal intent at time of deliberate self-harm
- Intensity, frequency, and duration of self-harm thoughts
- Behaviour at time of overdose/self-harm
- Impulsivity or planned nature of the self-harm episode
- Help seeking or help avoiding behaviour
- Ongoing plans for further self-harm or suicide
- Previous history of self-harming behaviours.

Current level of functioning
- Psychosocial functioning
- Peer relationships
- History of bullying
- Education ability and attainment.
- Evidence of other risk taking behaviour
- Drug and alcohol abuse.
- Conduct problems.
- Early adversity
- Significant life events including trauma, abuse and bullying.

A full mental state assessment should be completed.

Clinical interview with the parents which will include:
- A corroborative history of events surrounding self-harm episode
- An exploration of parental response to the episode of self-harm
- An assessment of current family functioning and available support for the child or adolescent
- Identification of a history or symptoms suggestive of an underlying psychiatric disorder.

Differential diagnosis

Consider if the harm could have been caused by someone else.

Co-morbid disorders

There are several disorders commonly associated with increased rates of self-harm:
- Mood disorder
- Alcohol and substance abuse
- Anxiety disorder
- CD or ODD
- Physical health problems.

Clinical example

Amy is a 12-year-old girl who was admitted to paediatrics after she had taken an overdose of 6 paracetamol tablets. She had taken the tablets following an argument with her mum. The argument started when mum refused Amy's request to spend her birthday weekend with her dad and his new partner. Amy described being angry with her mum and storming up to her room. She saw the paracetamol tablets on her dressing table and started taking them. They were in her room as she suffered inter-mittently from headaches and taking paracetamol helped.

She remembered briefly thinking that she had had enough of the argu-ments and she would be better off dead. When she calmed down she was worried about what she had done. She did not want to tell her mum as she thought she would be angry. Instead Amy phoned her older sister who was able to get Amy to tell mum. Mum then called an ambulance.

At assessment Amy described regretting taking the overdose and being embarrassed about the trouble she had caused. She was thoughtful about how upset her mum, dad, and sister were. She had no previous history of self-harm and was adamant that she would not do anything else to harm herself having seen the upset she had caused.

Amy's psychiatric assessment did not identify any underlying psychi-atric disorder.

When Amy was asked about mum getting angry, Amy said that since her dad had left 6 months previously her mum was angry a lot of the time. When mum got really angry Amy got scared. Amy was scared because sometimes mum would slap her across the face. On one occasions Amy's face was bruised and Amy had not gone to school for a week in case anyone asked her what had happened. Amy said that she was worried about her mum; since dad left she thought she was sad.

Amy had always had a good relationship with her dad and wanted to spend more time with him. Amy found it difficult when her mum was angry with her dad and when her dad was rude about her mum.

Amy's parents were upset about the overdose and wanted to know how to help Amy. They were aware that she had been very upset when they separated. Amy was able to tell them how sad she was about how they were behaving towards each other and that she felt stuck in the middle.

Amy's mum was seen separately to explore the incident when Amy was hit by mum and Amy's concern about Mum being sad.

Mum said that she had not been coping since dad left. She was worried about money. She felt her mood was low and that she was not coping. She had meant to see her GP, but was worried about what would happen to Amy if he knew she had hit her. She was afraid Amy would be taken away and sent to live with her dad.

At this point it was clear that there were ongoing child protection concerns. Referral to social work was discussed with Amy and her parents. All were in agreement with this. Amy's mum said that she knew she needed help, but did not know where to start.

Amy was seen for follow-up by the self-harm team.

Amy's parents engaged with social work to ensure Amy's needs were met.

Parents agreed to attend family mediation to find ways of working together to help Amy. Mum received treatment for depression. She was also getting advice on her financial circumstances

Social work arranged a child protection case conference. At the meeting it was decided not to put Amy's name on the child protection register as there was an appropriate plan in place to meet her needs and she was not thought to be at significant risk.

Management

Initial intervention should be to treat physical effects of the self-harm episode and to arrange a mental health assessment.

Emergency psychiatric assessment should be arranged for children and adolescents who have:
- Taken an overdose
- Ongoing suicidal ideation or risk of significant self-harm
- Significant symptoms of mental illness, which contributed to an act of self-harm.

Initial risk management

Following risk assessment it is important to make sure that appropriate levels of supervision are in place.
- Consider access to medication and other means of self-harm
- If there are significant concerns re young person's ongoing suicide risk, consider admission to an inpatient unit
- If there are concerns about child protection and or care issues a referral should be made to social work.

Co-morbid psychiatric disorder should be managed as outlined in relevant chapters.

Management options for deliberate self-harm

Treatment may be provided on an individual or group basis. Aims of intervention are to:
- Address self-esteem issues
- Improve interpersonal skills and address relationship difficulties
- Improve communication skills
- Learn more helpful ways to communicate emotions.

Family work

This may include family support and counselling. More structured and intensive family therapy may be appropriate where family functioning is a contributing factor.

School-based interventions include:

- Entire school programmes focusing on self-esteem peer relationships
- Peer support programmes
- Development and implementation of anti-bullying policies in school.

Prognosis, course, and outcome

Suicidal ideation or a suicide attempt in adolescence is associated with:
- An increased risk of subsequent self-harm or suicide attempts
- Ongoing problems with depression, anxiety disorders, and substance misuse.

The risk of ongoing mental health problems is higher in young people who have actually self-harmed than those who have had thoughts of self-harm, but not acted on them.

Some of the increased risk for mental health problems can be accounted for by the shared risk factors for deliberate self-harm and mental health problems.

Recommended reading

Hawton, K., Rodham, K., Evans, E., et al. (2006) By *Their Own Young Hand, Deliberate Self-harm in Children and Adolescents.* Jessica Kingsley Publishers, London.

Hawton, K., Rodham, K., Evans, E., Weatherall, R., et al. (2002) Deliberate self-harm in adolescents: self report survey in schools in England. *Br Med J* **325**: 1207–11.

National Institute of Clinical Excellence Guideline (2004) *Self-harm: The short-term physical and psychological management and secondary prevention of self-harm in primary and secondary care.* Available at: http://www.nice.org.uk/guidance/CG16 (accessed 24 March 2008).

Anxiety disorders

Definition, epidemiology, aetiology, differential diagnosis, and co-morbidity

Definition

The general term 'anxiety disorder' covers a number of disorders where excessive fear and worry, triggered by internal or external events, interferes with normal daily activity, and leads to impairment of functioning. Anxiety disorders tend to be associated with a specific cognitive processing style in which the person:

- Over-estimates risk
- Under-estimates their own personal coping skills
- Under-estimates the availability of helpful interventions from others. Several anxiety disorders will be discussed in greater detail:
- Generalized anxiety disorders:
  - General anxiety disorder
  - Panic disorder
- Situational anxiety disorders:
  - Separation anxiety
  - School refusal
  - Social anxiety
  - Selective mutism
  - Specific phobias.

Epidemiology

Prevalence of all anxiety disorders in children and adolescents is 5–10%. Male: female ratio is equal in childhood; prevalence increases in girls after adolescence from when the female to male ratio is around 2:1. This gender imbalance is particularly significant for specific phobia, panic disorder, agoraphobia, and separation anxiety disorder.

Aetiology

Genetic factors

Twin studies have demonstrated that genetic factors play a significant role in the development of anxiety disorders with heritability estimated at approximately 30%.

Several parent– child interactional styles are associated with increased rates of anxiety disorders

- Insecure attachment is linked with low level of confidence in a child's ability to cope with threat, and confidence that others will be able to provide necessary support and help
- Over-controlling maternal behaviours and the use of a critical behavioural management style have both been linked with an increase in anxiety disorders in the child. This may be mediated by the tendency of such styles of parenting to limit a child's opportunities and willingness to explore their environment with a subsequent lack of opportunity to develop confidence in their own abilities and coping skills
- Lack of reassurance and support from parent to child.

Parental anxiety disorder

- Anxious behaviours may be learnt from behaviours that have been modelled by parents, who are themselves suffering from an anxiety disorder
- Parental anxiety can also increase or reinforce a child's or adolescent's anxieties or avoidant behaviour.

Differential diagnosis

Psychiatric disorders

- Disorders secondary to life events or stressors:
  - Adjustment disorders
  - Acute stress reaction
  - Post-traumatic stress disorder (PTSD).
- Obsessive compulsive disorder (OCD)
- Depression
- Psychosis.

Physical disorders

- Hypothyroidism
- Prescribed and non-prescribed drugs
- Hypoparathyroidism
- Caffeine
- Migraine
- Asthma.

Co-morbid disorders

Co-morbidity with other anxiety disorders is common; 60% of children and adolescents diagnosed with an anxiety disorder will meet diagnostic criteria for at least one other anxiety disorder, in Generalized Anxiety Disorder this increases to 90%.

Children and adolescents with a mood disorder often also have a coexisting anxiety disorder. It is less common for children and adolescents with an anxiety disorder to develop a mood disorder.

Co-morbidity also occurs with other psychiatric disorders including:

- OCD
- Oppositional defiant disorder (ODD) and conduct disorders (CD)
- Attention deficit hyperactivity disorder (ADHD)
- Drug and alcohol abuse.

General prognosis of anxiety disorders

Anxiety disorders in childhood are likely to remit, but there is an increased likelihood of developing a subsequent anxiety disorder. The more disabling disorders are thought to be associated with a higher risk of recurrence. Overall, anxiety disorders in childhood and adolescence are associated with a significantly increased risk of anxiety, depression, or substance misuse in adulthood. 50% of adults with depression will have had an anxiety disorder in adolescence.

General management principles both psychological and pharmacological

A general care pathway is described in Fig. 19.1.

Psychological treatment

Cognitive behavioural therapy (CBT)

CBT is the treatment of choice for anxiety disorders. It can be delivered in several ways as either individual or group programmes. Treatment programmes should, however, all contain several specific components:
- Psychoeducation about anxiety
- Techniques to improve symptom control such as relaxation techniques
- Cognitive restructuring
- Exposure to anxiety provoking situations or events
- Social skills training
- Relapse prevention.

Parental involvement in therapy

Clinical experience suggests that involving parents in treatment programme for anxious children should be beneficial; the evidence, however, is conflicting. It is currently considered good practice to involve parents in the treatment process. Group therapy can be used to deliver programmes to children or adolescents, and their parents.

Pharmacological

Medication is usually reserved for when there is either no response or only an incomplete response to psychological therapy, or for situations where the child or adolescent is either unable or unwilling to participate in a psychological therapy. The selective serotonin reuptake inhibitors (SSRIs) have been shown to have short-term benefit in the treatment of anxiety disorders, including selective mutism, in children and adolescents. A systematic review of current studies suggests good efficacy with a number needed to treat (NNT)* of 3 for adolescents and 4 for children (compared with a NNT for SSRIs in adolescent depression of 8). Research does not currently suggest superiority for any particular SSRIs; longer-term outcome studies are required. The prescribing guidelines for SSRIs described in the chapter on depression should be followed. There is no strong evidence to support use of other anxiolytics in children or adolescents. The use of benzodiazapines are not recommended and may cause irritability and behavioural dysregulation and disinhibition.

---

* Number needed to treat is an estimate of the number of patients that would need to be treated for one genuine response to treatment (smaller the number the better the treatment).

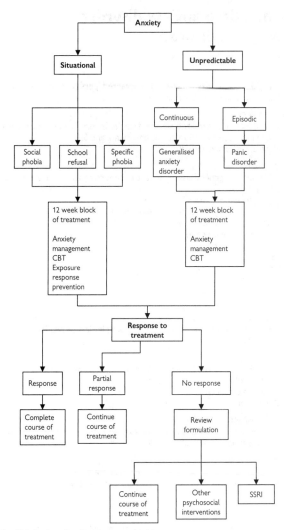

Fig. 19.1 Anxiety disorder treatment algorithm.

Generalized anxiety disorder and panic disorder

Generalized anxiety disorder

Definition

The key feature is anxiety, which is generalized, persistent, impairing, and not specific to any particular circumstance.

Epidemiology

The incidence of generalized anxiety disorder is very low in children; incidence in adolescents is reported as between 2 and 5%.

Mean age of onset 16 years.

Assessment

In addition to a general assessment it is important to explore common themes for anxiety:

- Threat to self or others
- Fears of sleeping away from home or alone
- Fears being alone at home
- Events that will cause separation
- Performance anxiety
- Fear of failure
- Quality of relationships
- School work
- Worries about appearance.

It is also important to assess:

- Social and problem-solving skills
- Somatic symptoms, including the ruling out physical causes for symptoms.

Co-morbidity

- About 90% of those with generalized anxiety disorder also have evidence of another anxiety disorder
- School reluctance/refusal
- Depression.

Specific aspects of treatment

CBT does not usually need to include exposure work, as avoidance is not usually a feature of generalized anxiety disorder.

Outcome

Generalized anxiety disorder often persists into adulthood. This is, in part, due to the high incidence of co-morbid anxiety disorders.

Panic disorder

Definition

Recurrent attacks of severe unpredictable anxiety (panic attacks). This anxiety is accompanied by physical symptoms:

- Increased heart rate
- Shortness of breath
- Choking sensation

- Sweating
- Depersonalization
- Derealization.

There is often a feeling of impending doom and worry that the sufferer is about to die. Panic attacks may subsequently become associated with places or events, and therefore become associated with anticipatory anxiety.

Epidemiology

- Incidence of panic disorder in children and adolescents is between 0.5 and 5%
- Onset is most frequent in late adolescence
- More common in girls than in boys.

Assessment

In addition to a general assessment a careful history of physical symptoms and a physical examination to rule out physical illness.

Co-morbidity

Panic attacks may occur in combination with all other anxiety disorders.

Differential diagnosis

Physical illness.

Specific aspects of treatment

- Exposure work may be appropriate if panic attacks become related to specific places or events
- Cognitive techniques, such as self-monitoring of anxiety/panic symptoms, cognitive restructuring to correct catastrophic misinterpretations of bodily sensations
- SSRIs or tricyclic antidepressants may result in a transient increase in anxiety prior to a reduction.

Outcome

Panic attacks in adolescence are associated with an increased incidence of anxiety disorders in adulthood.

Separation anxiety and school refusal

Separation anxiety

Definition

Fear of separation from attachment figure that interferes with daily activities and developmental tasks. Onset prior to age 18 years.

Epidemiology
- Incidence of separation anxiety is 3–5%
- Onset commonly occurs pre-adolescence
- More common in girls.

Assessment

In addition to a general assessment common worries should be explored including:
- Worries about own or others' health and/or safety
- Fears of abandonment by parent or carer
- Worries about potential traumatic events leading to loss or separation.

An assessment of temperamental style, and of social skills and problem solving skills is also important.

Co-morbidity

Separation anxiety disorder is associated with social phobia and general anxiety disorder in approximately 60% of cases. Many children display oppositional and defiant behaviours on separation.

Differential diagnosis
- Other anxiety disorders
- Mood disorder.

Specific aspects of treatment
- Parents of younger children may benefit from parental strategy training to manage oppositional behaviour associated with anxiety
- There is some evidence that systemic family therapy, alongside an anxiety management programme, is beneficial in older children and adolescents.

Outcome

Significant separation anxiety disorders are associated with further episodes of anxiety disorders in adolescence and adulthood.

School refusal

Definition
- A persistent refusal to attend school associated with anxiety
- May initially present with somatic symptoms.

Epidemiology
- Incidence in children and adolescents reported as 1–5%
- School refusal is a common problem for children with separation anxiety disorder and/or social phobia
- School refusal occurs more frequently at transition points, such as starting primary or secondary school. It is also more frequent after breaks from school, such as holidays or illness. Parents are more likely to be able to ensure school attendance of children than adolescents.

Assessment

In addition to a general assessment it is important to assess:
- Common worries in children and adolescents with school refusal:
  - Fear of leaving home
  - Being bullied
- Social skills and problem solving skills
- Temperament
- Somatic symptoms and physical causes for somatic symptoms
- Parental management techniques (in particular those relating to the refusal to attend school).

Co-morbidity

Anxiety disorders particularly:
- Separation anxiety disorder
- Social phobia
- Specific phobia, for example, public transport
- ODD.

Differential diagnosis

- Non-attendance at school due to truanting
- Parental physical or mental illness requiring the young person to be at home to provide care or support.

Specific aspects of treatment

- Liaison with school and early reintegration where possible
- Address any bullying issues
- Social skills programmes
- The use of circle time to promote classroom integration and support.

Outcome

- 70% will successfully reintegrate into school, but a significant minority will not
- Social anxiety and communication problems may persist.

Social anxiety disorder and selective mutism

Social anxiety disorder (sometimes called social phobia)

Definition
Significant anxiety in social situations despite a desire for social interaction. This anxiety impairs functioning in most settings.

Epidemiology
- Incidence 1–2% in children and adolescents
- Social anxiety disorder occurs in childhood and adolescence
- More common in girls than in boys.

Assessment
In additional to a general assessment it is important to assess:
- Common worries about being:
  - Scrutinized
  - Ridiculed
  - Humiliated
  - Embarrassed
  - Inadequate in social skills and interactions.
- Avoided activities such as:
  - Asking for something in shop or restaurant
  - Speaking in school
  - Eating in public
  - Attending social events.

Co-morbidity
- Other anxiety disorders
- Depression.

Differential diagnosis
- Autism or other pervasive developmental disorders
- Mood disorder.

Specific aspects of treatment
- CBT including anxiety management and exposure work.
- Social skills training.

Outcome
An earlier age of onset is associated with a poorer prognosis.

Selective mutism

Definition
Children demonstrate normal language skills in some situations, but fail to speak in others. Typically, the child speaks with familiar people in familiar surroundings, e.g. at home, but fails to speak at school or with strangers.

Epidemiology
- Incidence reported as around 0.4 in 1000
- Onset is in pre-school years, although it is often not identified until starting school
- It is thought to be more common in girls.

Assessment
In additional to a general assessment it is important to exclude autism, or other pervasive developmental disorder and to assess:
- Temperament: children often socially anxious or withdrawn
- Formal speech and language assessment, using tapes if necessary
- Developmental assessment
- Parental management
- Social communication skills
- Psychosocial development
- Assessment can include observation of video material of the child's patterns of communication in situations where they are perceived as communicating normally.

Specific worries associated with selective mutism have been difficult to define due to lack of verbal communication; it is proposed that one fear may be that of a stranger hearing one's voice. Worries associated with social anxiety disorder may also be present.

Co-morbidity
Anxiety disorders
- Separation anxiety
- Social phobia
- ODD.

Differential diagnosis
- Autism or other pervasive developmental disorder
- Specific developmental disorders of speech and language
- Psychosis.

Specific aspects of treatment
- A behavioural approach with positive reinforcement techniques aimed at increasing the frequency of talking and decreasing the frequency of non-communication
- General anxiety management techniques.

Outcome
- Most children will become able to communicate more widely, but persistence of social anxiety and or phobia is common
- Children may also develop other anxiety disorders in later life.

Specific phobias

Definition

Phobic disorder is defined as a marked unreasonable fear of a specific object or situation that occurs every time it is encountered. Such an encounter evokes clinically significant distress, or affects normal activity by avoidance of feared situation or object.

Epidemiology
- Incidence is estimated at around 5%
- Phobias are more common in girls
- Onset is common in childhood.

Assessment

In additional to a general assessment it is important to assess for:
- Common phobias
  - Animals
  - Environment, e.g. water, thunderstorms, darkness
  - Medical or dental treatment
  - Situations involving height, e.g. bridges, flying, lifts, transport
- Difficulties with social skills and problem solving skills
- Temperamental predisposition
- Family history of phobias.

Co-morbidity
Other anxiety disorders.

Differential diagnosis
- Psychosis
- PTSD.

Specific aspects of treatment
- Exposure is essential
- Anxiety management is essential prior to exposure work
- Imaginal exposure can be used with adolescents.

Outcome

Phobias are, in general, the anxiety disorder that respond best to treatment and have a fairly good prognosis.

Clinical examples

Example 1

Adam is a 4-year-old only child who has just started pre-school nursery. His mother has been taking him for 1 week and is extremely concerned about how upset he becomes when she tries to leave and the fact that he was not playing with the other children.

He lives with his mum, dad and two younger brothers. Mum reports to staff that he is normally a happy boy who gets on well with his cousins who are around the same age and live near by. Mum does not work and Adam is used to her being with him all the time.

He has not been to mother and toddlers group, or play group.

All health assessments by GP and health visitor indicated that he was developing normally and was securely attached to his parents.

It felt that Adam was slow to adapt to the change in his environment, which was very different to his previous experience.

Following discussion with mum, it was agreed that Adam's mum would spend time in the nursery with Adam until he was settled. With mum present Adam engaged in activities—tentatively at first returning to mum regularly for reassurance. After 1 week he was playing happily and confidently in the nursery. It was then agreed that mum would decrease the time gradually that she spent with Adam in nursery, initially, by ensuring that Adam was settled and waiting in the staff room in case she was needed. As she was not needed at any point for the following week she then was able to ensure that Adam was settled and leave.

After 4 weeks Adam was able to go into nursery with minimal support from mum.

Example 2

Sinead is a 14-year-old girl who has a phobia of spiders. This has become problematic as she would like to go camping with her friends, but is too afraid of a spider getting into her sleeping bag to do this. She feels she is missing out on fun and wants to do something about this.

Sinead was referred for CBT, she was motivated to address her fears and engaged well in therapy.

Therapy consisted of relaxation techniques, and exploring the basis of her thoughts and fears about spiders. Subsequently, Sinead agreed to an exposure response prevention programme. Exposure was to pictures of spiders, then a spider in a covered jar, the therapist holding a spider, then Sinead holding a spider. Once Sinead was able to tolerate holding a spider she was encouraged to practice exposing herself to spiders outwith sessions to maintain her ability to be around spiders and not experience fear.

Sinead confessed to still being afraid of poisonous spiders, but she was aware that she was unlikely to encounter a poisonous spider in the UK.

She thought she may need further sessions if she ever wanted to go to Australia where spiders are dangerous, but that she had achieved what she wanted at this time, which was to go camping with her friends.

Example 3

Katie is an 11-year-old girl who is unhappy at school, since her best and only friend changed school 1 month ago. Her GP was concerned that she may be becoming depressed and referred her for assessment.

Assessment highlighted that she had longstanding social anxiety, which had increased significantly since her friend left school, she was sad at times, but not depressed.

Treatment options of individual or group therapy were discussed with Katie and her parents. Katie was initially very anxious about attending a group, but thought it would be helpful to talk to others with the same problems. The therapist also felt that Katie would benefit from group treatment, but might struggle with getting started in the group. It was, therefore, agreed that Katie would benefit from 4 individual sessions prior to the group to help her manage her anxiety about attending.

Katie's difficulties were discussed with her class teacher who was aware of Katie's isolation, since her friend had left. The class were about to start a new project and the teacher was organizing the groups thoughtfully so that Katie would be in a supportive peer group. She would also encourage Katie to attend structured supervised groups at lunchtime so she could practice what she was learning in group therapy.

Katie responded well to therapy and her anxiety decreased significantly. She was able to form new friendships at school and was more confident. She was discharged from therapy and was made aware that if anxiety was causing her problems in future that coming back for some more sessions would be a good option.

Recommended reading

AACAP Official Action (2007) Practice parameters for assessment and treatment of children and adolescents with anxiety disorders. *J Am Acad Child Adoles Psychiat* **46:** 2.

Rutter M, Kim-Cohen J, Maughan B, *et al.* (2006) Continuities and discontinuities in psychopathology between childhood and adult life. *J Child Psychiat Psychol* **47**(3–4): 276–95.

Obsessive compulsive disorder

Definitions and epidemiology

Classification

Definition of obsessions

Obsessions are recurrent persistent thoughts, images, or impulses that are distressing, time-consuming, and functionally impairing. Young people recognize these thoughts as their own, and perceive them as unhelpful and at times senseless.

Definition of compulsions

Compulsions are mental or physical behaviours that are completed in an attempt to neutralize anxiety caused by the obsessional thoughts or images.

ICD-10 classification: requires obsessional symptoms or compulsive acts, or both, to be present on most days for at least 2 successive weeks, and be a source of distress or interference with activities.

DSM-IV classification: requires the presence of obsessions or compulsions unrelated to another axis 1 diagnosis. Symptoms must be distressing, time-consuming (more than 1 h/day), and must interfere with activities or relationships. The person must recognize that the obsessions are excessive and unreasonable.

Diagnostic issues in children

Rituals and habits are present in 2/3 pre-school children. They are similar in form and content to compulsions in obsessive compulsive disorder (OCD), but:
- Are less frequent and intense
- Do not impact on functioning
- Do not cause distress.

Children are not required to have insight into the nature of their thoughts to meet the criteria for a diagnosis of OCD.

Epidemiology

Prevalence of OCD in children and adolescents is estimated as 0.5%. This is lower than in the general population where estimates of prevalence vary between 1 and 3%.

30–50% of adults who have been diagnosed with OCD will have had symptoms before age 18 years.

A prepubertal onset is more common:
- In boys
- In the presence of a family history of OCD or Tourette Syndrome.

Childhood onset OCD has a ratio of 2 boys to every girl, whereas an onset of OCD post-pubertal is more common in girls.

As a consequence the ratio of males to females with OCD equalizes in adolescence, and remains equally into adulthood.

Aetiology

The risk of developing OCD is associated with genetic and biological vulnerability, and the influence of external stressful stimuli.

Genetic component

A hereditary component has been demonstrated in family and twin studies. Ongoing research is addressing a possible overlapping genetic link with tic disorders.

Pathophysiology

Serotonin hypothesis

Serotonin transporter or re-uptake deficits have been demonstrated in the basal ganglia-cortex circuits in people suffering from OCD. This is supported by the response of OCD symptoms to treatment with the serotonin reuptake inhibitors (SSRIs) and clomipramine.

Brain infection or injury

- OCD can occur following meningitis or encephalitis
- Head trauma associated with basal ganglia damage can also result in OCD.

Autoimmune disorders

Post-streptococcal autoimmunity paediatric autoimmune neuropsychiatric disorders (PANDAS)

OCD and tic disorder can develop after group A ß-haemolytic streptococcal infection. This is associated with autoimmune damage to the basal ganglia. (also Tics and Tourette's, 📖 Chapter 13, p. 191).

Neuropsychological and neuroimaging evidence of basal ganglia dysfunction has been demonstrated in PANDAS and Sydenham's chorea. 75% of children and young people with Sydenham's chorea also have OCD symptoms.

Environmental influences

Stress or trauma preceding onset of OCD symptoms is present in 1/3 cases. High expressed emotion may exacerbate symptoms. Family pathology, however, has been shown to be neither necessary nor sufficient to explain the onset of OCD.

Assessment, differential diagnosis, and co-morbidity

Assessment

Detailed history of current and past obsessions and compulsions, including information on:

- Frequency, intensity duration of obsessions and compulsions
- The response of others to obsessions and compulsions
- Their impact on functioning
- The presence of suicidal thoughts and self-harm
- Recent stressful or traumatic events
- Premorbid temperament, including perfectionist traits
- An assessment for co-morbid disorders is essential
- Past medical history
- Family history and family functioning.

Rating Scales may be used to complement the assessment, e.g. Children's Yale-Brown Obsessive Compulsive Scale (CY-BOCS).

Common themes for obsessions in children and adolescents

- Contamination and dirt
- Infections, illness, and death
- Causing or having caused harm or danger to self or others
- Something dreadful happening
- Sexual thoughts
- Religion
- Obsessional slowness.

Common behaviours for compulsions

- Checking
- Washing
- Counting
- Repeating activity
- Arranging objects
- Seeking reassurance
- Content and behaviour.

Co-morbidity

- Anxiety disorders
- Depression
- Tic disorders
- Learning difficulties
- Body dysmorphic disorder
- Trichotillomania.

Differential diagnosis

- Normal developmentally appropriate rituals
- Tourette's syndrome/tic disorder
- PANDAS
- Sydenham's chorea
- Trichotillomania
- Autistic spectrum disorders
- Neurological damage
- Dermatological problems.

Clinical example

Emily is a 14-year-old girl who presented to her GP with concerns that she had contracted bird flu after visiting a nature reserve. When this was explored further it was apparent that she was constantly worried about being in contact with germs or viruses, becoming unwell and dying. She had developed compulsive hand-washing behaviour. The thoughts and behaviours were significantly impairing. She was unable to complete school work and her grades had fallen significantly.

She was able to identify that the death of her grandmother from pneumonia 3 months previously occurred at the time she started to become concerned about her health.

Initially she thought 'if I touch something that someone who is unwell has touched, I will become ill and die'. In response to these thoughts she had instituted a regime of hand washing, which involved washing her hands with soap three times or if unable to wash her hands cleaning them three times with disinfectant wipes. This initially reassured her and allowed her to continue with her daily activities.

Over the following 3 months the frequency of the thoughts increased, and she was washing or disinfecting her hands more frequently. She also gradually increased the number of times she was washing her hands on each occasion, and was now washing her hands or using wipes ten to twelve times.

She was aware that her thoughts were irrational and was afraid she was going insane. She was too embarrassed to tell anyone, but was finding it harder to keep her hand-washing a secret. Emily agreed to be seen with her mother for assessment. Emily was assessed as suffering from OCD with no co-morbidity. Emily and her mum received two sessions of psychoeducation about OCD and treatment approaches.

Emily attended 12 sessions of cognitive behavioural therapy (CBT) in which she was able to explore her thoughts about her grandmother's death. She learned cognitive techniques to challenge her obsessional thoughts.

She responded well to a response prevention intervention programme to decrease her hand washing. Having gained an understanding of OCD, Emily's mum was able to support her in this.

On completion of treatment Emily had occasional intrusive thoughts about illness. She was able to challenge these thoughts and did not need to wash her hands in response to them.

Management: psychological

Psychoeducation

Age and developmentally appropriate psychoeducation regarding both the psychological and biological perspectives of OCD is an essential component of treatment for all children and young people. Parents or carers should be included in this (with the young person's consent) to facilitate treatment and to prevent inappropriate symptom maintaining behaviours.

Guided self-help

Guided self-help works on the principle that understanding the thought process and behaviours associated with OCD promotes change.

Key themes
- Performing rituals, compulsions, and reassurance decrease anxiety only in the short term
- Completing compulsions strengthens the belief that the compulsive actions stop bad things from happening and increases the need to respond to obsessions with compulsive behaviour
- Guided self-help therefore encourages young people to resist performing compulsions, but not thinking obsessional thoughts.

Where the young person is unwilling or unable to use guided self-help, treatment outlined for moderate to severe symptomatology should be used.

Family based interventions

Parents or carers should be included in all aspects of treatment (with the young person's consent where appropriate) as this encourages and facilitates them in helping the young person combat their OCD symptoms, and helps avoid inappropriate reinforcing and/or maintaining behaviours.

Management of moderate to severe OCD in children and young people

Cognitive behaviour therapy (usually conducted in a 12-week block of weekly therapy).

Key targets/strategies
- Challenging false beliefs, the reality of obsessions, and the need for performing compulsions
- Exposure and response prevention
- Anxiety management with relaxation techniques.

Day patient admission may be required to allow for more intensive sessions. Admission to an inpatient facility may occasionally be required if there is a significant risk of suicide.

Management: pharmacological

Reasons for prescribing

- If the young person is unable or unwilling to engage in psychological therapy
- If there is no or poor response to treatment following a 12-week block of psychological therapy.

If psychological therapy is initially refused, it should remain a treatment option as children and young people may be more motivated and able to participate in therapy following a response to medication.

Prior to prescribing

Check for:
- History of unipolar or bipolar depression in parents and grandparents
- Symptoms correlating to side effect profile of recommended antidepressant, which may include:
  - Physical symptoms, such as nausea, vomiting, abdominal pain, sweating, headache, insomnia, tremor, and sexual dysfunction
  - Suicidal behaviour and self-harm
  - Hostility.

Recommended medication for OCD (NICE guidelines).

- Fluvoxamine and sertraline are licenced for treatment of OCD in children and adolescents, and should be prescribed as per BNF guidelines
- Fluoxetine is recommended for OCD in young people with significant co-morbid depression
- Clomipramine may be used as an alternative when SSRIs are not tolerated or there is no therapeutic response. Electrocardiogram (ECG) should be carried out prior to commencing treatment
- Neuroleptic medication may be used for co-morbid tic disorder.

Monitoring of side effects and response to treatment

- Time for OCD symptoms to respond to SSRI's is up to 12 weeks. Depressive symptoms improve more quickly
- Patients should be seen weekly at the beginning of treatment and when the dose of medication is changed
- Potential side effects to check for are suicidal behaviour, self-harm, or hostility, and physical symptoms as described above.

Duration of treatment

Antidepressant medication should be continued for 6 months after symptoms are not clinically significant and the young person has been fully functional for 12 weeks. Review for 12 months following completion of treatment. Symptoms may return after medication is stopped. If there is an increase in obsessive compulsive symptoms when withdrawing medication, CBT top-up sessions should be used to consolidate the skills gained in therapy and to prevent relapse. When relapse occurs early treatment intervention is recommended.

Prognosis, course, and outcome

Prognosis

The course of OCD may be acute or chronic and can have a variable impact on various aspects of functioning including:
- Social functioning
- Interpersonal relationships
- Ability to reach academic potential
- Employment status.

Course and outcome

On recovery from an illness episode, people often experience some residual symptoms. Longitudinal studies of adults who have had a diagnosis of OCD suggest that prognosis is variable, but that most people fall into one of three patterns:
- 40% will recover and experience only mild symptoms, not fulfilling diagnostic criteria. These symptoms will have little if any impact on their ability to function
- 40% will experience a fluctuating illness course with symptoms remitting and relapsing. When severe, symptoms will have a significant effect on functioning
- 20% will develop a chronic illness pattern, with ongoing impact on functioning in all areas.

Recommended reading

National Institute of Health and Clinical Excellence Guideline (2005) Obsessive-compulsive disorder: core interventions in the treatment of obsessive-compulsive disorder and body dysmorphic disorder. Available at: http://www.nice.org.uk/CG031 (accessed 10 March 2008).

Rapoport J, Inoff-Germain G. (2000) Treatment of obsessive compulsive disorder in children and adolescents. *J Child Psychol Psychiat* **41**: 419–31.

Somatoform disorders

Definitions

Somatoform disorders

The terminology surrounding the somatoform disorders is complex, poorly operationalized, and standardized, and many issues relating to definition remain unresolved. In many ways, this is a reflection of the limitations of the physical/psychological dichotomy that continues to pervade medical thinking. To add to this lack of operationalization, many of the terms in common usage appear to be somewhat interchangeable. These include terms such as 'functional', 'psychosomatic', 'medically unexplained physical symptoms' ('MUPS'), 'abnormal illness behaviour', and occasionally the more old fashion terms 'hysterical' and 'neurotic'; This wide nosological variety complicates an already complex field.

However, as we continue to develop an increasingly sophisticated understanding of the physical processes that underpin psychological functioning, and increasingly recognize the relevance of the multiple psychosocial factors that can contribute to in the presentation of physical symptoms, then the separation of 'the physical' and 'the mental' becomes increasingly difficult to either justify or achieve.

A basic current definition of somatoform illness is one that characteristically presents with *prolonged physical symptoms* in the absence of *demonstrable physical cause*, with significant associated functional impairment and often (but not always) in the *setting of an identifiable stressor*.

ICD-10 defines somatization disorder as:

• A history of at least 2 years complaints of multiple and variable physical symptoms that cannot be explained by any detectable physical disorders. If some symptoms clearly due to autonomic arousal are present, they are not a major feature of the disorder, in that they are not particularly persistent or distressing
• Preoccupation with the symptoms causes persistent distress and leads the patient to seek repeated consultations or sets of investigations with either primary care or specialist doctors
• Persistent refusal to accept medical advice that there is no adequate physical cause for the physical symptoms, except for short periods of up to a few weeks at a time during or immediately after medical investigations
• A total of six or more symptoms from the following list, with symptoms occurring in at least two separate groups.

Gastro-intestinal symptoms

• Abdominal pain
• Nausea
• Feeling bloated or full of gas
• Bad taste in mouth, or excessively coated tongue
• Complaints of vomiting or regurgitation of food
• Complaints of frequent and loose bowel motions, or discharge of fluids from anus.

Cardio-vascular symptoms

• Breathlessness without exertion
• Chest pains.

Genitor-urinary symptoms

- Dysuria or complaints of frequency of micturition
- Unpleasant sensations in or around the genitals
- Complaints of unusual or copious vaginal discharge.

Skin and pain symptoms

- Complaints of blotchiness or discolouration of the skin
- Pain in the limbs, extremities or joints
- Unpleasant numbness or tingling sensations.

Conversion and dissociation

Refer to 'sensory symptoms' and 'states of altered awareness', respectively. These are, however, still genuine *physical symptoms*, which are generated, at least in part, by psychological processes. By definition, therefore, both conversion and dissociation symptoms are somatoform in nature.

In common usage, conversion disorder usually applies to a person who is perceived to be expressing something psychologically intolerable via physical means, where dissociation (or a dissociative state) suggests a more generalized loss of control, involving fear, confusion, or even aggressive behaviour, again in response to intolerable or inexpressible feelings or emotions.

When and only when, symptoms are deliberately and voluntarily fabricated or feigned should the terms *factitious disorder* or *malingering* be considered. It should be noted, however, that it is very uncommon for children to entirely manufacture symptoms for premeditated gain.

Diagnoses of irritable bowel syndrome, abdominal migraine, chronic fatigue syndrome, neurasthenia, etc., will usually involve a greater or lesser degree of somatoform elements, and therefore continue to be sources of debate.

Presentation

Any system may be involved. However some are more frequently implicated than others:

- **Gastrointestinal:** including recurrent pain, nausea, loss of appetite
- **Neurological:** headache, seizure, motor dysfunction, sensory
  dysfunction, fatigue, memory, altered consciousness
- **Musculoskeletal:** joint pains, muscle weakness.

An inconsistent (in terms of accepted disease process) and/or changing
pattern of symptoms is often seen.

There are also developmental and gender trends in presentation:

- Younger children generally display more headaches and recurrent
  abdominal pain, with limb pain, aching muscles, fatigue
- Neurological symptoms occur more in older children and adolescents
- Neurological symptoms are also more common in females than males
- It is not uncommon for a child to present with symptoms that are
  similar to those experienced by a family member who is unwell.

The child's own response to the problem may be far more muted than that
of their family. The reasons for this 'Belle indifference' are not clear.

Other presentations, such as chronic fatigue type problems have been
described as having overlaps with eating disorders in their apparent
long term pattern of 'pervasive refusal'. However, the term pervasive
refusal syndrome more correctly applies to the long term refusal to eat,
drink, communicate or even more, seen in some children. This has been
associated with early above in some, and can result in inexplicable sudden
recovery with return to normal functioning.

Impact

Somatoform disorders often have a significant negative impact on a child or young person's life. This may increase over time as a self-perpetuating cycle becomes established. This cycle may be fuelled by:
- Increased family impatience and expressed emotion as the problem persists, so further increasing the stress on the child
- Persistence in the face of increasing questions about cause, making it increasingly difficult for the child to recover without appearing to have been 'putting it all on', to recover with dignity.
- Uncertainty raised by ongoing investigations, many of which may have mildly abnormal results
- Secondary gain from the persisting and disabling symptoms
- New symptoms resulting from inactivity: muscle pain and stiffness, loss of exercise tolerance, insomnia, increased somatic over-focusing.

Epidemiology and aetiology

Epidemiology

In view of the heterogeneous and overlapping nature of the somatoform disorders, it is not surprising that estimates of prevalence are difficult to pin down and tend vary greatly. In addition to the nosological issues noted earlier it is also likely that somatization and the associated impairments will vary on a spectrum that extends well into the 'healthy' population. Most children (and adults) will have had at least one physical symptom, which was related more to stress than to a strictly organic process at some point in their lives.

There are, however, some figures available.

- It is estimated that in around 25% of children who present with headaches, this relates to a somatoform disorder
- Similar estimates suggest that around 23% of children with low energy, 21% with sore muscles, and 17% with abdominal discomfort are, in fact, presenting a somatoform disorder.

A Dutch study of adults visiting a primary care physician suggested that 16% of visits were due to a somatoform disorder that was associated with significant impairment. Similar figures are not available for children but are likely to be in the same sort of region.

Aetiology

Somatoform disorders are certain to be heterogeneous and to have multiple causal relationships.

Whilst, in part, these will relate to the generation of the subjective experience of illness, they will include many other factors, including those that govern an individual's sensitivity to and interpretation of symptoms.

In children it has been speculated that the generation of a somatoform response in could be conceptualized as:

- Either, a general phenomenon by which children communicate their distress through physical symptoms, which arises as a consequence of their not yet having developed a level of sophistication that enables them to express these stresses verbally (or because the stress is unspeakable or the result of an intolerable situation)
- And/or a tendency to overly focus on or misinterpret the significance of somatic processes, which results in a cycle of anxiety and symptom monitoring.

Studies into somatization suggest that personal, family, and social factors combine in varying ways to result in a somatoform presentation. Somatoform disorders can arise in a variety of settings and, although a stressor of some type may be present, it may not be clear or known to the child, their family, or the clinician.

Examples of these factors are presented subsequently. It is important to note, however, that in general these are neither required nor sufficient to explain a somatoform disorder; their presence can, however, add to diagnostic suspicion.

Factors associated with increased likelihood of somatoform response

Child factors

- Older child/adolescent
- Females
- Lower IQ
- Pre-existing mood or anxiety disorder
- Certain predisposing personality factors, such as anxiety traits, perfectionism and conscientiousness (these traits will be heritable to some extent – somatoform disorders cluster in families)
- Previous abuse.

Family factors

- A family history of anxiety or depression
- A family experience of illness (there is a high incidence of chronic disease and disability in parents of somatizers)
- High expectations of the child
- Systemic family dysfunction, such as poor emotional communication.

Social factors

- Lower socioeconomic class
- Predisposition may vary culturally—according to norms (e.g. increased acceptability of physical response to stressors in non western cultures).

Assessment, differential diagnosis, and co-morbidity

Assessment

Nowhere is a biopsychosocial approach to assessment and management more relevant. Assessment should take place within the context of:
- The child and family's own understanding of the symptoms
- The child's temperament
- The family environment.

The aim is to arrive at an agreed consensus about the presentation and diagnosis, whilst acknowledging any diagnostic uncertainty.

A full physical and psychiatric history (including family and psychosocial information) plus physical examination with pertinent basic investigations will always form the basis of a good assessment.

There are several general guidelines that can facilitate the assessment process:
- Symptoms are symptoms, whether or not they have a physical cause, and it is therefore essential to *believe them*. (Pain and discomfort are, and will always be, subjective; it is not your task to decide whether or not they truly exist)
- Ideally, a 'not-medically-provable' or 'stress-related' cause for the presentation should be considered early in the process of assessment. However, this rarely happens
- As a result, as the mental health clinician is prepared to be perceived as 'the shrink who has come to see whether it is all in the mind after all' (and it is important to recognize the reality is that this usually *is* the case—you have most likely been asked to assess the patient as a last resort after a long list of negative investigations)
- 'Physical' and 'non-physical' symptoms can, and almost always do, co-exist (and it may be helpful to point out both to the patient and their physician that the two are often inseparable and can be conceptualized as being on a continuum)
- Whilst assessing the child, always keep trying to identify strategies that will eventually allow them to recover with dignity (rather than aiming to catch them out, e.g. avoid questions like 'Your pain seems to disappear when you play on the computer. How do you explain that?')
- Maintain an awareness of possible rare missed 'true' physical causes to allow yourself to 'recover with dignity', if nothing else
- Solutions are usually more important than causes.

Differential diagnosis

Usually a somatoform illness is seen as the differential of other disorders, but somatoform itself illness will clearly always have a very long list of differentials, many of which can often quickly be ruled out. In some cases, however, physical causes may exist that were not detected on initial medical investigation. Examples include:

- Recurrent abdominal pain:
  - Volvulus
  - Parasitic infections
  - Reflux
- Recurrent headache:
  - Childhood migraine (consider food triggers)
  - Visual inacuity
- Fatigue:
  - Sleep apnoea
  - Depression
- Atypical neurological presentations—epileptic syndromes including frontal lobe epilepsy.

Co-morbidity

Children who somatize have higher rates of several psychiatric disorders than the general population, including:

- **Depression:** this is important as the symptoms of depression include a wide range of 'somatic' symptoms. However, depression is not usually diagnosable on the basis of somatic symptoms alone
- **Anxiety disorders and related difficulties,** such as school refusal are frequently seen in association with somatic complaints. There may also be some overlap with the heightened awareness of body processes that is found in panic disorder.

Childhood epilepsy is frequently accompanied by *pseudoseizures*, which are seizures that are not epileptic in origin and are frequently triggered by emotional stressors. As such, these are a variant on the somatoform theme.

As with epilepsy, other chronic childhood conditions may provide a basis of experience of illness, and so also generate somatoform presentations, such as asthma (where anxiety overlay can generate true airway compromise) and diabetes.

Management

Basic psychoeducation

A clear explanation of processes of symptom generation, and reassurance of the low likelihood of serious or life-threatening illness are almost always required, and should form the cornerstone of management. These factors are, however, often neglected at the beginning of the treatment process. Techniques for enhancing communication and developing a strong a therapeutic alliance are important, as are those aimed at developing understanding, and increasing concordance with treatment. Problem solving strategies and involvement of the school can also make the therapeutic path a smoother one.

Family approaches

Adult family members will also benefit greatly from an explanation of the processes at work. For example, using well known parallels, such as 'butterflies' when nervous and the concept of 'tension' headaches. More in depth systemic family therapy may be indicated in some cases where it can focus on a wide range of issues, such as conflict resolution, exploring previously uncommunicated stresses or allegiances/rivalries within the family.

Physical approaches

Physical therapies are helpful in treatment of many somatoform conditions. Many, particularly those involving fatigue, involve a graded return to previous levels of activity and functioning. The use of exercise programs provided by physiotherapy can reduce muscle and joint problems

Cognitive behavioural therapy (CBT)

CBT is often a mainstay of treatment for somatoform disorders. There is increasing evidence supporting its usefulness in modifying illness behaviour. The link between thoughts, feelings, and bodily sensation can be explored in a number of ways that include externalization and visualization techniques.

Behavioural management

Behavioural techniques also play an important part in most therapeutic strategies for somatization. Their use largely focuses on positively rewarding improvements in health and with the removal of the reinforcers of sick role behaviours. They may also include self-management techniques such as relaxation training and chronic pain reduction techniques, which overlap with those used in cognitive behavioural therapy.

Pharmacological approaches

There is not a strong evidence base for the use of medication to treat somatization in children. However, although some drugs, such as the antidepressants, have been demonstrated to be efficacious in adult populations, there will remain a cautious role for analgesia and anxiolysis.

Clinical example

Amir was a 12-year-old boy who had been admitted to a paediatric ward for observations and tests, then referred for Child Psychiatric opinion whilst still on the ward. He presented with a 3-month history of progressive fatigue and arthralgia. He was complaining of tiredness, joint and chest pains that started during a flu-like illness, and have remained despite resolution of respiratory tract symptoms. These symptoms had become quite debilitating. On some days he was bed-bound for whole days, whilst on others he mobilized with difficulty. He had stopped going to school 2 months previously and his parents, fearful of the impact of this lost school time, had requested a wheelchair and were considering home tuition. Amir now slept downstairs because of fatigue, with his mother often sleeping beside him.

Amir had no significant past medical history; his premorbid temperament was described as 'thoughtful'. Prior to this illness he was doing well at school and enjoyed sports, particularly basketball. He came from a close, hardworking family. The family had suffered multiple bereavements in recent years, which were related to a genetic loading for cardiac disease. The most recent loss was of an older brother aged 30. Amir was particularly close to his mother. His father was described as being quite strict and 'traditional'.

Physical examination, blood tests, ECG, and echocardiography normal, apart from non-specific changes on ECG, which the paediatric cardiologist said should not raise any concerns.

Medical and nursing staff on the ward described a variable and inconsistent presentation, with mixed upper and lower limb weakness, and hyperaesthesia. His father had noticed that Amir moved his limbs normally when turning in his sleep.

At interview Amir was pleasant and appeared in good spirits. However, he did say that he was angry with himself for being unwell and adding further to his mother's burden.

Possible formulation

Predisposing factors
* Family closeness
* Difficult family circumstances
* Thoughtful nature
* Ethnic origin.

Precipitating factors
* Viral illness with chest pain
* Worry about possible causes in context of the family history
* Overly protective response from family (although understandable considering their experiences and losses).

Perpetuating factors
* Increasing symptoms as a consequence of prolonged inactivity
* Fatigue, joint, and muscle pains, exacerbated by renewed attempts at activity

- Clinician's concerns as to possibly missing a cardiac problem
- Family's and Amir's concerns as to possible missed cardiac problem
- Over-awareness of somatic factors (hyperaesthesia, arthralgia, may simply be stiffness in underused joints) with excessive levels of self-monitoring
- Secondary gain, from increased closeness to mother leading to a subconscious reinforcement of symptoms
- Prolonged absence from school progressively makes return more difficult due to missed work or stigma
- Amir's father suspected it was 'all in his head' and a ploy to avoid school. This would be 'confirmed' were Amir to recover without either a diagnosis or an intervention. Hence, a recovery with dignity became increasingly difficult.

Management points

The first stage would be to discuss the formulation candidly with Amir and his parents. Emphasizing that, whilst these symptoms are real, they are on balance, and in view of the history, examination, and investigations, more likely to have arisen via this mechanism than from a purely physical one, such as undiagnosed cardiac failure or another 'missed' medical condition.

Explanation in terms of the potential contribution of both psychological and physical factors should help with discussion of proposed management, which should include both physical (e.g. physiotherapy for joint problems, graded exercise programme for fatigue) and psychological (e.g. CBT-based therapy to deal with somatic focus, family/systems therapy to examine impact of elevated family risk and bereavements).

Recommended reading

Oster J. (1972) Recurrent abdominal pain, headache and limb pains in children and adolescents. *Pediatrics* **50:** 429–36.

Sanders MR, Shepherd RW, Cleghorn G, Woolford H. (1994) The treatment of recurrent abdominal pain in children: a controlled comparison of cognitive-behavioral intervention and standard pediatric care. *J Consult Clin Psychol* **62:** 306–14.

Lewis M. (2002) *Child and Adolescent Psychiatry: A Comprehensive Textbook*, 3rd edn. Lippincott Williams and Wilkins. Philadelphia.

Kirmayer L, Looper K. (2006) Abnormal illness behaviour: physiological, psychological and social dimensions of coping with distress. *Curr Opin Psychiatry* **19:** 54–60.

Taylor S, Nunn K, Lask B. (2003) *Practical Child Psychiatry: The Clinician's Guide*. BMJ Books, London.

Sharpe M, Mayou R. (2004) Somatoform disorders: a help or hindrance to good patient care? *Br J Psychiatry* **184:** 465–7.

Post-traumatic stress disorder

Life stresses and psychiatric disorder

The concept of post-traumatic stress disorder (PTSD) was first coined in relation to symptoms reported by war veterans from the Vietnam War, although it was subsequently recognized that the 'shell shock' experienced by soldiers in the First World War in Europe was the same phenomenon. Later, the term was used to describe symptoms experienced by patients who had experienced an 'event outside the range of usual human experience … that would be markedly distressing to almost anyone' (DSM-III-R, American Psychiatric Association). To begin with, it was believed that the diagnosis would not be relevant to children and young people. This view has now been discarded and it has been demonstrated that younger patients also display the symptoms associated with PTSD, although developmental differences must be taken into account.

The role of life events as important contributors to the aetiology of child and adolescent psychiatric disorder is now well established. Research shows that life events rated as significant by children do not always correlate with adult ratings. Parents and other adults can misinterpret the significance of particular events in the lives of children and young people. In child and adolescent mental health practice, single stresses are unusual, with a constellation of various stresses and life events being a much more common finding.

Chronic life stresses in childhood

- Deprivation
- Poverty
- Abuse:
  - Physical
  - Emotional
  - Sexual
  - Neglect
- Parental mental illness
- Parental alcohol and/or drug misuse
- Chronic family discord
- Exposure to conflict
- Refugee status
- Social discrimination, due to physical or intellectual difference, ethnicity, mental illness, etc.
- Chronic physical illness, particularly of a parent.

Acute life stresses in childhood

- Accident, e.g. road traffic accident (RTA)
- Bereavement
- Illness of a significant adult
- Separation from main carers
- Bullying
- Assault
- Death of a pet
- Change of school
- Loss of friends
- Physical illness.

Association between stresses and psychiatric disorder in children

- Severe adverse life events in children contribute to an increased risk of psychiatric disorder
- This risk is further increased if adverse life events occur against a background of psychosocial adversity
- Accumulation of stressors is important
- The significance of particular stressors is poorly understood
- Children's reaction to stress is strongly mediated by the responses of the adults around them
- It is important to recognize resilience effects in children. Good family functioning, supportive relationships, etc., often protect against the development of disorder.

Not all those exposed to severe traumatic events will develop PTSD. Indeed, most do not. Other reactions to stress are common and the majority of people will recover from stress reactions very quickly. In studies of adult victims of RTAs, only about 10% developed PTSD.

Definitions and epidemiology

Definitions

Diagnostic criteria for PTSD are the same for children and young people as they are for adults, with some consideration given to developmental issues.

ICD-10 criteria

Occurs as a response to an exceptionally threatening or catastrophic event. This leads to:
- Repeated reliving of the trauma, with flashbacks or intrusive memories of the event (in children may be demonstrated in play, drawings, etc.)
- Avoidance of reminders of the trauma

And either:
- Inability to recall, either partially or completely, some important aspects of the period of exposure to the stressor

Or
- Persistent symptoms of increased psychological sensitivity and arousal (not present before exposure to the stressor) shown by any two of the following:
  - Difficulty in falling or staying asleep
  - Irritability or outbursts of anger
  - Difficulty in concentrating
  - Hyper-vigilance
  - Exaggerated startle response
- Emotional 'numbness' is also often reported
- There is usually a delay between the trauma and onset of symptoms
- PTSD may run a chronic course.

DSM-IV

- Includes stricter criteria
- More emphasis on violent trauma
- Requires that symptoms cause significant distress or interfere with functioning.

Particular issues for childhood PTSD

In children, symptoms may begin almost immediately after the traumatic event. Emotional numbness as described in adults is difficult to elicit in children, although children are much more likely to experience dissociation in traumatic situations and when this happens repeatedly, as in abusive experiences, it has serious effects on future functioning.

Epidemiology

Studies have demonstrated that children and young people, as well as adults, can experience symptoms of PTSD following both individual and group traumas. Most research in childhood PTSD has involved tracing children following major disasters, such as war, earthquake, and more specifically following high impact events, for example, the Lockerbie plane crash and the sinking of the 'Jupiter' cruise ship.
- 30–60% of children develop PTSD following disasters

- Around 25–30% develop symptoms following road traffic accidents
- Lifetime rate of PTSD in older adolescents around 6%
- Follow-up of children involved in the Jupiter sinking showed:
  - 52% had PTSD in the weeks after the sinking
  - There were few cases of late onset PTSD
  - Around 30% recovered in the first year
  - 5–8 years later, 34% were still suffering.

Aetiology

Although not everyone develops PTSD following an extreme event, anyone exposed to such significant stressors can do. Whilst some children and young people appear to be more vulnerable than others this vulnerability by itself is insufficient to predict who will and who will not develop the disorder. There is also a group of children whose early childhood experiences have been so repeatedly traumatic that they remain in a chronic state of hyperarousal and display distorted responses to stress.

Risk factors associated with an increased likelihood of developing PTSD include:

Pre-disposing factors unrelated to the trauma

- A history of early neglect or abuse, including sexual abuse
- A family history of psychiatric disorder
- Low socio-economic class
- Poor education
- Female gender
- Previous exposure to trauma
- Lack of supportive adults.

Factors associated with the trauma itself

- Life-threatening event
- Proximity to the event
- Ability to get away or protect oneself
- Length of exposure
- Repeated traumas
- Seeing dead bodies or body parts
- Unexpected nature of the event.

Effects of stress on brain function

Neuroimaging studies have demonstrated that severe stress, such as child abuse, can impact on hippocampal development in children. This effect is mediated by the toxic effects of raised cortisol levels. This damage leads to inaccuracy of episodic memory and mismatches between what is current and what is remembered, which leads to hyperarousal of the behavioural inhibition system and excess stress reactions. Habituation to this increased stress is impaired due to the dysfunctional episodic memory evaluation and consolidation.

Children who have experienced prolonged deprivation and/or abuse in the first 3 years of life, where severe neglect is a feature have smaller brain volume than age equivalent peers.

Assessment, differential diagnosis, and co-morbidity

Assessment

Although there are a number of structured questionnaires and semi-structured interviews of relevance in assessing children and young people for PTSD, nothing substitutes for a thorough clinical assessment of the child and their family. This should include both family interviews and individual meetings with the patient. Most children, and even some older adolescents, can make use of drawing and toys to help them tell their story, and an appropriate range of materials should be provided. Assessing children and adolescents who have experienced traumatic events is a difficult and sensitive issue, and can take some time. Because of the nature of some of the histories that these young patients have, it is almost always helpful to have a team approach to assessment and clinical supervision for clinicians is essential.

Clinical assessment
- Full psychiatric assessment
- Family history
- History of the trauma from the perspective of the adult and young person (this may take some time to elicit)
- Developmental history
- History of functioning, adjustment, and mental health issues prior to the trauma
- History of exposure to previous traumatic events
- Psychosocial functioning
- Reports from school (and others such as social work if relevant)
- Observation of the family interaction with the patient
- Patient's response to the therapist
- Identification of resilience factors.

Structured assessments of PTSD
- The Clinician-Administered PTSD Scale for Children and Adolescents for DSM-IV
- The Anxiety Disorders Interview Schedule for Children for DSM-IV
- The Schedule for Affective Disorder and Schizophrenia for School age Children (K-SADS)
- The Children's Impact of Trauma Events Scale (revised).

Apart from the K-SADS, which is validated down to the age of 6 years, none of these measures is valid for children under the age of 8 years. Assessing PTSD in younger children is dependent on rigorous clinical assessment. There is some disagreement about the validity of the syndrome in very young children, although new, but as yet unvalidated criteria have been suggested. These emphasize the importance of regressed behaviour and the emergence of fear in this group of children.

Differential diagnosis

- Acute stress reaction
- Adjustment reaction
- Attachment disorder
- Depressive illness
- Other anxiety disorder
- Sleep disorder
- Oppositional Defiant Disorder (ODD)
- Attention deficit hyperactivity disorder (ADHD).

Co-morbidity

- Depressive disorder
- Attachment disorder
- Conduct disorders (CDs) or ODD
- Sleeping difficulties
- Self-harming behaviour
- Regressive behaviour
- Separation difficulties
- ADHD.

Management

There is currently no good evidence about the usefulness of medication in the treatment of PTSD symptoms in patients under the age of 18 and there are no drugs that are licensed for this indication. However, it may be necessary to use medication in the treatment of co-morbid depressive disorders and, in this case, fluoxetine is licenced and recommended.

Otherwise, the treatment relies on psychological therapies. Although much of the work on treatment of trauma in young people has been conducted with those who have been sexually abused, these experiences have been used to treatment plan for patients with other trauma histories.

Psychological therapies

- **Trauma focused cognitive behavioural therapy (CBT):** adapted to the age and developmental stage of the child or young person
- **Family therapy:** can address the young patient's need for support, but also identifies issues of secondary trauma within the family
- **Creative therapies** especially art therapy have been offered to young victims of trauma. Many clinicians use play and art materials in a therapeutic way, but this is not the same as formal therapy. It can be very useful for patients, especially a very young child, to have alternative means of expressing themselves apart from the spoken word
- **Eye movement desensitization reprocessing** (EMDR) has been shown to be a useful adjunct to psychological therapies for young victims of trauma in helping them to construct a 'safe space' where they can regain some control over their symptoms. It is not clear, however, whether it is the eye movement *per se* or the guided remembering that carries with it the therapeutic effects
- **Single session trauma focused de-briefing:** there is no evidence to support the use of this intervention with children and young people (see NICE Guidelines on PTSD)

Dealing with the legal system

Many children and young people who have been exposed to trauma, also have to face the further traumatic effects of making a formal legal statement, having a forensic examination, and appearing in court. These are experiences outwith the norm for the vast majority of young people.

The language used is outwith their knowledge and the formality of the process can be intimidating. Although investigations of abuse are now carried out with sensitivity by specially trained police officers and social workers, the requirements of evidence mean that young people often find they are not able to tell their stories in their own way and at their own pace.

Furthermore, young patients often do not understand the difficulty of bringing a case to court and securing a conviction. Investigations can be lengthy. Consequently, they often feel let down by the system and this secondary trauma can further compromise their recovery.

Therapists, too, can feel confused by the need not to be seen to be 'coaching' a child to give evidence, and this has sometimes led to children and young people being denied the treatment they need because of an ongoing legal investigation. This should not be the case and, whilst particular care should be taken, necessary treatments should not usually need to be withheld for these reasons

Assisting a young person with the legal process

- Answer their questions truthfully
- Do not make predictions or promises that you have no control over
- Do not use jargon unless necessary and if you do need to, always explain what it means
- Clearly explain who everyone is in the process and what role they play
- Explain fully what will happen if they have to go to court
- Liaise with solicitors or social workers in order to arrange a pre-trial visit to the court
- Arrange for them to give their evidence by video link if possible
- If they can, they should have a supportive adult with them and they should have met this adult beforehand
- Always tell them the outcome truthfully in language they can understand
- Use their own language to describe the people involved, such as their abuser (e.g. 'that man')
- Cross-examination can inevitably be very stressful and this needs to be communicated sensitively.

Planning for disasters

Most schools are aware of the likely need to support young people after traumatic events. These can range from large scale events involving the whole school, such as the school shootings in Dunblane and America, to events such as the death of pupils in RTAs, which may affect only a few pupils. Schools should have contingency plans to deal with such events and should know who will take responsibility for implementing these, and what services and supports are locally available.

The same advice is true for communities where similar circumstances may affect, for example, youth groups and sports clubs.

Prognosis, course, and outcome

- The majority of patients will recover within a year following a disaster
- The severity of symptoms is an important predictor of outcome
- Children, especially, and adolescents are very dependent on how their parents or other supportive adults are, themselves, coping to help them recover
- Effective treatment is important in influencing outcome
- Course of the disorder is complicated by pre-morbid experience and co-morbidity
- Effects on some can be very long lasting, even into adulthood
- The outcome for those that experience early, significant neglect and/or abuse is poor in terms of long-term adjustment.

Clinical example

Jodie was a bright and lively 6-year-old who was the youngest of 3 siblings. She lived with her mother, her siblings, and her mother's partner in a small village. They lived in a specially adapted house with a 'safe room' installed that had a direct link via a panic button to the local police station. Eighteen months previously, her mother had been seriously attacked by Jodie's father, and had spent several weeks in hospital with head and neck injuries and a ruptured kidney.

When they were referred by their GP, all three children had variable symptoms of PTSD. Jodie was not sleeping at night, was sharing her mother's bed, was oppositional, and would not go out to play with her friends from school. She had also begun wetting again. The family was all seen together and the maternal grandmother also attended the first meeting. It transpired that they were waiting for a date to go to court when all three children were expected to give evidence. The court date had already been put back four times.

Jodie's mum and grandmother were both very supportive of the children, allowing them space to tell their stories in a non-judgmental way with little interference. They stressed the successes the children had had without minimizing their symptoms.

Jodie was very chatty during the session, often talking over her brother and sister, whilst spending a lot of time drawing. She was very forthright and, unlike the other family members, did not try to hide her thoughts or feelings about the events.

As the assessment progressed, Jodie told how her father used to shut her in a cupboard when her mum was out and would hit her if she disobeyed. She was a feisty little girl who often got in to trouble with her father, but her mother was unaware of what went on when she was not around.

Her mother's previous partner had also been abusive to her, and the older siblings had already witnessed a lot of domestic discord and violence.

A social worker from the court was supporting the family and they had ongoing contact with the family police unit who had investigated the case. Therapy continued with various combinations of the family until after the court hearing.

Although the plan had been for all the children to be supported individually by members of their own family while they gave evidence, in the event, only Jodie was allowed to have her grandmother with her. The two older children had support workers allocated by the court. The defendant was found not guilty. The family was never told why he had not been convicted.

In the course of therapy, all three children's symptoms waxed and waned depending on mother's mental health, the proximity of the most recent court date, and how they were getting on at school.

Following the trial, Jodie's symptoms began to resolve. Despite the fact that there had been no conviction, she felt that she had told her story and been believed. She was well supported by her family and school, and 6 months after the event was sleeping in her own bed again and had ceased wetting.

Recommended reading

National Institute for Clinical Excellence, Clinical Guidelines 26, PTSD The management of PTSD in adults and children in Primary and secondary care (March 2005). Available at: http://www.nice.org.uk/nicemedia/pdf/CG026NICEguideline.pdf (accessed 5 April 2008).

Anorexia nervosa

Definitions

Anorexia nervosa in children and young people shares many of the features defined by ICD-10 and DSM-IV for an adult population (Table 23.1). However, there are some differences that need to be taken into account in a growing child and especially in pre-pubertal children. Eating disorders in children and young people also include a broad variety of patterns of disturbed eating that are not generally seen in adults. Hence, in a younger population one may include:

- Anorexia nervosa
- Atypical anorexia nervosa
- Bulimia nervosa
- Atypical bulimia nervosa
- Food avoidance emotional disorder
- Selective eating
- Restrictive eating
- Food refusal
- Fear of food or phobia
- Pervasive refusal disorder.

Nevertheless, the concepts of the eating disorders that are formally defined in classification systems remain clinically useful.

Table 23.1 Definition of anorexia nervosa

ICD – 10	DSM-IV
Body weight maintained at a BMI <17.5	Refusal to maintain body weight above a minimal level (85% of expected for height)
Weight loss is self-induced by avoidance of 'fattening' foods, vomiting, exercising purging, etc.	Intense fear of gaining weight
Body image distortion with dread of fatness	Disturbance of perception of body image
Endocrine disturbance of hypothalamic-pituitary-gonadal axis	The absence of at least 3 consecutive menstrual cycles in post-menarchal women
In pre-pubertal patients, delayed or arrested growth	

ICD-10 recognizes 'atypical anorexia nervosa', as well as 'eating disorder, unspecified', whilst DSM-IV describes restricting and binge eating/purging sub-types of anorexia and also 'Eating disorder not otherwise specified'.

Body Mass Index (BMI) is a measure of height to weight ratio used to assess healthy weight. It is a ratio of weight (Kg) divided by height (m), squared:

$$BMI = Weight\ (Kg)/Height\ (m)^2$$

For example, for Height = 1.65 m, Weight = 50 Kg,

$$BMI = 50/(1.65)^2 = 50/2.72 = 18.3$$

Normal BMI is considered between 20 and 25 for adults, but is lower and more flexible in children and adolescents. The use of age- and gender-standardized BMI centile charts is recommended.

Epidemiology

- Anorexia nervosa has a prevalence of 19 per 100,000 per year for females and 2 per 100,000 per year for males
- The highest prevalence is amongst teenage girls
- Peak age of onset between 15 and 19 years, but can occur from age 8 upwards
- Females consistently outnumber males by a factor of up to 40 in clinical studies
- There are higher reported rates of anorexia nervosa in Western civilizations
- Epidemiological studies do not support the clinical impression that anorexia nervosa is associated with higher social class.

Anorexia, together with all eating disorders, has long had an association with culture. It is seen only rarely amongst African and Asian populations, although is common in Japan in the more affluent classes. There is some emerging evidence from cross-cultural studies that the adoption of western lifestyles and aspirational ideals may be contributing to a rise in anorexia in non-western populations.

Aetiology

Like many mental disorders, the aetiology of anorexia nervosa is far from straightforward. Indeed, there is no single explanation for the genesis of this disorder, despite an emphasis in the media on dieting and excessively thin role models as the cause in young women. Rather, it is considered to be of multifactorial aetiology with a range of factors leading to the end pattern of symptoms.

Genetic factors

- Family studies: for the full anorexia nervosa syndrome, the risk to female relatives of those with the disorder is 11 times that in the general population
- The results of twin studies are variable, but the estimated range for the heritability of anorexia nervosa is between 58 and 76%.

Environmental risk factors

- Obstetric complications
- Very pre-term delivery
- Early feeding disturbances
- Childhood obesity
- A history of dieting behaviour
- Severe adverse life events.

Neurobiological factors

- Neuropsychological, neuroimaging, and other techniques have implicated a variety of processing deficits and cognitive profiles in the aetiology of anorexia nervosa
- In addition, it is now recognized that, for a proportion of young people, impaired social functioning, which in extreme cases can look like autistic spectrum disorder (ASD), may be present. There remain questions, however, about how much of this is pre-morbid, and how much is a consequence of the disorder and amenable to treatment.

Temperament

Temperamental traits associated with anorexia nervosa include:
- Low novelty seeking
- Harm avoidance
- High persistence
- Low self-directedness.

Family factors

- 'High concern' parenting style
- High rates of major depression in first degree relatives
- Family pre-occupation with eating, feeding, weight, and body image.

Socio-cultural factors

The debate about the role of social pressures on young women, and increasingly young men, to conform to an overly thin 'ideal' body shape on the development of eating disorders has yet to be resolved. Whilst it is unlikely that the impact of the media preoccupation with thinness will cause healthy people to develop eating disorders, for those with other vulnerabilities, it may be a contributing factor.

There is evidence that cultures newly exposed to media influences do change their attitudes to shape and size, and acquire dieting habits not previously seen.

In cultures undergoing change to a more western lifestyle, with greater affluence and availability of food, there is evidence of increased incidence of eating disorders, although bulimia nervosa appears to predominate. In contrast, there seems to be some protection offered to young women in African societies by the acceptance of a different pattern of body image.

At the same time as the ideal of an extremely thin body image is being promoted, there is, in most industrialized countries, a super-abundance of cheap high calorie food available. This creates a tension that, for some people, may result in persistent dieting behaviour with the subsequent risk of developing anorexia.

Assessment

Early identification and treatment of anorexia nervosa is important in the prevention of long-term complications. It is, therefore, vital that clinicians in primary care are aware of the potential for eating disorders in the young population. Parents, school teachers, school nurses, and others in the helping professions can all play an important part in encouraging young people to seek help if they have concerns about their eating.

In primary care, screening instruments such as the SCOFF Questionnaire (📖 p. 354) can be useful in helping to identify those at risk. This short questionnaire of 5 questions has been shown in patients over 18 years to have good validity. Its use with younger patients has not been demonstrated, but nevertheless, the questions can help guide primary care physicians. Early referral to a CAMHS should be facilitated.

History of disorder

- Duration and extent of weight loss
- Rate of weight loss
- Current food and fluid intake, including avoidance of food, mealtimes and attitudes to eating
- Onset of amenorrhea or not
- Extent of exercise
- Purging.

Psychiatric/psychological assessment

- Full psychiatric history
- Attitude to body shape and size
- Cognitive distortion about weight gain
- Developmental history
- Psycho-social adjustment, including educational history
- Attitude to treatment and recovery.

Family assessment

- Family's thoughts and feelings about the patient's weight and physical health
- Family coping mechanisms and problem-solving ability
- Assessment of family dynamics
- Family history of eating disorders
- Family mental health history
- Attitudes of family members to treatment.

Physical health assessment

- Measure height and weight, and calculate BMI, charting on appropriate children's BMI centile charts
- Measure pulse and blood pressure (sitting and standing)
- Assess pubertal status
- Assess nutritional state and hydration.

Possible physical signs

- General listlessness
- Dry hair and skin
- Sallow complexion
- Brittle nails and hair
- Thinning scalp hair
- Lack of subcutaneous fat
- Wearing baggy, disguising clothing
- Lanugo hair
- Bradycardia
- Hypotension with postural hypotension
- Cold extremities
- Cyanosis
- Failure of development of secondary sexual characteristics
- Eroded tooth enamel caused by persistent vomiting
- Russell's sign (callused skin over finger joints)
- Swelling of the parotid glands.

Physical investigations

- **ECG:** check for prolonged QT interval
- **Full blood count (FBC):** raised Hb may indicate dehydration
- **Urea and electrolytes**: including magnesium, phosphate. Check for signs of dehydration, alkalosis from vomiting or acidosis from laxative use
- **Blood glucose**
- **Liver function tests:** including proteins, clotting factors and Vitamin K
- **Endocrine tests:** T4, T3, TSH
- **Iron, folate, and B12**
- **Other physical examinations may be undertaken:** ECHO cardiogram, bone scan.

Standardized questionnaires

- Eating Disorders Examination (EDE) child version
- Eating Disorders Inventory for Children (EDI-C)
- Children's Eating Attitudes Test
- Kids' Eating Disorders Survey.

Differential diagnosis and co-morbidity

- Severe depressive illness
- Obsessive compulsive disorder (OCD)
- Chronic debilitating physical illness
  - Brain tumours
  - Intestinal disorders, e.g. Crohn's disease
  - Chronic debilitating disease
  - Post-viral syndrome.

Co-morbidity

- Mood disorder, especially depression
- Anxiety disorder
- OCD
- Social interaction difficulties similar to autism spectrum disorder
- Body dysmorphic disorder.

Management: psychological

Management of anorexia nervosa in children and young people requires a team effort, and virtually all cases will require intensive treatment with more than one therapeutic modality. Working with the parents, as well as the child is essential. The majority of anorectic patients will be able to be treated as outpatients or day patients, but occasionally inpatient treatment cannot be avoided. Any admission other than for a short period to stabilize physical health should be to an appropriate unit dealing with children and young people. Very rarely, it may be necessary to use legal detention, under the Mental Health Act, in cases of young people under the age of 18.

Individual psychological treatment

The key to success in individual treatment is the engagement with the therapist, rather than the type of therapy provided, which is often determined by availability, rather than recommendations. Although cognitive behavioural therapy (CBT) would be the first choice, interpersonal therapy is also used, and individual psychodynamic psychotherapy can have a part to play in carefully selected cases. The use of motivational interviewing techniques can also be useful. Success is more likely if continuity of the therapist can be assured even if a patient is admitted to a day or inpatient facility.

Family therapy

Working with the family is crucial to the success of treatment. The style of family therapy is generally supportive, educative, problem solving, and facilitating. Any pre-morbid issues can be addressed as therapy continues, but in the initial stages, most families will need help to reinforce boundaries around eating and exercise in order to prevent further weight loss.

On some occasions as resources permit, a multi-family approach to treatment has been used. This involves a number of families meeting together over the course of at least 1 day and sometimes more. Therapy involves the sharing of meals, as well as discussion groups and problem-solving sessions

Dietetic input and re-feeding

Assistance from a dietician helps families to feel reassured about diet and balance. In severe cases, where there is a threat to health or life, it is essential to have input from dietetics in order to minimize the risks associated with re-feeding, particularly the risk of cardiac decompensation. In severe cases, hospitalization should be sought.

Indications for hospitalization
- Body weight <75% expected weight for height
- Dehydration
- Severe bradycardia (<50/min daytime)
- Cardiac complications
- Severe hypotension
- Acute medical complications
- Psychiatric emergency
- Refusal to eat or drink
- Failure to stop weight loss with outpatient treatment.

Re-feeding in children and adolescents

- Higher risk of re-feeding syndrome than in adults; therefore, do not use adult type re-feeding programmes
- Careful planning is vital
- Team approach required
- Calorie need is greater in children and young people to allow for growth
- Avoid enteral feeding if at all possible
- Set target weight at 100% expected weight for height
- Onset of menses is a good indicator of adequate nutrition in adolescent girls.

Re-feeding syndrome

This is a high risk condition associated with cardiac decompensation and sudden death. It occurs when re-feeding is undertaken too quickly without adequate attention being paid to electrolyte balance. The first 2 weeks of a re-feeding programme are especially high risk. Children and young people are at higher risk of re-feeding syndrome than adults and at very low weights, it is recommended that re-feeding of younger patients takes place in hospital.

Symptoms of re-feeding syndrome include:

- Excessive bloating
- Oedema
- Congestive cardiac failure.

Ethical issues in the treatment of anorexia nervosa in young patients

The issue of re-feeding against the patient's wishes is particularly difficult with young patients, where parental and, indeed, staff anxiety is high, and where a child or young person is critically ill and at risk of dying. The collaboration of the patient should be obtained if at all possible even if that extends to permission to nasogastrically feed. However, where the patient is refusing permission to feed, NICE recommends the use of the appropriate mental health or children's legislation.

Management: pharmacological

- Pharmacological treatment is not appropriate for the core disorder
- If there are co-morbid disorders, then treatment with an SSRI may be appropriate. However, there are considerations in using these drugs in an under-18 population. Only fluoxetine is licensed for the treatment of depression. Sertraline and fluvoxamine are licensed for the treatment of obsessive compulsive disorder
- Tricyclic drugs are not recommended because of the possibility of cardiac complications
- Vitamin and mineral supplements can be useful
- Food supplements on the recommendation of a dietician can help support eating in the early stages.

All medications must be used cautiously, staring with a low dose and building up over a number of weeks. It is wise to check out physical status before commencing any drug treatment.

Prognosis, course, and outcome

Anorexia nervosa is a serious psychiatric disorder that carries a significant risk of mortality as well as considerable morbidity. Although some cases of anorexia in children and young people are mild and resolve without intensive treatment programmes, many will go on into adult services with chronic eating problems. Whilst the quoted long-term outcomes for anorexia generally accept that a third will recover fully, a third will make a partial recovery, and a third will have chronic symptoms, this is taking into account the lifetime course of the illness. Predicting the course from a child perspective is more difficult and, in all cases, it is safer to assume that intensive treatment will be needed.

The risks to physical long-term health are greater without early attention to malnutrition and long-term problems include:
- Growth retardation
- Delayed or arrested puberty
- Reduced bone density
- Higher likelihood of low birth weight baby.

Risk factors for poorer outcome
- Late onset
- Excessive weight loss
- Vomiting and purging as part of the clinical picture
- Poor social adjustment
- Poor parental relationships
- Male gender
- Chronic course of illness.

Clinical example

Fiona presented to her GP aged 15 with a 6-month history of low mood and weight loss. At that point her GP measured her BMI at 18.5 and, after discussion about strategies to improve mood and exhortation to increase her food intake, she agreed to review Fiona in 2 weeks time. At that point, her BMI had dropped only slightly to 18.4 and she claimed to be eating better. She was seen alone on both occasions.

One month later, Fiona was brought to the surgery by her mother who complained that she was very moody, tearful, and withdrawn. Her school work was suffering and she had no appetite. She had lost more weight and her BMI was now 18.1. The GP gave further advice about eating, referred her to the community dietician, and prescribed fluoxetine giving a diagnosis of depressive illness. As Fiona's parents were both doctors themselves, she asked them to monitor Fiona's weight at home and arranged to see her again in 2 weeks time.

When Fiona returned to the surgery, she looked ill and tired. She had not yet seen the dietician, her weight had decreased again, and her BMI was now 17.7. She continued to complain of low mood and was not sleeping well. The GP took blood tests for FBC and U&Es, and asked Fiona to return the following week with her mother. Blood results showed a mild dehydration pattern and when Fiona returned to the surgery, her weight had once again dropped. At this point, the GP asked about Fiona's attitude to eating and gaining weight, and began to suspect that she may have an eating disorder. She increased her antidepressants dose and made a referral to the local CAMHS for assessment.

Fiona and her mother attended the clinic 3 weeks later. A full history revealed a 1-year history of increasingly restricted eating following remarks at school that Fiona was 'fat' with 'thick legs'. Fiona was an excellent hockey player and, as a result of these remarks, had not only restricted her eating, but had started going to extra athletic training and had been swimming 5 times a week for up to 2 h at a time. Her menstrual cycle had stopped 6 months ago. Her low mood had only begun about 1 month prior to seeing her GP for the first time. An excellent student at school, her work had been suffering because of poor concentration and she complained of chronic fatigue, but poor sleep for the past 2 months.

At the clinic, she was weighed and measured again, and her BMI was 17.2. Arrangements were made for Fiona and her mother to see the clinic dietician the next day and she was asked to return the following week with her family for an extended assessment session. A tentative diagnosis of anorexia nervosa was made, and explained to Fiona and her mother. She was asked to reduce her exercise to essential activity only, to increase her fluid intake to at least 2 L/day, and to follow the dietician's advice regarding food intake. She was advised that the antidepressants were probably not helping her, but pressure from both Fiona and her mother meant that she stayed on them for the time being.

Over the next few weeks, the diagnosis of anorexia nervosa was confirmed, and both individual and family treatment programmes were commenced. Fiona was seen regularly, both alone for individual cognitive behavioural therapy (CBT) and together with her family. She had an individual diet schedule composed by the dietician, which included a recording diary. Despite this, Fiona's weight continued to fall and 1 month later, her BMI was 15.9 and blood tests showed signs of malnutrition.

At this point, a referral was made to the CAMHS Day Service for Adolescents and the paediatric service was asked to assess Fiona's physical state. This precipitated a crisis with Fiona refusing to eat anything and severely restricting her fluid intake. An emergency appointment was arranged for Fiona and her family at which it was revealed that Fiona had been accessing 'pro-anorexia' sites on the Internet and was being encouraged to refuse food by a girl with whom she was corresponding in America. Fiona's parents were appalled and determined to supervise her access to the computer. This also helped them to accept their role in taking charge of Fiona's eating at home and the need to be more vigilant in monitoring her exercise. Admission to the Day service was accepted and Fiona attended for 6 months, during which time her physical health improved, her weight increased, and her family were able to re-direct their efforts to support her eating and appropriate social interactions. Her fluoxetine medication was withdrawn with no ill effect. When she was discharged from the Day Service, Fiona's BMI was 18.9 and she was attending school full time, but not playing any sports.

Although her weight dropped slightly on discharge, Fiona remained relatively well for a while until a further crisis was precipitated by her older brother going off to University and her father being admitted to hospital with a suspected heart attack. Fiona once again stopped eating and her weight plummeted rapidly until he was dangerously ill with a BMI of 14.5, a severe bradycardia, and disordered blood results. She refused admission to hospital and consideration was given to detention under mental health legislation. She was admitted briefly to a general hospital ward for stabilization of her physical health, while options were considered. During this time, Fiona was offered an opportunity to go to Africa with a school party some 8 months ahead if her physical state allowed. This provided some motivation for Fiona to re-engage in treatment and she once again commenced individual CBT sessions with concurrent family support work. Fiona made slow progress initially, but as her physical health improved, and her cognitive function with it, she was increasingly able to join in the activities associated with the forthcoming expedition. With ongoing support from her family and extra support from her school, Fiona was well enough to go on the trip with a BMI of 19.3. During this time she struck up a relationship with one of the young men going on the trip and also made a decision to train in medicine herself, like her parents. When she returned, her plans had been further confirmed by what she had seen in Africa and she settled into her final year at school enthusiastically.

Fiona remained relatively well and continued contact with the clinic until after she had left school. In her first term at University she struggled to maintain her eating and her weight started to fall again. She was referred to the student counselling service and saw a psychologist regularly. She managed to stabilize her condition and continue with her course. She continues to be vulnerable, but has successfully completed her course and is now practicing medicine.

Recommended reading

NICE Collaboration for Mental Health. (2004) *Eating Disorders; Core Interventions in the Management of Anorexia Nervosa, Bulimia Nervosa and Related Eating Disorders.* Gaskell, London.

Lask B, Bryant-Waugh R. (2007) *Eating Disorders in Childhood and Adolescence,* 3rd edn. Routledge, London.

Rome ES, *et al.* (2003) Children and adolescents with eating disorders: the State of the Art. *Pediatrics* **111**: 98–108.

Bulimia nervosa and other eating disorders of childhood

Definitions and epidemiology

Definitions

Bulimia nervosa is an eating disorder that seldom presents before the age of 14, and is thus much rarer in child and adolescent psychiatric practice than anorexia nervosa. On the other hand, it is common for adult patients with a diagnosis of bulimia nervosa to describe a pattern of disordered eating and preoccupation with body shape from a young age. Bulimia nervosa is characterized by loss of control of eating, with periods of intense over-eating, preoccupation with food and body shape, and attempts to get rid of the food consumed by vomiting, purging, or exercising (📖 Table 24.1).

Table 24.1 Definitions of bulimia nervosa

ICD-10	DSM-IV
Persistent preoccupation with eating craving for food with episodes of consuming large quantities of food in a short period of time	Recurrent episodes of binge eating with a sense of lack of control during the episode.
Purging of food by self-induced vomiting, laxative abuse, appetite suppressants, and other drugs	Recurrent use of vomiting, laxative, diuretics, etc., to prevent weight gain
Morbid fear of fatness	Self-image is preoccupied with body shape and/or weight
	Binging and compensatory behaviour at least twice a week for 3 months

ICD-10 also recognizes atypical bulimia nervosa, whilst DSM-IV subdivides the disorder into purging and non-purging types.

Epidemiology

- Although onset of the disorder is generally in the mid to late teens, it is unusual to present for help before the early twenties
- Distributed right across the social classes
- 90% + of cases are female
- There is a lower prevalence in developing countries and rural areas
- Rare before the age of 13
- In adult women, the incidence is 1–1.5%
- There may, but does not need to be a preceding history of anorexia nervosa
- In teenagers, bulimia may be seen alongside other externalizing teenage behaviours, such as sexual promiscuity, drug-taking, drinking, and self-harming
- There was probably a true increase in incidence in the 1980–1990s, but it is not clear if this has now slowed down or not
- Associated with westernized lifestyle.

Aetiology

Similar factors contribute to the aetiology of bulimia nervosa as are found for anorexia nervosa (📖 p. 338). Additional risk factors particularly in adolescence include:

- Adverse family life events
- Family history of obesity
- Parental substance misuse
- Family history of affective disorder
- Poor social network
- Critical parents.

Temperament

In contrast to anorexia nervosa, bulimia is associated with high expression of emotions, impulsivity, and a chaotic lifestyle.

Neurobiology

The involvement of endogenous opiates and serotonin in satiety regulation has been postulated as contributing to the aetiology of binge eating.

Assessment

Primary care

Young people commonly approach adults outwith health services for help with eating issues. Hence, a school teacher or youth leader may often be the first to hear about the problem. Adolescents should be encouraged to seek a consultation with their GP, preferably in the company of a parent. The SCOFF questions are recommended to assist GPs in determining which patients should be further investigated. Although these are designed for adults, the general principles are useful for adolescents and are a good starting point.

SCOFF Questions

- Do you make yourself **S**ick because you are uncomfortably full?
- Do you worry about having lost **C**ontrol over what you eat?
- Have you recently lost more than **O**ne stone in a 3-month period?
- Do you believe yourself to be **F**at, when others say you are too thin?
- Would you say that **F**ood dominates your life?

Morgan JF, Reid f, Lacey JH (1999) The SCOFF questionnaire assessment of a new screening tool for eating disorders. *BMJ* **319**: 1467–8.

If further investigation suggests a possible eating disorder, then the young person should be referred to a specialist CAMHS.

Secondary care

Assessment of bulimia nervosa, or of any child or young person who presents with a binge eating disorder should follow the same general protocol as for anorexia nervosa. Because of the high risks associated with anorexia nervosa, it is essential to exclude this diagnosis as part of the assessment process. The family should be involved in the assessment process. Hence, assessment of bulimia nervosa needs to include:

- History of the disorder including a detailed eating history
- Full psychiatric assessment of the individual
- Developmental history
- Psychosocial history, including school attendance and attainment
- Family interview with family history included. This should cover the family mental health history, as well as any history of eating disorders
- Assessment of physical health
- Appropriate physical investigations.

Possible physical signs

- Particular issues related to bulimia:
  - Cardiac; arrhythmias/bradycardia
  - Electrolyte disturbances
  - Oesophageal/gastric ulceration or perforation
  - Constipation/diarrhoea
  - Erosion of tooth enamel
  - Russell's sign (callused skin over finger joints)
- Others more generally related to eating disorders
  - General listlessness
  - Dry hair and skin
  - Sallow complexion
  - Brittle nails and hair
  - Thinning scalp hair
  - Lack of subcutaneous fat
  - Wearing baggy, disguising clothing
  - Lanugo hair
  - Hypotension with postural hypotension
  - Cold extremities
  - Cyanosis
  - Failure of development of secondary sexual characteristics
  - Swelling of the parotid glands

Physical examination will indicate which investigations are required. The potential range is the same as for anorexia nervosa.

Most patients with bulimia nervosa will be at or near the normal expected weight for their height.

Differential diagnosis and co-morbidity

Differential diagnosis
- Eating disorder not otherwise specified (EDNOS)
- Upper gastrointestinal disorder with repeated vomiting
- Depressive disorder
- Brain tumour or other space occupying lesion
- Substance misuse.

Co-morbidity
- Anorexia nervosa
- Impulsive externalizing behaviours, e.g. self-harm, excessive consumption of alcohol, drug taking, sexual promiscuity
- Depressive disorder
- Anxiety disorder
- Family dysfunction
- Body dysmorphic disorder.

Clinical example

Eva was a 20-year-old art student, in the 3rd year of an honours degree and was living away from home in a flat with 3 other young women. She had spent much of her first 2 years at University having a good time, and had consumed a substantial quantity of alcohol and experimented with recreational use of drugs, mainly cannabis and ecstasy. She was in a relationship with a young man of 24 who was an up and coming fashion designer. Eva was viewed enviously by her friends who considered her mature, attractive, and slightly 'edgy'. She rarely visited her family home, but when she did, her parents were critical of her friends and frequently raised the issue of how much they expected from Eva in the future.

Eva developed toothache 2 days before a significant assignment was due in and was forced to make an appointment with the campus dentist. At the consultation it was discovered that she had a dental abscess and required further treatment. As an incidental finding, the dentist noticed that the enamel on Eva's teeth was seriously eroded. She asked Eva about her eating and recommended that she made an appointment to see the student health service.

When Eva attended, the practice nurse administered the SCOFF questions and arranged for Eva to see the doctor for further assessment. The GP asked Eva about her eating history and discovered that she had been inducing vomiting as a means of controlling her weight from the age of 14 years. She gave a history of childhood obesity and being taken to see the doctor by her mother at an early age. She was put on a strict diet monitored by the dietician and lost a significant amount of weight. However, she had soon found that her appetite was getting out of control and had resorted to binging on large quantities of sweets, crisps, and biscuits. Soon Eva was binge-eating up to 4 times a week and controlling her weight by vomiting.

Eva's mother was delighted with her daughter's weight loss and began to put pressure on her to achieve in other areas. Although she was an intelligent girl, Eva found studying difficult, but was talented in Art so concentrated on this instead. To Eva's parents this was always second best and Eva was constantly compared unfavourably to her older brother, who had gone to Oxford to study engineering.

Soon Eva was spending more and more time away from home with a group of 'cool' friends who were into experimenting with alcohol and drugs. As the pressure mounted on Eva, she began cutting herself, but managed to stop this after a few months with support from her school guidance teacher.

Eva left home to go to university at the first possible opportunity and from the outset rarely went home. She continued her previous pattern of behaviour, and managed to conceal the binge-eating and vomiting from everyone until she attended the dentist.

Eva's doctor recommended that she attend the psychologist at the student counselling service for advice with her eating problem. Bloods taken by the GP indicated a degree of electrolyte disturbance and by this time Eva was beginning to realize that she may be seriously damaging her health, and so agreed to the referral being made.

The psychologist who saw Eva took a full history and uncovered the unhappiness and poor self-esteem that had led to Eva embarking on her eating disorder path in the first place. The psychologist used motivational interviewing techniques to engage Eva in the process of change and recommended a structured cognitive behavioural therapy (CBT) self-help manual that Eva could use to assist her regain control over her eating. One month later, Eva had reduced her binges to once weekly and was vomiting only occasionally. The psychologist decided to have a few sessions face to face with Eva before sending her off with her self-help material again.

Eva did well, and as well as gaining control over her binge-eating and vomiting, managed to reduce her alcohol intake. She was able to apply herself better to her work and achieved a first class degree. She remained distant from her family who were not able to accept her chosen career as a fabric designer.

Management: pharmacological

Although high dose SSRI antidepressants have been licensed for the treatment of binge eating disorder in adults, this is not the case for children and young people under the age of 18. The evidence base for the use of antidepressants to treat bulimia nervosa in young people has not been established. Pharmacological treatment should therefore only be considered in the context of treatment by a specialist multi-disciplinary team. As presentation of young people under the age of 18 is extremely unusual, it follows that the use of antidepressant medication will be even more so.

Nevertheless, SSRIs (fluoxetine) are licensed for use in specific circumstances in patients under the age of 18 if recommended by a specialist. Within the context of a CAMHS multi-disciplinary team treating a young person with bulimia nervosa, it may on occasion be appropriate to use medication as an adjunct to psychological therapy.

Management: psychological

Although bulimia nervosa is much less dangerous to health and development than anorexia nervosa, its relative rarity in child and adolescent practice means that it is usually best managed within a multi-disciplinary team, with the appropriate range of skills to deliver a comprehensive treatment programme. As with all other young patients with an eating disorder, the family should be involved in the treatment from the start. Some older adolescents who present for treatment may not wish their family to be involved, but the team should still do their best to try to persuade them. Nevertheless, if the young person is adamant, this should not debar them from treatment.

Bulimia nervosa can almost always be managed on an outpatient basis, and a treatment package generally consists of a combination of individual and family therapies.

Appropriate individual psychotherapies

- Motivational interviewing
- Structured self help manualized CBT
- CBT
- Interpersonal therapy.

Like anorexia nervosa, the crucial factors in success of treatment are engagement and continuity of the therapist.

Family therapy

Families should be engaged in education about bulimia and in supporting the young person in their efforts to overcome their difficulties. A problem-solving approach is often useful. If family dynamic issues that are interfering with the progress of treatment are encountered, then intervention should be negotiated with the family as part of the treatment package.

Prognosis, course, and outcome

There are few outcome studies for bulimia nervosa that focus on the younger age group. Studies of community samples of women with bulimia nervosa often describe early symptoms of the eating disorder and some describe a move from an adolescent anorexia to bulimia in later years.

Outcomes from adult studies

- Full recovery in up to 50%
- 66–75% show at least partial recovery at 10-year follow-up
- Longer follow-up leads to lower relapse rates
- Bone density follow-up shows no osteopenia or osteoporosis in recovered bulimic patients.

Other eating disorders of childhood

Although anorexia nervosa and bulimia nervosa represent the commonest eating disorder diagnoses in childhood and adolescence, many young patients have disturbances of eating that do not fit neatly into these categories. Although not all are recognized in classification systems, these are very useful in describing the variety of eating difficulties encountered in CAMH clinics.

Eating disorder not otherwise specified (EDNOS)

- Includes around 40% of young patients with an eating disorder
- Have core cognitive distortions associated with anorexia and bulimia nervosa
- Do not meet full ICD-10 or DSM-IV criteria for diagnosis of anorexia or bulimia
- Assessment and treatment is as for the above.

Food avoidance emotional disorder (FAED)

- Primary emotional disorder
- Food is a central issue in the disorder
- Do not have the cognitive pre-occupations of anorexia or bulimic
- Often very physically unwell.

Selective eating

- Narrow range of foods
- Often consume mainly carbohydrate
- Usually normal growth
- Calorie intake usually within normal range
- Commoner in boys
- High impact on social development
- No pre-occupation with body image
- Usually stops in adolescence due to peer pressure.

Restrictive eating

- Small food intake
- No emotional difficulties
- May be small for their age and can be a problem at puberty.

Food refusal

- Normal behaviour in pre-school children
- Usually underlying worry or misery
- Not consistent in pattern of eating. Usually resolves once the underlying problem is addressed.

Specific phobias

- Often has a clear precipitant, e.g. a choking incident
- Can generalize to other foods rapidly leading to extremely low intake leading to very low weight
- None of the cognitive features of anorexia nervosa.

Pervasive refusal syndrome

- General, and often complete, refusals to eat, drink, manage self-care etc.

- Can often be very ill and can be mistaken for anorexia nervosa
- Can be life-threatening
- Do not have the fear of fatness and body image distortion associated with anorexia
- Not a depressive illness
- Very rare
- Usually requires hospitalization.

As a general rule, assessment and treatment of any of the disorders should follow that already outlined for anorexia and bulimia in child and adolescent patients. Families should always be involved in the consultations and in treatment planning. Attention should be paid to physical health issues, especially in the growing child and at puberty to ensure an optimal health outcome. Treatment is usually multi-modal and involves a team approach. Occasionally, these disorders can raise child protection issues and, in these cases, advice should be sought from the local social work department.

Recommended reading

NICE Collaboration for Mental Health. (2004) *Eating Disorders; Core Interventions in the Management of Anorexia Nervosa, Bulimia Nervosa and Related Eating Disorders.* Gaskell.

Lask B, Bryant-Waugh R. (2007) *Eating Disorders in Chilhood and Adolescence,* 3rd edn. Routledge.

Treasure J, Schmidt U, van Furth E. (2005) *The Essential Handbook of Eating Disorders.* Wiley.

Obesity

Definitions

Obesity in children and adolescents is not, by itself, a psychiatric disorder, indeed in our current climate it is more of a public health issue. However, certain conditions have to be excluded in the investigation of obesity and, without doubt, obesity in childhood is the cause of much misery, and can be a precursor to psychological problems and, indeed, to psychiatric disorder.

Body Mass Index (BMI: 📖 p. 336 for definition and sample calculation) is now widely used in the calculation of healthy body size and defines both obesity and underweight. Although BMI is a reliable measure in adults, it is of more variable application in growing children and young people. It is therefore important when treating a young population to always refer to the appropriate BMI centile chart that allows comparisons of the calculated BMI against that expected for age and gender. Figure 25.1 shows a sample centile chart for boys in the UK. The girls' chart is very similar.

Defining obesity in children using BMI centile charts

Clinical obesity	≥98th centile
Epidemiological use	
Overweight	≥85th centile
Obese	≥95th centile

In older adolescents who have completed puberty, adult definitions of obesity using BMI calculations are more applicable. Table 25.1, published by the World Health Organization (WHO), shows the BMI ranges for healthy weights in adults.

Table 25.1 The international classification of adults underweight, overweight, and obesity according to BMI.[*]

Classification	BMI (kg/m^2), principal cut-off points
Underweight	<18.50
Severe thinness	<16.00
Moderate thinness	16.00–16.99
Mild thinness	17.00–18.49
Normal range	18.50–24.99
Overweight	≥25.00
Pre-obese	25.00–29.99
Obese	≥30.00
Obese class I	30.00–34.99
Obese class II	35.00–39.99
Obese class III	≥40.00

[*] Reproduced from the WHO Global Database on Body Mass Index

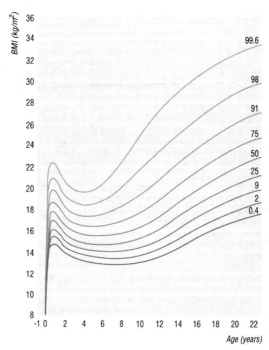

Fig. 25.1 BMI centile chart. Reproduced with permission from Prentice, A. M. (1998) *BMJ* **317**: 1401–2.

Epidemiology and aetiology

Epidemiology

Obesity in childhood has become a major international public health concern. Studies, particularly those conducted in developed countries, but also some from developing countries, have consistently demonstrated rising rates of obesity amongst children, adolescents, and adults, and much public funding has been devoted to health education and promotion in an attempt to reverse this trend.

Current published prevalence figures for obesity in children show:
- 1991: 1 in 5 children in the USA was overweight
- In England: 2006/07 school year, 1 in 4 children in reception classes was either overweight or obese, and 1 in 3 in Year 6 classes
- At least 10% of all 6-year-olds and 17% of all 15-year-olds in the UK are now clinically obese
- Whist the percentage of overweight boys and girls is almost equal, the prevalence of obesity is significantly higher in boys
- Prevalence is higher in urban than rural areas
- In developed countries, obesity levels are higher in lower socioeconomic groups
- Prevalence rates in England are highest in the North East, the West Midlands, and London
- Recent prevalence rates are higher than predicted from earlier studies, numbers of obese children have tripled in the last 20 years
- 2004: 10% of children in China were obese, rising by 8% per year
- The vast majority of cases are simple obesity
- Less than 1% of cases of obesity are due to an underlying medical condition.

Aetiology

Lifestyle

There is little doubt that lifestyle choices make the largest contribution to the genesis of obesity. These include:
- Excess consumption of high calorie food especially highly processed, high fat, 'fast' foods
- Too little physical exercise—not taking part in sport, avoiding physical education classes, and not going out to play
- A sedentary lifestyle—spending lengthy periods watching television, playing video games and using computers
- Snacking between meals
- Bad family eating habits—not sharing meal times, eating while watching the television or other activity.

Genetics

Although obesity *per se* is not genetically determined, genes controlling appetite and satiety have been identified, and may contribute to patterns of inheritance to a tendency to obesity in some families.

Medical causes

Medical causes of obesity in children are rare, but important.

- Hypothyroidism
- Overproduction of steroids
- Prader–Willi syndrome
- Certain drug treatments, including steroids and some psychoactive drugs, such as atypical antipsychotics and antidepressants.

Assessment

In most developed countries, and many others in the third world, children are screened from birth onwards in relation to their physical health and development. Indeed, screening for obesity should begin antenatally with assessment of the parents' weight, lifestyle, and eating habits. Given that preventing obesity is much more effective than treating, attention paid to mothers' eating and feeding regimes for infants is the first step in assessing the risks of obesity in their children.

Screening

Children are normally regularly screened by health visiting staff, general practitioners, and school nurses. Those who are gaining weight more quickly than they should be need to be identified early. It should be remembered that there is a great deal of individual variation in growth and it is important that mothers do not feel persecuted by overzealous attention to their child's weight. However, children identified as potentially obese should be assessed more thoroughly and their weight and height measured over a period of time to monitor changes in their BMI. If this shows evidence of significant increase or if it exceeds the recommended limits, then a more in depth assessment should be undertaken.

Detailed assessment

- Medical history
- Eating history including a diet diary if necessary
- Full physical examination
- Measurement of height and weight
- If indicated, then referral to a paediatrician for further investigation may be indicated.

Paediatric assessment

The most important reason for such a referral is to exclude any medical cause for obesity, and its most important function will often be to reassure the parents that there is nothing physically wrong with their child and to better engage them in attempts to treat the obesity.

However, a medical assessment should also identify any physical complications of obesity, such as cardiac problems.

Co-morbidity and consequences of obesity

Co-morbid conditions

- Some learning disability syndromes, such as Prader–Willi syndrome in which obesity plays a central part
- Endocrine disorders
- Rarely, specific brain tumours (pituitary, hypothalamus).

Physical consequences

Although many of the consequences of childhood obesity do not manifest until adult life, clinicians are increasingly seeing young people with early onset of cardiovascular disease and endocrine disorders. Complications of obesity include:

- Raised blood pressure
- Abnormal blood lipids
- Increased risk of type 2 diabetes
- Atherosclerosis
- Coronary artery disease
- Poor fitness leading to breathlessness
- Painful joints
- Abnormalities of foot structure.

Psychological and social consequences

- Poor self-esteem
- Depression
- Anxiety disorders
- Disordered eating
- Bulimia nervosa
- Bullying
- Stigmatization
- Social exclusion and isolation.

Management

Prevention

In recent years, resources have been committed to intervention programmes designed to reduce rates of obesity in children. Many, although not all, of these have focused on school-based programmes. Public education programmes, such as the campaign to get people to eat 5 portions of fruit and vegetables a day, have promoted healthy eating habits. Initiatives such as the 'Healthy Schools' and 'Healthy Eating Schools' programmes in the UK, and interventions involving whole town approaches in France, have adopted large population methods to try to reduce obesity. Supermarkets and other food suppliers are labelling food with calorie content and offering lower calorie alternatives. Even some of the fast food chains are now promoting 'healthier' options on their menus.

Increasingly governments are encouraging populations to pay attention to exercise, as well as eating. Investment in play parks and sports facilities, as well as increasing availability of physical education in the school curriculum is evidence of a commitment to this agenda.

As yet, little evidence has been accumulated about the effectiveness of these interventions in the long term in preventing or treating obesity in children and young people.

Primary care

The vast majority of obese and overweight children and young people will be treated in the community, either within a school or local health context. Treatment should only be undertaken with children after careful consideration as it can further stigmatize children who may already be isolated and feel depressed about their size. Scottish Intercollegiate Guidelines Network (SIGN) Guidelines (2003) suggest that treatment should only be offered to children when:

- A child is defined as obese (BMI >/= 98th centile) and
- The child and family are perceived as ready and willing to make the necessary life changes.

Aims of treatment

- Weight maintenance, rather than weight loss, with the expectation that the child will 'grow into their weight'
- Educating the child and family about eating awareness and parenting
- Encouraging small incremental changes in lifestyle
- Stressing the importance of monitoring eating and activity to prevent lapsing into old habits.

Families need to be regularly supported, especially in the initial stages of treatment, and positive reinforcement to the child or young person is especially important. The role of dieting classes in treatment for children is controversial. Most classes are aimed at an adult audience and particular skills are needed in working with children. Generally, this is not an avenue advocated for children and young people.

Secondary care

On occasion, it may be necessary to refer to a paediatrician for a small number of cases.

- The main purpose is usually to exclude underlying medical causes, but can also include
  - treatment of co-morbidity
  - management of severe obesity
- Weight management may include an expectation of very gradual weight loss (up to 0.5 kg per month)
- Referral to a CAMHS or psychologist for assessment and treatment of co-morbid psychological symptoms may be indicated.

Psychological management

If a co-morbid psychiatric diagnosis is made, then the patient should be offered the appropriate treatment. Otherwise, cognitive behavioural techniques may be helpful in the management of self-esteem, low mood, or other distress associated with obesity. Behavioural approaches can also be helpful to parents who are trying to help their child manage their weight problem.

Other treatments

Other physical treatments for obesity are generally contra-indicated in this population. No medications are licensed for the treatment of obesity in children or adolescents in the UK.

Prognosis, course, and outcomes

- There is an association between obesity in childhood and obesity in adulthood
- The risk is higher if one or both parents are obese
- Obesity in childhood tends to predispose to co-morbid complications in adulthood, such as diabetes and hypertension
- Stigmatization of overweight children tends to discriminate against them in school, and later employment leading to underachievement and poor self-esteem
- Successful treatment of obesity in childhood is largely dependent on the motivation and commitment of both the patient and their family.

Clinical examples

Public health initiative

A secondary school decided to remove vending machines from the concourse to promote healthier eating choices. The school senior management met with the Pupil Council to discuss this. The whole school already had healthy eating information as part of their Citizenship lessons so the pupils have quite a high level of knowledge in this area. The pupils were reluctant to do away with all the vending machines as they are a congregating point during break periods. As a compromise, the staff agreed to install free water dispensers in the same area for pupil use and to allow pupils to bring water bottles to school to fill.

The pupils then asked to discuss the idea of healthier options on sale in the school tuck shop. The staff agreed that, for a trial period, the shop would stock a range of fruit, nuts, and cereal bars, and limit the choice of sweets available. They all agreed that senior pupils would monitor this and report back after one term on the popularity of the move.

Primary care

11-year-old Emma was taken to her GP by her mother. She had been teased at school because she is overweight, a problem since early childhood. Emma's mother is very slim, but her father is overweight. Emma had only just begun puberty and had not had her menarche yet. After a brief consultation, the GP asked Emma and her mother to keep a food and exercise diet over the next week, and come back to see him. When they returned the next week, it was clear that Emma was exceeding her daily requirement of calories considerably. Her BMI was on the 96th centile and she was of average height for her age. The GP suggested a number of ways for Emma to increase her exercise and gave advice about weight maintenance. He suggested that Emma have weekly visits to the practice nurse to help keep her motivated and stressed the importance of family support. One month later, Emma returned and had successfully managed to keep her weight steady. She had joined the local swimming club and was enjoying the competitive aspect of her new sport. Her father had also begun to change his diet and they were both determined to be in better shape for their summer holiday in France.

Secondary care

Peter, a 14-year-old boy with Prader–Willi syndrome, was mildly learning disabled and attended a support base in a local school. He was generally happy, but tended to get very down because he could not play football with the boys in his class due to breathlessness. After an assessment at the paediatric clinic, Peter was found to be hypertensive and the risks of his obesity were explained to his mother. She explained that the family had tended to use food to placate Peter from an early age, partly because of his huge appetite, but also because he appeared to have little motivation for anything else. The football interest was a new thing for him. Peter's difficulties were managed by a combination of referral to the dietician, who recommended a special low calorie, but satisfying diet for him; and referral to a physiotherapist to help him with an exercise programme. Peter's mother was given advice on management strategies from the clinical psychologist and this helped her find other ways of managing Peter's behaviour.

Recommended reading

BMA (2006) *Childhood Obesity in Scotland*, member's debate in Scottish Parliament, February 2006. Available at: http://www.bma.org.uk/ap.nsf/content/obesity (accessed 2 April 2008).

Department of Health *heapital improvement information*. Available at: http://www.dh.gov.uk/en/Publichealth/Healthimprovement/Obesity/index.htm (accessed 2 April 2008).

Scottish Government. (2005) *Childhood Obesity Statistics*. Available at: http://www.scotland.gov.uk/News/Releases/2005/12/12124143 (accessed 2 April 2008).

Scottish Intercollegiate Guidelines Network (SIGN) (2003) *Management of obesity in children and young people*, No. 69. Available at: http://www.sign.ac.uk/guidelines/fulltext/69/index.html (accessed 2 April 2008).

Treasure J, Schmidt U, van Furth E. (2005) *The Essential Handbook of Eating Disorders*. Wiley, London.

Substance abuse

Definitions

In developed countries, the majority of adolescents will, at least once, experiment with illegal and potentially harmful substances. Clearly, not all of them will require psychiatric help and, hence, a definition or threshold for intervention is required.

- Various terminologies exist, including unsanctioned use, hazardous use, dysfunctional use, harmful use, and dependence. These definitions are at times overlapping and often confusing
- Whilst it is sometimes helpful to separate dependence from non-dependence, this is more relevant to adult populations. For adolescents, it may be better to consider defining stages of substance use, not all of which are necessarily harmful.

Curiosity → Experimentation → Regular Use → Harmful Use → Dependence

It is also important to remember that:

- The amount of substance use that is socially acceptable varies considerably across different cultural contexts
- Any drug, prescribed or illicit, can meet this definition, as well as pastimes such as gambling
- The impact of a drug can be related to both the direct effects of intoxication and to indirect effects, such as the illegal nature of the use
- The resulting harmful effects of a drug will therefore vary according to several factors beyond simple quantity and type of drug, such that a threshold of amount 'drug required to cause harm' is not easily definable.

An overall definition that covers most of the above issues is that from The Advisory Council on the Misuse of Drugs, who define someone with problem drug use as:

Any person who experiences social, psychological, physical or legal problems related to intoxication and/or regular excessive consumption and/or dependence as a consequence of his own use of drugs or other chemical substances.

Epidemiology

Although substance abuse peaks in the twenties the vast majority will have begun abusing prior to the age of 18. The nature of substance abuse means that reliable data is difficult to achieve, particularly as many studies rely on self-report. Data is often difficult to disentangle, which can make it problematic, for example, to know whether a substance has simply been tried once or is being used regularly. Current trends are summarised overleaf posite.

However, it must be noted that many types of drug use vary with local or national sociocultural trends, and as a consequence the availability and acceptability of particular drugs may increase or decrease within particular areas or peer groups.

Current substance abuse prevalence and trends in young people

Estimates can vary and subjective questioning can be inaccurate—in one study of a group admitting cocaine use, 42% then denied use when re-questioned. However, description of overall patterns is possible:

Alcohol

The most commonly abused substance by adolescents with up to of 30% of 13-year-olds admitting to the use of alcohol at least once a week. Binge drinking patterns continue to predominate, with little evidence of adult patterns of dependence. In the UK, the current trend is towards a smaller number of school age children using alcohol, but of increasing levels of consumption in those who do drink.

Tobacco

Tobacco use via cigarettes in young people is decreasing in Western societies. This trend is perhaps partly related to increasing legislation and the increasing unacceptability of public smoking in all age groups.

Cannabis

In one study, 5% of 11–16-year-olds in the UK had used cannabis at least once, with rates increasing significantly in the late teens. Prevalence is probably higher in the US, but overall trends towards increased rates of use globally. This is concerning in view of the increasing evidence for the contribution of cannabis to schizophrenia aetiology.

Inhaled solvents

Exact prevalence figures for use are difficult to find, but UK deaths from inhaled solvents (all ages) were stable at around 60 p.a. in a 2001 survey, most of these were due to inhalation of lighter fuel, and half were under 17 years of age. Death rates were higher in the early 1990s.

Heroin

Use in under 18's has increased in the past decade in many countries including the UK. Increased availability, including of inhalable and smokeable forms, together with cultural changes may be partly responsible. At least 15% of users will switch to IV use within 1 year, with its attendant additional risks.

Cocaine

A 2004 US national survey suggested that 2.4% of the 12–17-year-old age group used cocaine at some point in their life. 0.5% of 11–15-year-olds in the UK admitted to use between 2004 and 2005. There is a trend for increased use in the USA and UK partly because of increasing availability and cultural acceptability.

MDMA (ecstasy)

This along with the other 'party' drugs (GHB, ketamine, rohypnol) do not account for a large proportion of child and adolescent substance problems, but are being experimented with at increasingly young ages.

Metamphetamine (MA, speed)

A US review of 12th graders indicates a downward trend of life-time MA use from 1999 to 2005 (4.7–2.5%); however local areas of higher levels of use exist.

Other stimulants

Frequently concerns are raised as to the illicit use of stimulants used in the treatment of ADHD/hyperkinetic disorder. 'Diversion' of stimulants can range from swapping/buying tablets in the playground to use by adult carers in an attempt to lose weight or improve concentration. The difficulty in truly abusing the drug [only intravenous (IV) use can produce a high truly mimicking amphetamine] means that in practice stimulant abuse is rarely problematic.

Benzodiazepines and other anxiolytics

There is little reliable data. Use may be mainly as 'downers' to counteract their 'upper' effects or deal with the 'come down' associated with speed and ecstasy.

Steroids

Only US data is available. There between 4 and 12% of male adolescents have used anabolic steroids to improve performance at sport or alter body size. No UK data is available, but the rates are almost certainly less than the US.

LSD/hallucinogens

Use is down since a peak in the 1990s, and now used only by a small minority. Reliable data regarding hallucinogenic (magic) mushroom are not available.

Aetiology

If drugs are common why do they only cause problems for some young people?

Psychological, social and biological risk factors are all important; their interplay dictates the initiation, quantity and impact of substance use. The strength of genetic factors (which will include temperamental, metabolic and central response differences) in particular is emphasized by twin study findings, for example, where the presence of alcohol dependence in the biological father raises the risk of the same in adopted-away male offspring.

Psychopathological factors
- Temperamental factors, such as impulsivity (little thought given prior to substance use) and insecurity (the substance allows escape or temporarily improved self-esteem)
- Cohort studies show that aggressive and antisocial behaviour in young boys raises risk of substance abuse, which is likely to result from a combination of the temperamental factors (above) and social factors.

Social factors
- The social acceptability of substance use and availability of drugs within cultures and subcultures has a strong bearing on the initiation of substance abuse
- Personal experiences of individuals may increase or reduce their risk – for example:
  - **Risk increased by:** a overly strict tee-total parent triggering rebellion and experimentation
  - **Risk decreased by:** an abusive alcohol-abusing parent triggering a revulsion or fear of alcohol.

Biological factors
There is increasing research interest in the biochemical differences between individuals with regard to response to various substances. This includes:
- **Pharmacodynamic variation**: e.g. differential response of craving and reward systems (such as those located in the amygdala)
- **pharmacokinetic variation:** e.g. variability in metabolic drug clearance (which may also alter the profile of unpleasant effects associated with the drug).

Prevention strategies

Prevention strategies range from community or school-based educational schemes, on the one hand, to the treatment of psychopathology in young people at increased risk of substance abuse on the other. This would include, for example, treatment of early onset behavioural disorders, attention deficit hyperactivity disorder (ADHD) and mood/anxiety disorders.

Educational prevention programmes are difficult to evaluate. There is, however, some evidence that targeting programmes on high risk groups and the use of peer-delivered messages may be effective strategies.

Peer pressure aside, it should be noted that, in the case of alcohol, the manufacturers' advertising budgets consistently dwarf those allocated to prevention and education schemes. At the time of writing, the 'do it' message may remain stronger than the 'don't do it' for many young people.

Screening

Substance abuse problems appear to be one of the more frequently missed child and adolescent mental health presentations, particularly in primary care. This may, in part, relate to the difficulties clinicians have in defining who does and doesn't have a problem. These can be significantly reduced by the use of structured screening methods prior to a full assessment.

The use of screening in this population remains somewhat controversial Questions include:

- **Who should be screened?** All school children? All primary care attendees? Those at high risk only?
- **When should one screen?** At all primary care visits? At all secondary care visits?
- **How best to screen?**
  - Subjective tests (such as self-completed/clinician completed questionnaires)
  - Objective tests, such as urine screening? With/without consent? (Voluntary, but with automatic suspicion if refused?)

For many authorities, a validated, but very brief and simple screening tool is recommended as the first step. However, those that are used in the adult population, such as the 'CAGE' and the Alcohol Use Disorder Identification Test may be less appropriate for child and adolescent populations.

Validated alcohol and drug abuse screens for adolescent populations include The Substance Abuse Subtle Screening Inventory, Adolescent version (SASSI–A) and the CRAFFT (☐ opposite), both of which (although developed in the USA) may be a suitable for use in young people in the UK. Longer screening instruments are also available.

Although there is no clear evidence on which to make a decision, screening is probably best used with a young person in a primary care or initial secondary care assessment situation for whom there is reason to suspect problem drug use or who is in a high risk population.

Possible reasons to consider screening for substance abuse:

- Sudden drop in academic performance and/or motivation
- Sudden increase in school disciplinary action
- Recent unexplained loss of interest in sports/pastimes
- Rapid changes in mood—low mood, irritability
- Early drinking (under 15 years old)
- Onset of antisocial behaviour, association with peers with known substance abuse.

The CRAFFT substance abuse screening questionnaire

Score of >2 indicates likely problem use.

C   Have you ever been in a **c**ar driven by someone (including yourself) who was 'high' or had been using alcohol or drugs?

R   Do you ever use alcohol or drugs to **r**elax, feel better about yourself, or fit in?

A   Do you ever use alcohol or drugs while you **a**lone?

F   Do you ever **f**orget things you did while using alcohol or drugs?

F   Do your **f**amily or **f**riends ever tell you that you should cut down on your drinking or drug use?

T   Have you ever been in **t**rouble while you were using alcohol or drugs?

Assessment

General assessment

Assessment is often usefully initiated by recording current amount and frequency of use.

Broader issues

- Assessment of the family environment and functioning is of particular importance
- Denial of drug use is very common on the part of both parents and children
- Degrees of confidentiality and use of information must be clear to the clinician and the child/young person
- Other sources of information may be required, which may also risk conflicts of confidentiality, for example, urine toxicology
- A non-judgmental approach is vital to ensure accurate and effective evaluation.

Assessing for dependence

Although dependence is less common in young people, the presence of a dependence pattern is important both in management planning and prognosis, as it suggests that the use may be less likely to reduce at the end of adolescence (as substance use often does) and, instead, persist into adulthood.

Signs of dependence:

- **Tolerance:** a need for markedly increased amounts of the substance to achieve intoxication or the desired effects, or a markedly diminished effect following continued use of the same amount of the substance
- **Withdrawal:** manifested by either a withdrawal syndrome for the substance or the taking of either the same, or a closely related substance in order to relieve or avoid withdrawal symptoms
- The substance is frequently taken in larger amounts or over a longer period than intended
- The presence of a persistent desire to take the substance or unsuccessful efforts to cut down or control its use
- Spending a great deal of time in the activities required to obtain the substance, use the substance, or recover from its effects
- Either giving up or reducing participation in important social, occupational, or recreational activities as a result of substance use
- Continuing to use the substance despite knowledge that it is causing or exacerbating persistent physical or psychological problems.

Assessing for additional and related impairments

Many of those with substance misuse are also impaired within the following domains and an assessment should be comprehensive enough to identify:

- Mood/cognitive/behavioural problems
- Educational difficulties
- Social/recreational difficulties (including risk taking behaviours)
- Forensic issues
- Problems with physical health.

Urine toxicology testing

Urine testing in the UK usually occurs after the sudden onset of erratic behaviour in an adolescent, and is often in the setting of admission to an accident and emergency department or an inpatient unit. This acute diagnostic use is perhaps less complex than the use of urine testing in a more routine out-patient setting. Under these circumstances, coercion, or coversion should be avoided.

There is often confusion as to how long a specific drug may remain detectable, which as shown in Table 26.1, can vary significantly:

Table 26.1 Urine toxicology testing—applicability in terms of time elapsed since drug used*

Substance	Half-life (h)	Time detectable (days after last use)
Amphetamine	10–15	1–2
Benzodiazepine	20–90	2–9
Cocaine	0.8–6	0.2–4
Opiate	2–4	1–2
Phencyclidine	7–16	2–8
Cannabis, acute use	10–40	2–8
Cannabis, chronic use		14–42

*Source: AACAP Practice parameter on assessment of child and adolescent substance abuse 2005. *J Am Aced Child Adolesc Psychist* **44**:6.

Co-morbidity

Substance abuse is frequently co-morbid with other psychiatric conditions. Some will predate the substance abuse, some will be as a consequence of it, and some will allow it to perpetuate.

Estimates of co-morbidity in adult substance misusers range between 30 and 60%. It is likely that the rates in adolescents are the same or higher. Therefore, co-morbidity should be suspected until proven otherwise.

Behavioural/conduct disorders

Probably the greatest risk factor for developing substance misuse in the young is the presence of conduct disorder, particularly when associated with deprived social circumstances. These factors are also associated with increased rates of family discord and parental substance use.

ADHD/hyperkinetic disorder

Impulsivity and the frequent existence of social difficulties for an untreated ADHD sufferer may place them at higher risk of initiating and perpetuating drug use. However, evidence suggests that much of the association between ADHD and substance misuse is mediated by co-morbid conduct disorder. Appropriate treatment of ADHD in childhood can, however, reduce the risk of future substance abuse by a factor of two, bringing it down to that of the normal population.

This is contrary to the notion that the use of stimulant medication could raise the risk of future substance abuse because of a 'priming' effect or through the increased availability of stimulant drugs. As described elsewhere, the 'abuseability' of even immediate release prescribed stimulants is low.

Mood and emotional disorders

May both predispose to and be a consequence of substance abuse.

Psychotic disorders

Most frequently psychosis occurs as a consequence of drug use. This can be either as an acute short-lived psychotic episode or as the initiating event in a chronic psychotic illness, such as schizophrenia. Predisposed individuals may precipitate psychosis even by single use of a substance, with cannabis and metamphetamine being the most common precipitants.

Management

It is important that the clinicians approach to those with problem drug use should be *non-judgemental* and *unconditionally accepting*, with *positive regard*, and attempts to support the user in making their own decisions. Without this *Rogerian* stance, intervention is likely to meet 'intense and entrenched resistance'.

In the UK there are very few specialist substance abuse treatment centres for the under-18 age group. Services in the US are much better developed. In some ways, however, generic child and adolescent mental health services (CAMHS) may be better equipped to deal with substance abuse in this age group because of their skills in managing the extensive co-morbidity associated with substance misuse, and their experience at involving families, schools and social services in packages of care. However, generic CAMHS staff will often feel deskilled when faced with managing a young person's substance misuse problems. It is therefore likely that the ideal situation will involve co-working arrangements

There is little data to support a preference of inpatient over community-based treatment approaches. Indeed, the importance of addressing community pressures, and the problems that may be caused when 'importing' a heavy drug-using young person into an existing inpatient community, suggest the latter approach may be preferable.

Some data suggest that misuse and abuse of harder drugs, like heroin and cocaine are more amenable to intervention than 'everyday' stuff like alcohol and cannabis.

Cognitive and behavioural approaches

The nature of substance abuse means that the patient usually needs to make the decision to stop use for their own reasons before further treatment approaches can be instituted. This, together with the principles described above, forms the goal of motivational interviewing. Motivational interviewing involves using techniques that will, for example, help the user understand the costs associated with their substance use and challenging their perception of substance misuse as a relatively positive aspect of their life.

By encouraging the benefits vs. the drawbacks of particular behaviours, and by enhancing the *cognitive dissonance* arising from current substance abuse activity, the patient is encouraged to progress through the *stages of change* required to allow substance reduction. These stages are usually referred to as *precontemplative*, *contemplative*, and *action* stages.

Summarized principles of motivational interviewing

- An empathic approach allows the therapist to share their understanding of the patient's perspective with the patient
- To help patients appreciate the value of change by exploring the discrepancy between how they want their lives to be vs. how their lives are currently
- To accept a patient's reluctance to change as natural, rather than pathological
- To support self-efficacy, embrace patient autonomy.

Relapse prevention

Relapse prevention is a key principle in the management of substance misuse—simply stopping is easier than stopping and not re-starting, especially if the circumstances surrounding the initiation of substance misuse are recurrent.

Techniques, which should be routinely included in relapse prevention programmes, include cognitive and behavioural strategies for dealing with:

- **Cue avoidance:** avoidance of circumstances and acquaintances related to substance misuse
- **Social pressures** may be more important in adolescents than in adults, and being around a substance abusing peer group is one of the commonest routes to relapse
- **Development of alternative coping strategies for stressful situations**: restructuring of misconceptions and maladaptive thoughts, relaxation, and distraction techniques.

Family involvement

It is important to seek the right balance of family involvement. Barriers to achieving the much needed mobilization of family support will vary from anger and intolerance, through indifference to grief and self-blame. Systems and behaviourally-based family interventions can all help to address these issues.

Harm reduction

Where strategies to reduce substance use fail, strategies to reduce harm associated with continued use can have a positive impact. These include provision of information about reducing risky substance use techniques and first aid, and the availability of clean needles/safe needle disposal.

Recommended reading

AACAP. (2005) Practice parameter on assessment of child and adolescent substance abuse 2005. *J Am Acad Child Adolesc Psychiat* **44**: 6.

Fendrich M, Yun Soo Kim J. (2001) Multiwave analysis of retest artifact in the national longitudinal survey of youth drug use. *Drug Alc Depend* 62.

Fournier M, Levy S. (2006) Recent trends in adolescent substance abuse. *Curr Opin Pediat* **18**: 352–8.

Greydanus D, Patel D. (2003) Substance abuse in adolescents: a complex conundrum for the clinician. *Pediat Clin N Am* **50**: 1179–223.

Kaye D. (2004) Office recognition and management of adolescent substance abuse. *Curr Opin Pediat* **16**: 532–41.

Knight JR et al. (2002) Validity of the CRAFFT substance abuse screening test among adolescent clinic patients. *Arch Pediat Adolesc Med* **156**: 607–14.

St George's Hospital Medical School (2003) *Trends in Death Associated with Abuse of Volatile Substances 1971–2001*. St George's Hospital Medical School, London.

Therapeutic interventions

Behavioural therapy

Behaviour therapy is based on the principle that patterns of behaviour can be altered by changing their consequences or by changing the environment in which the behaviour occurs. Behaviour therapy can be used alone to facilitate behavioural change or as a component of CBT.

Behavioural modification programmes

Behavioural modification is based on the principles of operant conditioning. Wherein patterns of behaviour are reinforced by the response they elicit. The aim is to:
- Increase desirable behaviours by positive reinforcement.
- Decrease undesirable behaviours by neutral response or ignoring
- Only use negative responses or punishment when behaviours are unacceptable.

The purpose and function of a particular behaviour is understood by exploring its 'ABC's;
- **Antecedents:** what triggers it
- **Behaviour**: the actual behaviour itself
- **Consequences:** of the behaviour.

Steps in a behavioural modification programme
- Identify a target behaviour to change
- Set an achievable goal
- Establish a reward system that is immediate tangible and sustainable. Examples are praise, positive attention, or stickers
- Once the target behaviour has been established, the expectation regarding the behaviour occurring is increased, and the level at which it must occur to elicit a reward is also increased (in other words the child needs to try harder in order to get a reward)
- The frequency of rewards is decreased
- Once the new behaviour is firmly established, it should continue without the need for further reward and a new behaviour may be targeted
- This is a time-consuming process and if reinforcers are withdrawn too quickly the child is likely to revert to previous patterns of behaviour.

Effectiveness of behaviour therapy
Behaviour therapy has been demonstrated to be effective in modifying behaviour patterns in:
- Children aged less than 8 years with oppositional defiant disorder (ODD)
- Children with anxiety disorders who are not able to understand and use a cognitive behavioural approach to treatment—typically this means children aged less than 8 years
- Children with mild/moderate attention deficit hyperactivity disorder (ADHD), and when ADHD is co-morbid with an anxiety disorder
- Children and adolescents with learning disabilities and autistic spectrum disorders (ASD).

Behavioural approaches used as a part of cognitive behavioural therapy (CBT)

Activity scheduling involves:
- Identifying activities that are likely to have a positive effect on mood
- Encouraging the child or adolescent to re-engage in pleasurable activities
- Timetabling pleasurable activities appropriately throughout the week
- Monitoring the effect of increased activity on mood

Relaxation training
Children and adolescents with anxiety symptoms will benefit from being taught relaxation techniques. This is of particular benefit when therapy involves exposure to anxiety proving tasks.

Systematic desensitization
Exposure and graded exposure works on the principle that a person's anxiety will eventually decrease in the presence of a feared situation or object, if they remain in the situation or in the proximity of the feared stimulus for long enough.

Graded exposure is frequently used in treatment of anxiety disorders with children and adolescents where anxiety is linked to a specific situation or object (📖 Chapter 19 on anxiety disorders).

Parenting programmes

Parent training programmes

Various parenting programmes have been developed over the past 20 years. These aim to improve parent–child relationships and alter children's behaviour by teaching parents techniques (mainly behavioural in nature) designed to reward and reinforce positive and socially appropriate behaviours, and ignore and extinguish negative and socially inappropriate behaviours. A significant number of programmes are now available. The key principles common to most programmes include:

- Improve both parenting skills *and* parental confidence
- Encourage play and positive parent child interactions
- Increase the use of praise and rewards
- Encourage the use of clear instructions
- Ignore unwanted behaviours
- Use appropriate limit setting and consequences
- Teach the appropriate use of time out
- Use discipline selectively and effectively.

Parent training programmes may be used alone or in combination with a social skills programme for children. Some commonly used programmes include the Incredible Years Programme, Triple P, and Mellow Parenting.

Evidence of effectiveness of generic parenting programmes

Parent training programmes are particularly effective in reducing oppositional behaviour in children. They are most effective when children are aged less than 8 years. Increased effectiveness has also been demonstrated for children with no co-morbid psychiatric disorder. Good psychosocial functioning within the family predicts better treatment outcome. There is also some evidence that suggests that parents with learning disabilities or mental health problems (including untreated ADHD) find parenting programmes very difficult.

There is clear evidence that parent training programmes are most effective when delivered within the local community, and where transport and child care facilities are provided.

Adolescents do not benefit from parent training programmes. There is evidence that ODD or conduct disorder (CD) behaviour in adolescents will benefit from multisystemic therapy, which is a more intensive and comprehensive treatment package, involving marital therapy, family therapy, and individual CBT and case management.

Evidence for parenting programmes targeted at other specific disorders

Autistic spectrum disorders

Parenting programmes for parents of children with autistic spectrum disorders can modify target behaviours, such as wearing clothes at home or sitting at the table at meal times. However, these changes are limited to the environment in which the strategies are applied and there is no evidence for generalization either to other situations or behaviours.

ADHD

Parent training has been shown to be effective at increasing compliance with instructions by children with ADHD. Benefit is more significant in ADHD and co-morbid anxiety disorder, but there is some evidence that the skills learnt do not generalize to other settings. There is some evidence that parents with untreated ADHD find parenting programmes very difficult.

Anxiety disorders

There is currently conflicting evidence about whether running a parent group in addition to group therapy for children adds further benefits.

Cognitive behavioural therapy (CBT)

CBT in children and adolescents uses the same underpinning principles that form the basis of CBT in adults. Thoughts, feelings, and behaviour influence each other, and are themselves influenced by both short- and long-term environment factors. CBT aims to produce change in one or more of these areas of functioning to improve mental well being. CBT takes a collaborative approach with the therapist and patient working together towards a common set of goals.

For CBT to be effective, children and adolescents need to be able to (or be able to learn to):

- Identify their thoughts and think about their own thinking (metacognition)
- Identify and label feelings and emotions, both their own and those of others
- Reflect on the impact of their behaviour on themselves and others
- Identify problems, generate solutions, and identify that solutions are likely to have a positive outcome.

Once these skills are established as either present or able to be learnt, CBT can start to address the maladaptive thinking patterns that have a detrimental effect on how a child or adolescent is feeling and behaving.

CBT is of benefit for a significant proportion of children between the ages of 8 and 12 years, and for most adolescents within the normal range of intelligence.

Assessment for CBT (which should normally follow on from a diagnostic assessment)

Assessment will include:

- A description of symptoms and their effect on functioning
- The duration of difficulties
- The identification of precipitating contributing and maintaining factors
- The assessment of:
  - Interpersonal skills
  - Self-esteem
  - Problem-solving skills, emotional recognition
  - Ability to identify thoughts and recurrent patterns of thinking
- The identification of thinking patterns, e.g.
  - Current beliefs, attributions, and assumptions
  - Automatic thoughts and self-statements
  - Cognitive errors.

Information should be also be obtained from parents or carers, and school.

The completed assessment is then written as a formulation in language that the child or adolescent can understand, and contribute to, so that there is a mutual understanding of the difficulties and the focus for therapy. This provides the basis for an ongoing collaborative relationship.

CBT treatment phase

Duration of treatment

A contract is made for a specific number of initial sessions (4–6 on average). Sessions are often weekly. Response to treatment should be reviewed towards the end of this period, and further sessions are contracted as required. Validated questionnaires, completed before and after treatment, can also be used to monitor treatment response. The average duration of treatment is between 6 and 12 sessions. Complex and severe disorders may require active treatment for a 1–2-year period.

In the session

An agenda is set at the beginning of each session addressing areas highlighted in the formulation using the CBT model. Information should be provided in an age and developmentally appropriate format using illustrations or diagrams where appropriate.

Other activities include:
- Exploring skills and providing opportunities to learn new skills:
  - Emotional recognition using feeling charts and pictures
  - Problem-solving using modelling or role play
- Identifying maladaptive patterns of thinking, and promoting and exploring more adaptive thinking patterns
- Use of role play to explore alternative strategies.

Homework

As the term 'homework' is often perceived negatively, it may be described as 'detective work' or 'experiments' to increase compliance.

Tasks are identified that can be completed in between sessions to consolidate learning from the session and therefore maximize the learning experience.

Parents or carers can be enlisted to help with tasks between sessions.

Clinical effectiveness

Current evidence shows that CBT is an effective treatment for children and adolescents with:
- Mild to moderate depression
- Anxiety
- Agoraphobia and other phobias
- Social phobia
- Obsessive compulsive disorder (OCD)
- Post-traumatic stress disorder (PTSD).

Manualized treatment packages for treatment of anxiety and depression in children and adolescents have demonstrated clinically efficacy in randomized controlled trials.

Interpersonal therapy (IPT)

IPT was initially developed as a manual treatment for adults with depressive disorder. The underpinning theory of IPT is that difficulties in interpersonal functioning are a significant precipitating and maintaining factor in depressive disorders. The IPT model has been adapted for adolescents but to date has not been adapted for use with children.

Duration and structure of treatment

IPT is a very structured therapy that follows a clear timetable, consisting of weekly sessions lasting 1 h over a 12–16-week period.

Sessions 1–4

Involve the young person and may also include family members, if required, to provide additional information.

During these sessions there is assessment of:

- The symptoms of depression
- Family relationships
- Social context.

This is followed by a formulation of the patient's illness in interpersonal terms and psycho-education to the model of IPT.

Sessions 5–10

Involve the young person only.

Problematic relationship areas are addressed including:

- Interpersonal disputes and deficits
- Role disputes or transitions
- Grief
- Transitions
- Interpersonal conflicts
- Difficulties related to family situations.

Social problem-solving techniques are used to maintain and build on areas of current or previous positive social functioning.

Session 11/12

- Involves young person only
- Addresses and explores thoughts and feelings of loss related to the termination of therapy
- Asks what has been learnt in therapy?

Effectiveness

IPT has been shown to reduce symptoms of depression and improve self-esteem in adolescents. IPT is also an effective treatment for adults with dysthymic disorder, bipolar disorder, and bulimia, but there is little research in an adolescent group.

Family therapy

Theoretical perspectives

Most family therapy is based on systems theory. The underlying principle is that the behaviour of individuals is influenced and maintained by the way other individuals and systems interact with them. The family is a system and its functioning is influenced by the members of the family, and by individuals and systems that interact with the family. Family therapy is a way of working on problems by focusing on helping the whole family function in more positive and constructive ways. This is achieved by enabling families to explore and make sense of their experiences, and to use this understanding to change their functioning in a positive way. There are a number of schools of family therapy, but all tend to focus on a number of key issues:

- Family functioning, roles, and relationships
- Attitudes and beliefs within the family
- Patterns of communication and interaction
- Problem-solving abilities
- Strengths within the family
- Social and cultural backgrounds.

Delivery of therapy

In general, the therapist attempts to maintain maximum neutrality during the therapeutic process. For good practice, the team will have a minimum of two therapists. Family sessions may be screened and if numbers allow, a reflecting team may be used. The purpose is to allow reflection on the process of therapy by therapists external to the therapy system, and then feed this back to the therapist and the family.

In clinical practice, family therapy is frequently provided alongside individual treatment for a child or adolescent with:

- Emotional disorders
- OCD
- Psychosis
- PTSD
- Somatic disorders with unexplained medical symptoms.

Effectiveness of family therapy

The effectiveness of family therapy as a treatment has not been well studied. The strongest evidence is for families of adolescents under 19 years of age with eating disorders. There is also some evidence that family therapy is of benefit for adolescents with depressive disorders, in particular where family discord is a contributing factor.

Psychodynamic psychotherapy

Theory

In psychodynamic psychotherapy, the aim is to understand internal thought processes that influence a child or adolescent's behaviour. The underlying principle is that past events influence patterns of emotional and behavioural responses in the present. Emotions and behaviours are seen as being driven by unconscious defence patterns and memories formed by previous experiences. This can result in a child or adolescent using patterns of interaction that may have been adaptive previously, but that are not related to current situations or relationships, and are therefore maladaptive. These can have a significant negative effect on interpersonal functioning and behavioural responses.

Therapy aims to facilitate improvement in current function, and interpersonal relationships by enabling the child or young person to explore these issues in a safe therapeutic environment. As in adults, transference (how the child or young person makes the therapist feel) and counter transference (how the therapist then feels about the child or young person) are used to develop an understanding of the child or young person. The therapist provides feedback on all these to help the child or adolescent gain an understanding of themselves, and their previous experiences that will facilitate more adaptive patterns of functioning in the present and future.

Stability and security in present care situation are necessary before a young person or adolescent will feel safe and able to reflect on past experiences in a meaningful helpful manner, and therefore should be seen as a prerequisite for entering into psychodynamic psychotherapy.

Psychodynamic psychotherapy in children and adolescence has been significantly influenced over the past 50 years by the work of Anna Freud, Melanie Klein, Donald Winnicot, Wilfred Bion, and Carl Jung.

Psychodynamic psychotherapy in practice

For assessment, it is necessary to meet with the parents or carers, as well as the child. It is important that they understand the process of therapy, and that they are aware that therapy may be anxiety provoking for the child or adolescent. This can result in periods of challenging behaviour out with sessions.

Consistency within therapy is a key theme. The same room is used, and the child or young person will have a number of play or drawing materials that will be kept safely for them, and only them to use in sessions. Sessions are at the same time, on the same day(s) each week. Frequency is between 1 and 5 sessions per week. In the NHS, frequency of therapy is usually 1–2 times weekly. Duration of therapy can be between 3 months to 2 or more years.

For therapy to be effective, parents or carers need to be able to provide a supportive and containing environment out with sessions. Regular meetings between the parents or carers, and another therapist, while the child or young person is in therapy can be used to support this process.

Effectiveness

There is little systematic research regarding effectiveness of psychodynamic psychotherapy in children and adolescents. There is, however, some evidence that psychodynamic psychotherapy can be effective in:
- Treatment of anxiety disorders
- Treatment of mood disorders (intensive therapy x5 per week)
- Improvement in diabetic control in adolescents with brittle diabetes.

Further research is required to clarify the clinical and cost effectiveness of individual psychodynamic psychotherapy treatment in children and adolescents.

Group therapy

Group therapy can be a cost effective way of delivering a range of different psychological treatment interventions, and skills-based social communication and problem-solving training for children and adolescents.

Benefits of group over individual therapies

Working in groups facilitates:
- A mutual understanding and acceptance of others
- Decrease in feelings of isolation
- A safe environment to explore issues with peers
- Feedback and understanding by peers, which can be more meaningful than therapist interpretations or feedback
- Opportunities to practice skills using role play and modelling.

Limitations of group over individual therapies

Group therapy process may be disrupted by:
- Severe psychotic disorder
- Suicidal behaviour
- Significant conduct disorder and acting out behaviour.

There is evidence that many skills gained within the group setting do not readily generalize to other areas.

Psychological therapy treatment groups

Manualized programmes are available for group therapy treatments of anxiety and mood disorders in children and adolescents. These use CBT principles and approaches to treatment. There is good clinical evidence for their effectiveness in treatment of mild to moderate disorders.

Skills-based group programmes

Skills-based social communication and problem-solving groups are of benefit for children with oppositional behaviour and poor social problem-solving skills. Benefit is increased when the principles of the group are also applied in the home and school setting.

Group sessions focus on:
- Problem-solving
- Emotional recognition
- Social skills
- Co-operation
- Friendship skills
- Teamwork
- Concentrating and listening.

Play and art therapies

Play therapy

Play therapy uses play as the primary method of communication for the child; speech is secondary in this process. Play facilitates the development of healthy social relationships, communication skills, creativity, and cognitive and emotional skills, and is therefore seen as being therapeutic in its own right.

Play therapy is defined by the British Association of Play Therapists as: the dynamic process between child and play therapist in which the child explores, at his or her own pace, and with his or her own agenda, those issues, past and current, conscious and unconscious, that are affecting the child's life in the present. The child's inner resources are enabled by the therapeutic alliance to bring about growth and change.

Through play, the child may re-create difficult or traumatic past experiences in order to make sense of these. This understanding is thought to promote more healthy functioning in the here and now.

Play therapy aims to help children to:
- Find better ways of communicating
- Modify maladaptive behaviour
- Form healthy relationships
- Increase resilience and self-esteem
- Decrease anxiety.

Play therapy is used in children where there are issues surrounding abuse, disability, separation, loss, and trauma.

Unfortunately there is little systematic research regarding the effectiveness of play therapy.

Art therapy

Art therapy is a form of psychotherapy that uses arts and crafts as a medium through which a child or young person can express their thoughts, feelings, and experiences. The process of producing a piece of art is seen as therapeutic its own right. The thoughts, feelings, and experiences represented in the art form then provide a focus for exploration within the therapeutic relationship.

Art therapy is thought to be useful for children and adolescents with poor emotional language, for example, those with ASD or with learning difficulties. However, when a child or adolescent does have the ability to verbalize their emotions, the art work can be used as a focus for verbal exploration of the art work and its meaning.

While art therapy and art in therapy have been used widely with children and adolescents with mental health difficulties, there is a lack of systematic research about the effectiveness.

Self-help

There are a wide range of self-help materials about mental health problems available for children, adolescents, parents, and professionals. Material can be in leaflet, book, or computer-based format. Children and adolescents often prefer interactive computer programmes.

Self-help material, in particular psychoeducation material, can also be used alongside other therapeutic interventions.

Self-help can be used by individuals or groups, and may be a beneficial part of support groups.

Components to self-help

Psychoeducation

Understanding the causes and effects of disorders or illness can have a positive effect on:
- The individual's ability to function within the constraints of their illness
- The parent's or carer's ability to understand why a child or adolescent is behaving in a certain way.

Life style advice

Advice on life styles that can promote good mental health, healthy diet, exercise, and sleep hygiene.

Cognitive behavioural self help approaches

Teaches strategies for self-help and the mastery of illness, the most commonly used have both behavioural and cognitive components.

Parental management

Parental management self-help programmes using similar techniques to those outlined in the parent training section (📖 p. 398).

Self-help parental management materials are commonly used by parents for assistance in managing:
- ADHD
- Autism
- Anxiety
- Depression
- Eating disorders
- Parenting skills.

Clinical effectiveness

Psychoeducation and life style advice can be important components of treatment for all psychiatric disorders. Self-help interventions have not yet been well researched as stand-alone interventions for psychiatric disorders in children and adolescents.

Liaison

Liaison may be defined as two or more specialties working alongside or together to produce a better outcome. The most common area of liaison in CAMHS is paediatric liaison, joint working between paediatric and CAMHS staff.

Paediatric liaison facilitates the assessment and management of:
- Psychological aspects of physical illnesses
- Physical illness with co-morbid psychiatric disorder
- Physical aspects of psychiatric disorders
- Somatic disorders and unexplained medical symptoms
- Psychological aspects of non-compliance with medical treatments
- Impact on family functioning of physical illness.

There is evidence that this model facilitates acceptance of a psychological approach as part of treatment of a physical illness. It also can facilitate earlier recognition of significant mental health needs in children and adolescents.

Recommended reading

Bailey V. (2001) Application of CBT with children and adolescents. *Adv Psychiat Treatm* **7**: 224–32.

British Association of Play Therapists. Available at: http://www.bapt.info/aboutbapt.htm#bm4 (accessed 23 March 2008).

Robinson J. (2007) Child and adolescent individual psychoanalytic psychotherapy. In: Naismith J, Grant S.(Eds) *Seminars in the Psychotherapies*. Royal College of Psychiatrists, London, pp. 221–34.

Tagaret M, Fonagy P, et al. (2005) 'The psychological treatment of child and adolescent psychiatric disorders', What works for whom? In: Roth A, Fonagy P, et al. (Eds) *A Critical Review of Psychotherapy Research*, 2nd edn. Guildford Press, New York, pp. 385–424.

Child protection

Child protection: general issues

Definitions

Child abuse

Despite many attempts to develop one, there is no standardized definition of what constitutes child abuse and definitions vary amongst professionals, over time, and between social and cultural groups. The World Health Organization (WHO) has suggested that 'Child abuse or maltreatment constitutes all forms of physical and/or emotional ill treatment, sexual abuse, neglect or negligent treatment or commercial or other exploitation, resulting in actual or potential harm in the child's health, survival, development or dignity in the context of a relationship of responsibility, trust or power.'

Child protection

Whilst there are several definitions of child protection, most seem to agree that there are two approaches involved. The first involves a focus on the identification of children who are either being harmed or are likely to be harmed, whilst the second encompasses the actions that may be taken to prevent further harm occurring to these children. It is universally agreed that child protection is a responsibility shared by everyone, and that it is not the sole province any one person or professional group.

Identifying child abuse

In 1999, WHO estimated that 40 million children around the world aged 14 and under were suffering from abuse and neglect, and required health and social care services. Early identification of abuse and neglect should enable it to be stopped, and the child to receive the help and support they need. Research from the UK Department of Health (1995) demonstrated that child abuse comes to official attention in one of three ways:

- 51% are recognized when someone, usually the child or another member of the family, discloses their concerns to a professional
- 39% of cases are identified by professionals already working with the family
- 10% are recognized following an unrelated event, such as an arrest or home visit.

The identification of abuse is often difficult, since many of the signs and symptoms also indicate other problems or conditions.

Reporting child abuse and neglect

The Council of Europe has urged all countries to have mandatory reporting of child abuse, but the UK, along with several other European countries, still does not have laws requiring such mandatory reporting. Under UK law, only social workers and police have a duty to report suspicions that a child is in need of care and protection. Local child protection guidelines and professional codes of conduct do, however, expect other professionals, including health staff and teachers, to report abuse and suspected abuse as part of their professional duty. The UK General Medical Council (GMC), for example, recommends to doctors that:

Your first concern must be the safety of children and young people. You must inform an appropriate person or authority promptly of any reasonable concern that children or young people are at risk of abuse or neglect, when that is in a child's best interests or necessary to protect other children or young people.

Research in Europe, the USA, and Australia has indicated that medical practitioners are often reluctant to report even when they have a legal mandate to do so. Reasons include ideological and ethical concerns about confidentiality, family privacy, a desire for autonomy in practice, and a mistrust of state services. Doctors also often express ignorance about the reporting rules and procedures. Cases of sexual abuse are the most likely to be reported with physical abuse next, followed by physical neglect with emotional abuse, and neglect the least likely.

The GMC also points out that, whilst children, young people, and their parents may request that a health professional does not disclose information about them (particularly if they believe that they will be denied help, blamed or made to feel ashamed of what has happened), it is the role of the doctor to help them to understand the importance and benefits of sharing information. The doctor must not delay sharing relevant information with an appropriate person or authority if such delay would increase the risk to the child or young person, or to other children or young people. It is acknowledged that confidentiality is important and information sharing should be proportionate to the risk of harm. You may initially share some limited information, with consent if possible, in order to decide whether there is a risk that would justify further disclosures. Such a risk might only become apparent when a number of people with niggling concerns share them. If in any doubt about whether to share information, the doctor is advised to seek advice from an experienced colleague, a named or designated doctor for child protection, or a Caldicott Guardian, as well as from their professional body, medical defence organization, or the GMC.

Investigation and decision making

In most jurisdictions the main responsibility for investigating allegations of child abuse is held by the social work departments, the police, or both. Paediatricians also often have a responsibility for the physical aspects of investigation. These investigations are a highly skilled process and require specialist training. Others, including child mental health workers, should not attempt to investigate suspicions of abuse unless this is part of a clearly formulated plan supported by the relevant statutory agencies.

Health staff should, however, play a full role in child protection procedures, and should attend meetings whenever practical, and co-operate with requests for information about child abuse and neglect. They must make sure that have a clear understanding of their roles, local policies and practices, and the roles of other agencies and professionals with respect to child protection, including an understanding of the circumstances in which disclosure is justified.

Physical abuse and neglect

Definitions

Physical abuse

Physical abuse occurs when a child is exposed to actual or attempted physical injury, and where there is definite knowledge or reasonable suspicion, that this injury has either been inflicted or that it could have been prevented, but was not. As such, it can include one or more serious incidents, or a series of minor incidents involving bruising, fractures, scratches, burns or scalds, deliberate poisoning, attempted drowning or smothering, Munchausen syndrome by proxy, serious risk of or actual injuries resulting from parental lifestyle prior to birth (e.g. substance abuse), and physical chastisement deemed to be unreasonable.

Physical neglect

Physical neglect occurs where there is failure to provide for the development and needs of the child, and where this is likely to cause impairment to the child's physical mental, spiritual, moral, or social health and development. It includes all aspects of life—health, education, emotional development, nutrition, shelter, and safe living conditions, in the context of resources reasonably available to the family or caretakers. It includes a failure to properly supervise and protect children from harm as much as is feasible and a failure to secure appropriate medical treatment for the child, or when an adult carer persistently allows or encourages a child to follow a lifestyle inappropriate to their developmental needs, or which jeopardizes the child's health.

Prevalence

Whilst much of the data regarding the prevalence of physical abuse is derived from official statistics of reported cases, several studies that have questioned parents and adults suggest that physical child abuse is far more common than indicated in these official rates (i.e. not all physically maltreated children come to the attention of child protection agencies). In one well-conducted large scale UK study by the National Society for the Prevention of Cruelty to Children (NSPCC) it was reported that 72% of the 2869 18–24-year-olds questioned had experienced physical discipline (for example, hitting or slapping) in some form; 21% had experienced some degree of physical abuse by parents or carers, and 7% of these had been seriously physically abused. More males than females had experienced serious physical abuse and those from lower social classes were around 50% more likely to have experienced physical abuse than those from professional families. Overall, 7% now considered their experience amounted to child abuse.

Very few studies have attempted to measure the prevalence of neglect. In the NSPCC study mentioned above 18% of young adults indicated that they had experienced some absence of care in their childhood of which 6% indicated this was a serious absence of care and 2% considered their treatment amounted to neglect.

The consequences of physical abuse and neglect

As with other forms of abuse the psychiatric and psychological consequences of physical abuse and neglect are extremely varied. It is also difficult to be sure which of the problems faced by a child who has been abused are directly related to the abuse and which are related to other risk factors present in that child's life. However, studies have identified that children who have suffered physical abuse and neglect are also at increased risk for:

- **Interpersonal problems**: including insecure and disorganized attachments, peer relationship difficulties, and problems forming intimate relationships. These children are more disliked and less popular than non-abused peers. They exhibit more negative and conflictual behaviours even with close friends
- **Cognitive and academic impairments:** cognitive deficits are common, in particular, language skills difficulties (both receptive and expressive). Importantly, and contrary to popular beliefs, neglect seems to be associated with greater language problems than abuse. These language deficits have also been associated with subsequent aggressive behaviour in the child. Poor academic performance is also common with difficulties in both mathematics and language. Again, neglect seems to result in greater difficulties than abuse
- **Aggression and delinquency:** these are among the most common correlates of physical abuse. It has been hypothesized that an exposure to physical abuse results in increased aggression by increasing levels of irritability and aggression, engendering hypervigilance and paranoid thinking styles and reducing the recognition of pain in both the self and others
- **Self-harm, suicidal behaviour, and risk taking:** an association between a history of physical abuse and of self-harm and/or suicidal behaviours has been demonstrated in several studies, particularly those that have studied adolescents. Increased risk taking in the form of smoking, substance misuse and sexual risk taking is also seen. Physical abuse has been associated with teenage parenthood in both girls and boys
- **Psychiatric disorders:** children who have been physically abused are at increased risk for a wide range of psychiatric disorders including depression, anxiety disorders [including post-traumatic stress disorder (PTSD)], conduct disorder (CD), and oppositional defiant disorders (ODD), attention deficit hyperactivity disorder (ADHD), and substance misuse.

Emotional abuse

Definition

Emotional abuse occurs when there is failure to provide for the child's basic emotional needs, and this has a severe effect on the behaviour and/or development of the child. This can encompass a wide range of situations, such as those whereby children are persistently:

- Rejected, denigrated, or scapegoated
- Inappropriately punished
- Denied opportunities for appropriate play and socialization
- Are encouraged to engage in anti-social behaviour
- Are put in a state of terror or extreme anxiety by the use of threats or practices designed to intimidate them
- Isolated from normal social experiences
- Prevented from forming friendships.

Children who are left alone for long periods of time, who are under stimulated or suffer sensory deprivation, may also come into this category.

Prevalence

Emotional abuse is the least common cause of registration on child protection registers, but this does not mean that it is the least prevalent type of abuse as most cases are thought to go unreported.

The Audit Commission in England and Wales found emotional abuse to be a major form of abuse, but accurate figures are not known. This is the least well studied of all forms of child maltreatment and reliable prevalence data are almost non-existent. It would appear, however, that emotional abuse is much more common than is reported by official statistics. A UK study conducted by the NSPCC constructed a measure of emotional maltreatment and found that 6% of respondents had high scores indicating emotional abuse. Respondents were asked whether they thought the way they had been treated was child abuse, 3% said they had been abused, and 2% were unsure. Other research indicates that, whilst emotional abuse does occur in isolation from other forms of abuse it is also a factor in all forms of abuse, and that the overwhelming majority of physical abuse cases have also suffered emotional abuse. From this perspective one would expect emotional abuse to be the most frequent form of child abuse.

The consequences of emotional abuse

Although the impact of emotional abuse on psychological and psychiatric health has been poorly studied there are suggestions that emotional abuse may have a stronger association with long-term psychological functioning than other forms of child abuse.

Regression analyses of samples with physical and emotional abuse have suggested that the consequences of emotional abuse include internalizing and externalizing behaviours, social impairments, low self-esteem, suicidal behaviours, delinquency, substance misuse, and a wide range of psychiatric disorders. More research into this important determinant of child well-being is required.

Munchausen's syndrome by proxy

There is a growing awareness and medical literature concerning Munchausen's syndrome by proxy, the fabrication or induction of illness in a child by a carer. This is defined as occurring when an infant or child is presented to doctors, often repeatedly, with an illness or disability that has been fabricated by an adult, for the benefit of that adult. Such fabrications can occur in several ways:

- The fabrication of signs and symptoms and sometimes an inaccurate past medical history
- The falsification of hospital charts and medical records and specimens of bodily fluids
- The induction of illness by a variety of means, which can include poisoning or suffocation.

Data concerning incidence are sparse, but there were 128 confirmed cases of Munchausen's syndrome by proxy, non-accidental poisoning, and non-accidental suffocation recorded in the UK and the Republic of Ireland between 1 September 1992 and 31 August 1994. This suggests a combined annual incidence of at least 0.5 per 100,000 children aged less than 16 years of age. Most cases (around 75%) are aged below 5 years, meaning that the annual incidence for this age group was at least 1.2 per 100,000 children (for children aged <1 year annual incidence was even higher at 2.8 per 100,000). These figures are likely to be under estimates, as some professionals may have been deterred from notifying cases due to legal aspects, maintenance of confidentiality, or difficulties of diagnosing such an uncommon condition.

It should be remembered that, whilst some of these children will be presented with factitious psychiatric disorders, they are also at increased risk for suffering from a wide range of genuine psychiatric disorders. In such cases, assessment needs to be conducted and recorded particularly carefully.

Child sexual abuse: definitions and prevalence

Definition

Child sexual abuse occurs when a child is exploited either directly or indirectly by a person or persons who, either by design or neglect, directly or indirectly, engage that child in any activity intended to lead to the sexual arousal or other forms of gratification of that person or any other person(s), including organized networks. This definition holds whether or not there has been genital contact, and whether or not the child is said to have initiated the behaviour.

Sexual abuse may include such activities as:
- Incest, rape, sodomy, or intercourse with children
- Lewd or libidinous practices or behaviour towards children
- Homosexual practices towards children
- Indecent assault of children
- Taking indecent photographs of children
- Encouraging them to become prostitutes or to witness intercourse or pornographic materials.

Key indicators that any particular sexual activity (including those taking place between two children) may be abusive include:
- A lack of consent
- Inequalities in terms of chronological age, or developmental stage, or
- Actual or threatened force or coercion.

Prevalence

Child sexual abuse was considered rare before the late 1970s. Since this time recognition rates around the world have increased dramatically. Much of this increase is due to increased awareness and recognition rather than a true increased incidence. The number of people reporting having experienced some kind of sexual abuse varies considerably between studies and is dependent, at least in part, on the definition of sexual abuse used in the study. However, even if one accepts only the lowest reported rates, sexual abuse is relatively common in both boys and girls. In the UK NSPCC study:
- 1% of the sample of 2869 young people had been sexually abused by parents/carers, and almost all of this abuse involved physical contact
- 3% had been abused by other relatives (2% contact and 1% non-contact)
- Abuse by 'other known people' was the most common and was experienced by 11% of the sample (8% involving physical contact and 3% non-contact)
- Abuse by strangers or someone they just met had affected 4% of the sample (2% contact and 2% non-contact)

- Only a quarter of respondents with unwanted sexual experience had told anyone about the experience at the time of the study and when they had, their confidant was usually a friend, less often a family member, and very rarely the police or another professional person
- The person responsible for the sexual abuse was almost always male, very few respondents of either gender said that the person involving them in sex acts was female
- 6% of the total sample assessed themselves as having been sexually abused.

Other replicated findings include:
- More girls than boys report having been a victim of sexual abuse with a ratio of between 3 and 4:1
- Children may be abused from infancy onwards. Children who experience intercourse tend to be older with an average age of 11.4 years
- Children with disabilities are 2–3 times as likely to be abused compared with children with no disability
- Ethnicity, culture, and socioeconomic status do not alter the risk of sexual abuse
- Sexual abuse still appears to be generally under reported, and this seems to be particularly high for males due in part to their fears of being disbelieved and of being labelled homosexual
- Children are much more likely to be sexually abused by a male, but women do abuse
- Abuse can be perpetrated by people of any age (including by other children and young people)
- Approximately one-quarter to one-third of sexual abusers are themselves juveniles
- Prevalence studies show that sexual abuse is rarely reported to the authorities.

Theories of sexual abuse

There is no clear unitary theory to explain child sexual abuse. Current theories emphasize the responsibility of the abuser, and cite a wish for power and sexual gratification as the two central aspects. A sexual arousal to pre-pubertal children (paedophilia) is likely to be a driving force for those abusing younger children. Finkelhor described four preconditions necessary for abuse to occur:
- A motivation to sexually abuse children
- An absence of internal inhibitors to abusing children
- An absence of external inhibitors
- A child's vulnerability (or lack of ability to resist).

Once abuse has started proposed maintaining factors include;
- Secrecy
- Fear
- Helplessness
- Entrapment and accommodation
- Delayed or unconvincing disclosure
- Retraction of a disclosure.

Child sexual abuse: impact and intervention

There are certain 'impact issues' associated with child sexual abuse that are the expected consequence of having experienced such a traumatic experience. These are common to both male and female victims and are seen as a normative response to being abused. Sgroi described them as;
- The 'damaged goods' syndrome
- Guilt and self-blame
- Fear
- Depression
- Low self-esteem and poor social skills
- Repressed anger and hostility
- Impaired ability to trust
- Blurred role boundaries and role confusion
- Pseudomaturity, coupled with failure to accomplish developmental tasks
- Interference with self-mastery and control.

Other effects include:
- Sexualized behaviour
- Unwanted pregnancy
- Aggression and disruptive behaviours
- Deliberate self-harm
- Peer relationship difficulties
- Educational difficulties
- Post-traumatic stress disorder (PTSD) and dissociation
- Eating disorders.

Some of these effects continue into adulthood, whilst others may not emerge until adulthood. As a consequence, adults with a history of sexual abuse as children are more likely than those without such histories to suffer from:
- Depression
- Deliberate self-harm
- Anxiety
- Drug and alcohol abuse (more often in males)
- Difficulties in sexual functioning and intimate personal relationships
- Distrust of men
- Eating disorders.

Moderating factors
Several factors have been found to moderate the impact of sexual abuse.

Abuse variables
Factors associated with more severe psychological impact include:
- Prolonged duration
- Increased frequency
- Penetration of mouth, anus, or vagina
- Abuse associated with threats of or actual force
- Close relation between perpetrator and victim
- Multiple abusers.

Child variables

There is no consistent difference in the effects of abuse on boys or girls. Boys do, however, worry more about being homosexual, either as a result of their abuse or as a latent trait, which could have been detected by the abuser. Older children tend to be more symptomatic at presentation. Early abuse before the age of 7 years may be a risk factor for later inappropriate sexualized behaviour.

Pre-abuse circumstances and family factors

A wide range of pre-existing adverse family relationships may both increase the risk of abuse and increase the adverse impact of any subsequent abuse.

Post-abuse response

This includes:

- The way in which any investigation is handled
- **The response of the non abusive carer:** the support of the non-abusive carer is a significant predictor of a good outcome
- **The response of the abuser:** in cases where the abuser denies the abuse the victim's allegations are often seriously questioned and cross-examined with attempts to discredit them
- The protective steps taken following disclosure can also play an important role, particularly when either the child or the abuser is required to leave the home.

Therapeutic work

There is no single template for working with children who have suffered from sexual abuse. Indeed, not all victims of sexual abuse will require therapeutic work, but when assessing and formulating the response to any particular case, a systematic and systemic approach to planning is helpful taking into account the child's needs as an individual and a member of a family. It can be helpful to think of the individuals needs in relation to the three corners of 'the abuse triangle'—abuser, child, and non-abusing caregiver. An integrated multi-agency, multidisciplinary approach, including social work and other services, is often the most helpful.

Support for the victim should be given pro-actively and also be reactive to the child's needs. It should also be recognized that these needs will change over time. In the past, much emphasis was placed on play therapy as a response to abuse. Unfortunately, this work has never been properly evaluated and it is not possible to draw evidence based conclusions as to its effectiveness. More recently, group and individual cognitively-based therapeutic programmes have been demonstrated to be effective at reducing a range of problems faced by victims of abuse. Therapeutic work for the non-abusing carer and siblings may also be required. Recidivism is high amongst adult abusers, even following therapeutic work. Such work can, however, be helpful in reducing future risks. There is, however, no evidence to support work aimed at reintegrating an abuser back into the family and this should usually not be the aim of the therapeutic interventions.

Recommended reading

Finkelhor D. (1986) *A Sourcebook on Child Sexual Abuse*. Sage Publications, Thousand Oaks.

General Medical Council. (2007) *0–18 Years: Guidance for all Doctors*. GMC, London.

Scottish Executive. (2002) 'It's everyone's job to make sure I'm alright.' A literature review. Scottish Executive, Edinburgh. Available at: http://www.scotland.gov.uk/Publications/2002/11/15820/14009 (accessed 13 April 2008).

Sgroi S. (1981) *Handbook of Clinical Intervention in Child Sexual Abuse*. DC Heath, Canada.

World Health Organization *Child Abuse Prevention Report*. Available at: www.who.int

Forensic issues

Medico-legal assessments

Child and adolescent psychiatrists are asked to provide medico-legal assessments by a range of people:

- The local authority
- Parents via a solicitor
- A guardian *ad-litum* or safe-guarder
- A solicitor acting for the child
- The courts
- Insurance companies.

For many purposes these assessments include:

- An assessment of the adequacy of parenting
- Issues relating to parental responsibility, residency, and contact
- Issues relating to child abuse and neglect
- Educational issues
- Placement issues
- Criminal proceedings
- A child's ability to understand and participate in court proceedings
- Compensation issues.

Whilst the precise circumstances will vary depending on the situation, the jurisdiction, and the local laws, there are several guiding principles that can be applied in most circumstances.

Referral and pre-assessment

When conducting a specialist medico-legal assessment a clinician needs to have adequate information and clarity about what the person requesting the assessment is asking. The referrer can be asked to provide:

- Clear reasons for requesting the assessment
- Clear statements regarding the questions they wish to be addressed
- Details of the child's current situation, including how and why these arose
- Current and past involvement of social work, education, and other departments/services, with the child and other family members. Have there been any statutory decisions made by the authorities?
- What is the social work department (or other interested parties) considering recommending for the future?
- Relevant previous history for the child and family
- Copies of relevant previous reports
- History of developmental progress (including growth)
- Descriptions of current and past behavioural and emotional difficulties
- Descriptions of interpersonal relationships (within family, with peers, with other adults)
- Details of schooling, including attendance, academic performance, and attainments
- Details of previous placements.

Before making a firm commitment to conduct a medico-legal assessment the clinician should satisfy themselves that the questions being asked are appropriate, that they are the appropriate person to conduct such an assessment, and that they have the required skills and experience.

Having agreed to conduct an assessment, the clinician should consider who should attend for the assessment, and whether it should be carried out in one session or would be better spread over two or more meetings. In general, it is helpful if as many of the relevant parties, including the professionals, can attend for at least part of the assessment, although this may not be possible in all cases, e.g. where the parents have such an acrimonious relationship that it would not be advisable to have them in the same place at the same time or where a child has made allegations of abuse.

Assessment

The details of the assessment will depend on the questions being asked, but in general, a medico-legal assessment will follow similar principles to a comprehensive psychiatric assessment. The purpose of the assessment is usually to prepare an official report, which will often be widely distributed and may be read out in open court. Issues of confidentiality should be clearly addressed at the beginning of the assessment process, together with a clear explanation of what will happen to the information gathered at the assessment and to the report.

All relevant views should be obtained. This will usually require a combination of joint and individual interviewing. When there are conflicting views, opinions, or histories, these should be clarified and the differing points of view must be carefully document. The psychiatrist's task is to remain completely objective, impartial, and independent, irrespective of their own beliefs or by whom they have been instructed.

If, by the end of the assessment, the psychiatrist is clear about what his/her recommendation will be, it is often appropriate for this to be discussed at this point. Whilst this may be challenging in certain situations, it allows those involved to express their feelings and for these to be discussed.

Medico-legal reports and court work

Preparation of a medico-legal report

There are several templates available to assist with report writing. All stress the need for order, clarity, and impartiality. Whilst the specifics of the report will depend on the circumstances surrounding the request and the specific questions being addressed, there are several guiding principles that assist in writing a comprehensive and helpful report.

- Use a large typeface, double spaced on numbered pages with wide margins
- Write in short sentences and paragraphs with clearly labelled sections
- Avoid using technical language wherever possible.

Structure and content

- Introductory paragraph containing details of the nature of the report, subject's details, author's name, contact details, qualifications, position, experience, and areas of expertise
- Section referring to the letters of instruction, the reasons for writing the report
- The details of the assessment meeting and of other sources of information used to prepare the report
- A summary of the facts of the case
- The hypotheses guiding the assessment
- Details of the information gathered at assessment (described as they would be in a full psychiatric assessment including personal and family history, developmental history, psychiatric signs and symptoms, mental state etc.)
- Your opinion:
  - Diagnostic conclusions and formulation of child's difficulties
  - Answers to specific questions
  - Identification of the treatment/resources required to meet child's needs
  - Any recommendations regarding legal orders/processes that may be beneficial to the child
  - General recommendations, which should discuss the various options available and their pros and cons
- The report should conclude with any statements required by the courts (e.g. in the English courts this would read 'I declare that this statement is true to the best of my knowledge, information and belief, and I understand that it may be placed before the Court'), and be signed and dated on each page.

Appearing in court

The psychiatrist may be called to court as either a professional or an expert witness.

The professional witness is expected to give evidence based solely on their first hand knowledge gained from clinical contact with the child, young-person, and/or family, i.e. an account of their clinical work. As such, they can give opinions on matters such as the differential diagnosis, the reasons for certain treatments not working, etc., but are not expected to comment on general issues of relevance to the case that do not relate to their own clinical contact. The professional witness is allowed to refer to their notes in court, but can only quote from sections that were completed contemporaneously.

The role of the **expert witness**, who may not have even seen the child in question, is to comment on the more general aspects of the case and to provide expert opinion on the views of others.

In both cases, the evidence presented in court should be based in material contained in the reports previously submitted to the court.

On occasion, particularly in very complex cases, an expert witness is asked to sit in court and listen to the evidence of others in order to provide the lawyers with opinion as the case proceeds.

Whilst appearing in court can be very stressful, it is much less so if you are well prepared. Some general tips are:

- Arrive on time, but expect a long wait!
- Get advice from a more experienced colleague about what to expect
- Prepare well. Understand the case and the role you are being asked to play. Read your report and notes very carefully, and make sure that you understand each section well
- Take the files with you to court and re-read them whilst you are waiting
- Read the appropriate scientific literature carefully and ensure that you understand it well
- Try to anticipate lines of questioning that may arise in the cross-examination.
- Be clear about your own boundaries of expertise
- Dress appropriately (sober and smart), and present yourself well (sit and stand straight)
- Speak clearly and with confidence (remember, even as a professional witness you are an expert in your subject). Don't speak too fast as the judge may be taking notes
- Face the lawyer whilst they ask you a question but then turn to face the judge to give your answer
- Ask for advice on how to address the judge as it varies in different courts and different jurisdictions
- Become familiar with the order of questioning. First you are examined by the side that instructed you and then cross-examined by the other side, after which the first lawyer may ask a few more questions
- Remember that whilst the cross-examination is designed to be challenging it is not a personal attack and remain calm at all times
- Use your active listening skills during the questioning (especially the cross-examination). This will help you understand the direction of questioning and anticipate difficult questions
- Stick to your areas of competence.

The Royal Colleges and other organizations often run courses on witness skills that are usually very worthwhile and should be attended if possible.

Recommended reading

Black D, Wolkind S, Hendricks JH (1991) *Child Psychiatry and the Law* Gaskell, London.

Legal frameworks

Definitions and legislation

Whilst there are some UK-wide laws, most of the legislation covering children and the law in the UK varies between jurisdictions (England and Wales, Scotland, and Northern Ireland). The information in this chapter will focus on England and Wales, and Scotland. It is essential that clinicians working with children are familiar with the laws of the jurisdiction in which they work.

Definition of 'child'

In England and Wales a child is any person under 18 (except for certain financial transactions). In Scotland there is no one definition of a child, it depends on the legislation and/or circumstances:

- In general, 16-year-olds in Scotland can do most things legally except vote and buy alcohol (18) or drive (17)
- Parents are obliged to pay maintenance for their children until 16 and up to the age of 25 if the child is in full-time education
- When a child is 'looked after' by the local authority, care can last up to 18 and there should then be provision for after-care.

Main legislations

Child Welfare Law legislation covers:

- Private Law(arrangements within the family)
- Public law (involving the family and the state, usually the local authority).

The central themes of child welfare law are:

- The autonomy of the family with parental responsibilities and rights
- The provision of services by the state, particularly in support of children and families in need
- The protection of the child who may be at risk or has suffered significant harm
- Co-operation between professionals and families working in the best interests of the child.

General principles of the legislations

The Children Act 1989 (England and Wales)

Sets out 3 principles that should be applied in decisions.

Non-intervention

- The emphasis is on encouraging co-operation and negotiation between all parties in order to try and enable children to remain with their families
- It states that the court shall make no order unless it is better for the child to make an order, rather than not making an order.

Avoidance of delay

- Delay is not in the best interest of the child and should be avoided unless absolutely necessary
- The court uses 'direction hearings' to estimate the length of the full hearing, what evidence, and what witnesses will be called, in order to make full hearings as effective and economical as possible.

The welfare of the child is of paramount importance

When making decisions the court must take into account:

- The wishes and feelings of the child should be elicited (taking into account age and level of understanding)
- The child's physical, emotional, and educational needs
- The likely effect on the child of any change in his or her circumstances
- The child's age, sex, background, and any other characteristics that the court considers relevant to the child
- Any harm that the child has or is at risk of suffering
- How capable are each of the parents or anyone else who might have involvement in meeting the child's needs
- The range of powers available to the court under the 1989 Act
- Reference to this list when preparing court reports is not compulsory, but ensures that the report keeps in line with the principles of the act and will be welcomed by the court.

The Children (Scotland) Act 1995

Covers broadly the same areas as the English and Welsh legislation, but also includes the Children's Hearing system and Parental Responsibility Orders.

It sets out 4 principles that should be applied in decisions.

- **The child's welfare should be a paramount consideration**: in general, this refers to the duration of childhood, but in adoption cases it requires consideration for the welfare throughout the child's life
- **There should be consideration of the child's views:**
  - All children over the age of 12 years are presumed to have 'views', but there is no lower age limit and younger children may also be considered as having 'views'
  - Whilst it is necessary to consider the child's views this does not equate to doing exactly what the child wants
- **Minimum necessary intervention:**
  - Sometimes referred to as the 'no order' principle
  - The court/hearing must be sure that an order is necessary for the child's welfare, and the order it is making is the best one
  - If the child's welfare can be secured without an order or with a less restrictive order than was originally considered, then that is what should used
- **Consideration of religious persuasion, racial, cultural, and linguistic heritage**

In addition to these principles, there is an expectation that there will be co-operative working between all individuals and professionals. This extends to the parents where there is an expectation that parents will work together for the welfare of the child, even if they themselves do not get on.

Parentage, and parental responsibilities and rights

Parentage: legal mother and father

This refers to consideration as to who are the legal mother and father of a child. This has become a much more complicated question to answer with the development of new fertilization techniques and the diversity in what is considered to be a family.

Parental responsibility

Prior to The Children Act 1989 (England and Wales) and Children (Scotland) Act 1995, children were treated as the possession of their parents, but the emphasis has shifted and children are now seen as having their own rights.

In England and Wales, the term used is 'parental responsibility' whereas in Scotland it is 'parental responsibilities and rights'. Both give the legal basis for making decisions about a child.

Although there may be some jurisdictional differences the general principle are similar.

A parent's responsibilities are:
- To safeguard and protect the child's welfare
- To provide guidance
- To maintain contact if not living with the child
- To act as the child's legal representative if need be.

A parent's rights are:
- To have the child living with him or her
- To control, direct, or guide the child
- To maintain contact if not living with the child
- To act as the child's legal representative if need be.

These rights can be exercised by anyone having them without obtaining the consent of anyone else who also has them, with the exception that the child cannot be removed from the UK without the consent of everyone who has parental responsibilities, and rights of residence and contact, and is exercising these rights.

Parental rights and responsibility for a child are lost by death or adoption. In Scotland, the local authority must apply to the court for a Parental Responsibility order (PRO) to obtain parental responsibilities and rights.

In cases of surrogacy the individual or couple who commission the surrogacy are not the legal parents, and have no responsibilities and rights, but may acquire these with the consent of the legal parent(s) under the HFEA 1990.

Table 30.1 Summary of parentage and rights

Situation	Relationship	Legal mother	R&R	Legal father	R&R
Unassisted conception	Married any time between conception and the birth of the child, or anytime subsequently	Genetic mother	Yes	Genetic father	Yes
Unassisted conception	Not married any time between conception and the birth of the child	Genetic mother	Yes	Only if both he and the mother acknowledge him as the father, and the child is registered as his	Not generally, but can acquire these, e.g. if he marries the mother after the child's birth or, in Scotland, if he is named on birth certificate (after 2006)
Assisted conception	Uses her partner's sperm	Gestational mother	Yes	Yes	Only if married to the mother
Assisted conception	Anonymous sperm donor with partner's consent	Gestational mother	Yes	Yes	Only if married to the mother
Assisted conception	Anonymous sperm donor via registered clinic, partner does not consent	Gestational mother	Yes	The child has no legal father	
Assisted conception	Sperm from deceased donor	Gestational mother	Yes	The child has no legal father	
Surrogacy	If surrogate mother is married and partner agreed to surrogacy	Surrogate mother	Yes	Surrogate's partner	Yes
Surrogacy	If surrogate mother is married and partner did not agree to surrogacy	Surrogate mother	Yes	Genetic father	No

Table 30.1 Summary of parentage and rights (*continued*)

Situation	Relationship	Legal mother	R&R	Legal father	R&R
Surrogacy	Not married	Surrogate mother	Yes	Surrogate is the sole legal parent	
Marriage to a women with children from a previous relationship		Genetic mother	Yes	No	No

R&R: Responsibilities and rights.

Responsibility, capacity, and consent to treatment

Responsibility and capacity

In England and Wales and Northern Ireland the age of criminal responsibility (the age at which you can be legally tried for an offence in a court) is 10 years. In Scotland the age of criminal capacity in Scotland is 8 (the lowest in Europe). The age of civil capacity on Scotland is generally 16, but with some specific exceptions

A child under 16 years of age:
- Can carry out normal transactions, e.g. buy sweets and clothes
- Can make a will, if 12 or over
- Must be asked if he or she consents to adoption (unless deemed incapable)
- May instruct a solicitor in any civil matter if he or she has a general understanding of what it means to do so.

Consent to treatment

In England and Wales young people aged 16–18 have the right to consent or refuse treatment, but may be overruled by a person with parental responsibility or the courts. Those under 16 may have the right to consent to or refuse treatment if deemed capable by a medical practitioner, but may also be overruled as with older children. In general, the following points should be considered:
- Parental powers are for the protection of the child
- Parental powers dwindle as the child matures
- Parental powers depend on the understanding of the individual child, not on any fixed age (Gillick v. West Norfolk and Wisbech Health Authority and DHSS 1985).

In Scotland young people under 16 years of age are considered to be able to consent to and refuse treatment when deemed capable by a medical practitioner of understanding the nature and consequences of the treatment. When the young person is deemed capable they must be the person to consent, parental consent is not required, and *cannot* override the young person's decision. However, it is good practice to work with the family as a whole as this right to consent also includes the right to refuse treatment.

When emergency treatment is required practitioners must use their own clinical judgment about treatment if it is not possible to obtain consent from the young person or anyone with parental responsibilities.

It is important in these circumstances to document any attempts to consult with parents or those with parental responsibilities, and to outline why it has been necessary to proceed without consent.

Consent to psychiatric treatment

For treatment of informal patients, the same conditions apply as for medical, dental, and surgical treatment.

Detained patients

Both the Mental Health Act (MHA) (England) 1983 and the MHA (Scotland) 2003 have no lower age limit, and may be used for children and young people. The MHA (Scotland) 2003 includes a number of new provision to take into account the welfare and interests of the child.

Child protection legislation

There is guidance both from the Department of Health and the Scottish Executive requiring local authorities to have in place Child Protection Committees, with inter-disciplinary membership and clear local child protection policies. Everyone working with children and their families must be familiar with the policies and practices in their local area. Copies of policies should be readily available in the workplace and from the local social work department.

Legislation governing child protection clearly outlines threshold criteria that must be satisfied before any order is made. These are based on there being reasonable grounds to suspect harm has or may occur to the child, and specific measures are required. The particular grounds vary for each order.

Scotland

There are 3 orders in the Children (Scotland) Act 1995 that can be used for child protection. All require an application to the courts.

Child assessment order (CAO)

Only the local authority can apply to the sheriff for this order, which can last for a maximum of 7 days and allows 'for an assessment of the state of a child's health or development or for the way in which he/she has been treated'. CAOs are appropriate where attempts to achieve an assessment have been unsuccessful due to lack of parental or care co-operation.
- The order must specify the order start date, and length and the type of assessment to be conducted
- A CAO cannot be obtained on an emergency basis.

Consent and capacity to treatment issues are the same for CAO as for non-court directed assessments

Child Protection order (CPO)

Can be applied for by any person, including the local authority. Certain criteria must be satisfied. On granting of the order, the child becomes a 'looked after' child and must also be referred immediately to the Children's Reporter. Allows for the removal of the child from home or prevention of removal from a designated place.
- Can be applied for on an emergency basis
- Last for a maximum of 8 days.

Emergency Protection order (EPO)

This can only be granted under certain circumstances. This lasts for a maximum of 24 h, by which time an application for a CPO must have been made or the child goes home. The police have a similar power to give emergency protection for up to 24 h.

Exclusion order (EO)

Only the local authority can apply to the sheriff for an EO. This allows a named person to be removed from the home if the child is at risk, as an alternative to removing the child.

- It can be obtained on an emergency basis
- Lasts for a maximum of 6 months.

England and Wales

The Children Act 1989 describes several types of orders that can be used in cases of child protection.

Child Assessment order

The local authority or 'authorized person' apply to the court and the criteria to be satisfied are similar to Scotland.

Emergency Protection order

Anyone can apply to the court for this the criteria to be satisfied are similar to Scotland.

- Can be granted for up to 8 days
- Can be extended once by the court for up to 7 days
- The police have powers under the 1989 Act to take a child into police protection for up to 72 h. They do not acquire parental rights, but have a duty to safeguard and promote the child's welfare.

Care order

Only the local authority and/or an authorized person may apply to the court for this type of order. The court must be satisfied that the threshold criteria are met and, in addition, what plans the local authority has if the child is placed in care, and whether it would be possible to carry these out without a care order being made.

The local authority acquires parental responsibility, but the parent does not cease to have parental rights, and the implication is that the local authority and parents will work in partnership.

In addition, there are several private law orders also referred to as 'section 8 orders':

- Residence order
- Contact order
- Prohibited Steps order
- Specific issue order
- Family assistance order.

Specific details about the criteria for these orders can be found in the relevant section of the 1989 Act.

Duties and responsibilities of the local authority

Under child welfare legislation local authorities as a whole, not just social work departments, have a duty to provide services to children and families 'in need' and also to 'looked after' children. Local authorities are expected to have a co-ordinated plan for covering all the services they provide for children.

Children 'in need'

The Children (Scotland) Act 1995 has a clear definition of children 'in need' that are similar to the criteria in the England and Wales 1989 Act. This definition is broad and includes any child who is:
* Unlikely to achieve or maintain, or have the opportunity of achieving or maintaining a reasonable standard of health or development unless he/she receives services; or
* His/her health or development is likely significantly to be impaired or further impaired unless services are provided; or
* He /she is disabled; or
* He/se is adversely affected by the disability of any other person in the family.

Disability is this context also includes those suffering from mental illness as defined by the MHA (Scotland) Act 2003

'Looked after' children

The definition of a 'looked after' child differs across the UK. It is broadly defined as a child who is under the care of a local authority or provided with accommodation by the local authority. This may be on a voluntary or compulsory basis.

Children can be 'looked after' and remain within their own family, or they can be placed away from home if this is considered to be necessary within the principles of child welfare legislation.

In regards to parental rights and responsibilities, the position in England and Wales is that local authorities may acquire these for a child under a care order. However, in Scotland local authorities do not acquire parental rights and responsibilities unless they are granted a PRO following application to the courts.

Further details can be found in the relevant legislation for each country.

The Juvenile Justice System (England and Wales)

In England and Wales criminal proceeding relating to children 17 years or below are dealt with by a specialized for of magistrates court called the Youth Court under the (Criminal Justice Act 1991). This is similar to the arrangements in other European countries.

The Youth Court consists of 2 or 3 magistrates (including one man and one woman), drawn from a lay panel appointed by the Crown, who are not legally qualified, but have received special training. They sit with a legally-qualified clerk who advises them on points of law.

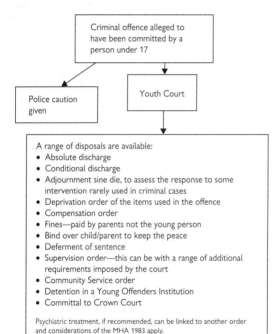

Criminal offence alleged to have been committed by a person under 17

Police caution given

Youth Court

A range of disposals are available:
- Absolute discharge
- Conditional discharge
- Adjournment sine die, to assess the response to some intervention rarely used in criminal cases
- Deprivation order of the items used in the offence
- Compensation order
- Fines—paid by parents not the young person
- Bind over child/parent to keep the peace
- Deferment of sentence
- Supervision order—this can be with a range of additional requirements imposed by the court
- Community Service order
- Detention in a Young Offenders Institution
- Committal to Crown Court

Psychiatric treatment, if recommended, can be linked to another order and considerations of the MHA 1983 apply.

Fig. 30.1 Juvenile Justice System England and Wales.

Antisocial Behaviour orders

Antisocial Behaviour orders (ASBOs) can be imposed by courts on young people and parents where there is persistent unacceptable behaviour. The details and regulation of these orders is beyond the scope of this book, and readers should refer to the relevant legislation in their jurisdiction for further details.

The Children's Hearing system (Scotland)

The children's hearing system is unique to Scotland, but is internationally highly regarded as a progressive approach to child welfare and juvenile justice. The Children's Hearing system was introduced by the Social Work (Scotland) Act 1968, based on findings of the Kilbradon Report and replaced the juvenile court system. The guiding principle of the child's welfare being paramount remains central to the hearing system.

Initially, the hearing system largely dealt with children who had committed crimes, but over the years more and more cases have concerned children with social problems and child protection. Despite having the lowest age of criminal capacity in Europe, only children charged with the most serious crimes, such as severe assault or murder, are dealt with in the adult court system. The Children's Hearing system deals mainly with those under 16 years of age, but once a child is subject to a supervision requirement, he/she can stay in the system until the age of 18.

Unlike the courts the hearing system is not concerned with guilt or innocence, but with the welfare principle—what is in the best interests of the child?

Structure of the children's hearing system

Each local authority in Scotland has a panel of specially recruited lay members (a children's panel) who are appointed by Scottish Government. A hearing consists of 3 panel members, of whom one must be a man and one a woman. One panel member, with appropriate training, acts as the chairman, but has no overriding vote. Decisions are made unanimously or by majority.

The reporter to the children's panel, who will have either a social work or legal background, acts as a clerk and advisor to the hearing, but has many other duties. The reporter system operates on a national basis, with one reporter for every local authority. The reporter system is independent and separate from the panel members system.

Anyone with concerns about a child may provide information or refer a child to the reporter if they have concerns about a child. The local authority and the Police have a duty to refer to the reporter, but they may also refer the case to the Procurator Fiscal (PF).

It is the reporter's duty to investigate referrals by seeking reports or further information from relevant persons, and arrange for a hearing to take place if the following criteria are met:

• The child needs compulsory measures of supervision

and

• There is sufficient evidence to establish one or more of the grounds for referral, which include:
  • The child being outwith control of any relevant person
  • The child being at risk of harm, such as abuse
  • The child having been abused
  • The child being likely to suffer from a lack of parental care
  • The child failing to attend school regularly without a reasonable excuse
  • The child committing an offence
  • The child misusing alcohol, drugs, or solvents.

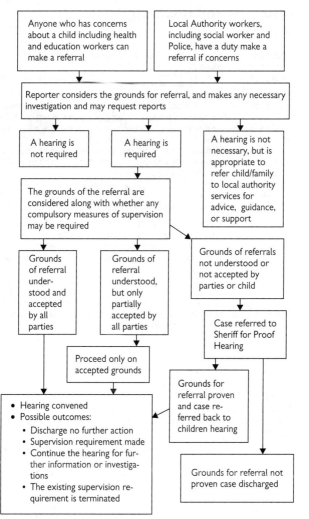

Fig. 30.2 Children's Hearing process.

Adoption and fostering

Adoption is regulated by a number of laws:
- Adoption (Scotland) Act 1978
- Adoption Allowance (Scotland) Regulations 1998
- Adoption (Intercountry Aspects) Act 1999
- Adoption and Children Act 2002.

Adoption is the legal process through which all legal ties and contact with a child's birth family are ended, and replaced in law by the new adoptive family.

In order for a child to be adopted, all of those with parental responsibilities and rights must either freely and unconditionally agree to the adoption, or have their agreement legally 'dispensed' with.

'Dispensation' with parental agreement refers to situations when a person whose agreement is required has refused to give it. It can take place under certain circumstances when the relevant person:
- Cannot be found or is incapable of giving agreement
- Withholds agreement unreasonably
- Fails to discharge parental obligations or ill treats the child in specific ways.

In dispensation the welfare of the child must always be considered. With respect to the parents, the issue to be considered is whether they are being reasonable, and not whether they are right or mistaken in their views. This issue of agreement is dealt with either in the adoption application or earlier, through a process known as freeing.

Freeing is a court application, which can only be made by the local authority, by which parental responsibility is transferred to the applying adoption agency, and thus enables parental agreement to be in place before a child is placed with an adoptive family. This process is not mandatory, but can avoid disputes between birth and adoptive parents.

Types of adoption

Agency adoptions

There are 2 types of adoption agencies:
- Local authority adoption agencies
- Registered adoption services.

These are voluntary agencies regulated and inspected in Scotland by the Care Commission, and in England and Wales under the Adoption Agencies Regulation 1983

Non-agency adoptions that include adoptions by relatives and step parents

Who can adopt?
- There is no legal upper age limit for those adopting, although agencies may impose one. The lower age limit is 21
- Adopters must either be domiciled in the UK or have been habitually resident in the UK for >1 year prior to the application (but only one member of an adopting couple needs to be domiciled in the UK)
- Adopters do not have to have British nationality to adopt
- Adoption by unmarried couples in England and Wales is allowed under the Adoption and Children Act 2002, and in Scotland under the Adoption and Children Act (Scotland) 2007
- Foster carers can also apply to adopt a child placed with them.

Who can be adopted?
- A child who is both unmarried and under 18 at the time of the adoption application
- A child of any nationality
- A child must have lived with one or both of the applicants before an adoption order can be granted
- A child must be at least 19 weeks of age, and have lived with one or more of the applicants for the previous 13 weeks
- In the case of children in foster care, the child must be at least 1 year old, and have lived with one or both of the applicants for at least 1 year.

Access to birth records by adopted children

Under the Adoption Act 1976, if a child was adopted through a court in England or Wales, and is aged 18 years or over they can apply to the Registrar General Office for information about their birth name, birth parent(s) name(s), and their district of birth with which to apply for a certified copy of their original birth entry. If the adoption was before November 1975 the individual is required to attend an informal meeting with an approved adoption advisor for confidential guidance. If the adoptions was between November 1975 and December 2005 there is no requirement to attend counselling, but it is available.

The Adoption Contact Register created in 1991 and held by the Registrar Generals Office exists to put adopted people, and their birth relatives in touch with each other if that is what they both wish.

The Adoption (Scotland) Act 1978 and subsequent legislation gives automatic access to birth record and adoption related court proceeding to any adopted person over 16. Counselling services are available, but optional

Fostering

This is the removal of a child either from home or from their current accommodation, and placement with a foster carer. Local authorities have a duty to inspect and approve all foster placements. In addition, in Scotland placements must be registered and inspected by the Care Commission.

Foster carers do not acquire parental rights and responsibilities, but have general rights of control because they are acting in place of the parents.

Disclosure checks

The Police Act 1997 introduced a system for disclosing criminal information to individuals and employers.

With the implementation of Protection of Children (Scotland) Act 2003 (POCSA) in 2005, disclosure checks are required for employees, prospective carers, and anyone else working with children or vulnerable adults, whether in a paid or unpaid capacity, including volunteers and instructors running sports or activity groups.

Disclosure Scotland is the body that arranges for checks.

There are 3 levels of disclosure:
- **Basic:** this shows only convictions that are unspent in terms of the Rehabilitation of Offenders Act 1974
- **Standard:** contains all disclosures whether spent or unspent in terms of the 1974 Act
- **Enhanced:** contains all convictions and 'police intelligence' about the individual. This type of disclosure is required for people working directly with or caring for children, such as foster carers and therapists.

In the rest of the UK, disclosure checks are carried out by the Criminal Records Bureau (CRB), an Executive Agency of the Home Office launched in March 2002. There are two levels of CRB check currently available, called Standard and Enhanced disclosures:
- **Standard:** available to anyone involved in working with children or vulnerable adults, as well as certain other occupations and professions, as specified in the Exceptions Order to the Rehabilitation of Offenders Act (ROA) 1974. Standard disclosures show current and spent convictions, cautions, reprimands, and warnings held on the Police National Computer. If the post involves working with children or vulnerable adults, the following lists of those considered unsuitable for work with children or vulnerable adults may also be searched:
  - Protection of Children Act (POCA) list
  - Protection of Vulnerable Adults (POVA) list
  - Information that is held under Section 142 of the Education Act 2002 (formerly known as List 99)
- **Enhanced:** this is the highest level of check available to anyone involved in regularly caring for, training, supervising, or being in sole charge of children or vulnerable adults; it contains the same information as the Standard Disclosure, but with the addition of any relevant and proportionate information held by the local police forces.

From February 2005, guidance issued the Department of Health requires that all NHS employers, including locums and agency staff, GPs, and dentists, volunteers, and students who have access to patients as part of their normal duties have a CRB disclosure.

The Independent Safeguarding Authority (ISA)

Following the murders of Jessica Chapman and Holly Wells in 2002, the Bichard Inquiry was commissioned. One of the issues this inquiry looked at was the way employers recruit people to work with children and vulnerable adults. Its recommendations included in Safeguarding Vulnerable Groups Act (2006) was the recognition for there to be a single agency to vet all individuals who want to work or volunteer with vulnerable people. The ISA was created to fulfil this role across England, Wales, and Northern Ireland (Scotland is developing its own similar system closely with the ISA.). The ISA will assess every person who wants to work or volunteer with vulnerable people. The ISA will work closely with the CRB and will maintain the ISA Barred Lists holding information previously contained in the POVA and POCA lists, and List 99 held by the Department for Children, Schools, and Families.

Children's Commissioners

In response to the Victoria Climbié Inquiry, the Government published the *Every Child Matters* Green Paper in September 2003, which proposed changes in policy and legislation to maximize opportunities, and minimize risks for all children and young people, focusing services more effectively around the needs of children, young people and families. The Childrens Act 2004 was produced in light of this report, and provides for the establishment of a Children's Commissioners in England, Wales, Northern Ireland, and Scotland to promote awareness of the views and interests of children (and certain groups of vulnerable young adults), and in certain circumstances initiate inquiries into individual cases that raise issues of public policy that would be relevant to other children. The commissioner reports to the Secretary of State.

Additional provisions under the Act apply only to England and lay out responsibility for key agencies duties to safeguard children and promote their interests. It also establishes statutory Local Safeguarding Children Boards to replace the existing non-statutory Area Child Protection Committees. In addition, it provides for regulations to require children's services authorities to prepare and publish a Children and Young People's Plan (CYPP), which will set out their strategy for services for children and relevant young people.

Recommended reading

All England Law Reports (1985) *Gillick West Norfolk and Wisbech Area Health Authority* 3, pp 402–37.

Black D, Wolkind S, Hendricks JH. (1991) *Child Psychiatry and the Law*. Gaskell, London.

Children Act. 1989. Chapter 41. HMSO, London. Available at: http://www.opsi.gov.uk/acts/acts1989/Ukpga_19890041_en_1.htm (accessed 13 April 2008).

Children Act. 2004. Chapter 31. HMSO, London. Available at: http://www.opsi.gov.uk/acts/acts2004/ukpga_20040031_en_1 (accessed 13 April 2008).

Children (Scotland) Act. 1995. Chapter 36. HMSO, Edinburgh. Available at: http://www.opsi.gov.uk/acts/acts1995/Ukpga_19950036_en_1.htm (accessed 13 April 2008).

Plumtree A. (2005) *Child Care Law: A Summary of the Law in Scotland*. British Association for Adoption and Fostering, London.

Service development and delivery

Child and Adolescent Mental Health Services (CAMHS): strategic issues

This chapter, of necessity, applies more to services in the United Kingdom, where much work has been done in the last decade looking at the shape of delivery of comprehensive services for children and young people with mental health difficulties.

The publication of the report *Together We Stand* by the NHS Health Advisory Service (often referred to as 'the HAS report') in 1995 began a process of systematic examination, strategic planning, and managed delivery of CAMHS that had previously been largely missing from these services.

Although much of this work will be applicable to other countries, it is in the context of the UK and its publicly funded National Health Service that this model was developed.

Historically, the development of CAMHS has been idiosyncratic and serendipitous, often depending of individual interest and influence, rather than sound planning, Thus, in England, many services developed mainly from a Child Guidance model, whilst in Scotland, it was often adult psychiatrists with an interest in young people working down the age range that caused services to evolve. The range of services provided to children and young people was often very variable in both quantity and quality, and issues of limited access to services were common. Nor was there any planning around the provision of inpatient beds for this population, with some areas having no access to beds and young people often being accommodated in adult psychiatry wards.

Tiered services

Together We Stand proposed a tiered approach to service delivery that is now widely adopted across the UK.

Tier 1

These include General Practice, Social Work, Education, and the Voluntary Sector, and indicates universal services to which all children and young people have access, whether or not they have a mental health problem.

Tier 2

This describes the situations where mental health workers of a variety of disciplines work independently with children and young people, or provide consultation to others who are doing this type of work.

Tier 3

This describes a multidisciplinary approach to more complex and specific difficulties, where members of a team work together to provide a service to children and young people. These professionals, who are likely to also be working at a Tier 2 level, usually belong to a comprehensive CAMHS.

Tier 4

Some young people have such special needs that they require a more comprehensive, all-encompassing service, such as an inpatient facility or a service for young people with severe eating disorders.

Whilst 'Together We Stand' gave a framework for the delivery of CAMHS, subsequent pieces of work have defined more clearly what should be delivered to meet the needs of children and adolescents with mental health problems.

The National Service Frameworks in England and Wales and the 'Framework for Metal Health Services for Children and Young People' in Scotland, describe the range and variety of provision that comprises a comprehensive mental health service for the young.

These documents make reference to:
- The composition of CAMHS teams
- The capacity required to deliver a comprehensive service
- Links with other agencies, emergency services
- Input to training and teaching, consultation work, and specialist services, such as inpatient beds.

Whilst this is by no means a comprehensive list, it illustrates the range of topics covered in these high level strategic documents. Implementation of the strategy is the business of local health providers in whatever way these are configured.

Implementation issues

Local health providers are charged with the task of implementing national strategies. In doing so, they clearly face a wide range of challenges.

Challenges facing service providers

- Enhancing capacity
- Training up the appropriate workforce
- Working across agencies in a collaborative framework
- Sharing information
- Improving access to services
- Increasing demand
- Transition to other services, e.g. adult psychiatry services
- Valuing the multidisciplinary nature of CAMHS work
- Understanding the stigma of mental health problems for young people
- Using information technology creatively
- Facing the challenges of specific groups
- Resistance to re-design and change.

Specific groups that present a particular challenge

- Looked after and accommodated children
- Children leaving care
- Children and young people with learning disability
- Young people who deliberately harm themselves
- Refugee and asylum-seeking children and young people
- Young people who misuse substances including alcohol
- Children from ethnic minorities
- Forensic services for children and young people who offend
- Children and young people with chronic physical illness
- Children with sensory impairments
- Young people with eating disorders
- Young people who need to move into adult mental health services.

The agenda laid out in the strategic documents cannot and should not be met by health alone. In order to meet these and other challenges, CAMHS have to work in partnership with other organizations, both statutory and voluntary, as well as making links with providers in the private sector. A commitment to developing CAMHS is now included in the health strategy of the different UK jurisdictions with timescales for implementation and all are on broadly similar lines.

Workforce issues

The strategic plans for CAMHS include ambitious targets for increasing the workforce in specialist CAMHS. However, there is a clear recognition that not all young people with mental health difficulties require intervention from a specialist service. The tiered model of service delivery relies on enhancing the skills of professionals working in Tier 1; this includes social workers, health visitors, school teachers, general practitioners, and youth workers, etc. In order to achieve this aim, staff within specialist services will need to be deployed in order that they can provide the considerable amounts of training and support that will be required in order to first up-skill the Tier 1 workforce and then to provide ongoing support.

In addition, there is no point in having a skilled Tier 1 workforce if there are not adequate specialist services for them to refer children into when required. Therefore, attention also has to be paid to the training, recruitment, and retention of specialist mental health professionals.

The new profession of Primary Mental Health Worker, which was outlined in *Together We Stand*, is starting to play a key role at the interface between universal services and specialist services. These workers can provide much of the training, consultation, and support to Tier 1 services, whilst retaining links to specialist services. However, as with any new professional grouping, it is not yet clear as to how primary mental health workers should be optimally organized and deployed.

Professional groups working in specialist CAMHS

- Psychiatrists
- Clinical and educational psychologists
- Mental health nurses
- Family therapists
- Specialist psychological therapists, e.g. cognitive behaviour therapists (CBTs) and interpersonal therapists (IPTs)
- Occupational therapists
- Child psychotherapists
- Primary mental health workers
- Creative therapists
- Speech and language therapists
- Social workers
- Dieticians
- Nursery nurses
- Administrative and support staff
- Management staff.

Inpatient services

The development of inpatient services for children and adolescents, like CAMHS themselves, have evolved from two different styles.

- The first is the therapeutic milieu idea, where the important therapeutic treatment is the ward environment itself. This was the most common model of inpatient unit for young people up until about 10 years ago
- The second model is an adaptation of acute adult psychiatric care often involving admission either to an adult ward or to a general paediatric ward with input from CAMHS staff. In this model the emphasis is on medical assessment and treatment rather than a therapeutic experience.

The 1950s and 60s saw a rapid expansion of child and adolescent inpatient beds. Whilst inpatient child and adolescent psychiatric facilities have remained common in much of mainland Europe, this had not been the case in the UK, where in the last two decades many units have been closed. This is particularly so for the children's inpatient units, but has also been the case for many adolescent units and there has been a subsequent rise in admission of young people to adult psychiatric wards. This has, to some extent, coincided with research evidencing the negative outcomes from residential care, particularly in the social care sector.

Inpatient beds for children and young people are now seen as a valuable if scarce resource and their use is more focused.

Legislation in the form of the Children Acts and Mental Health legislation actively discourage the admission of young people under the age of 18 to adult wards and CAMHS inpatient units have had to adapt to a greater demand for emergency admissions and a generally more unwell group of patients.

Reasons for admission to an inpatient unit

- Detailed assessment of complex cases
- Deterioration of symptoms despite the most intensive alternative outpatient/day-patient treatment that can be offered
- To allow the introduction of a new treatment, such as medication, to be observed
- To allow assessment away from the family environment.

Although this last reason may be seen as a contentious reason for admission to a health facility, it can be helpful when there is genuine concern that the family may be contributing in some way to the presentation.

Planning care

In most cases, the success of an inpatient admission is as dependant on good admission and discharge planning as it is on the care delivered whilst an inpatient. This can be very challenging in CAMHS where beds are few and units are often distant from patients' homes. Despite this, units generally make enormous efforts to plan admissions and discharges by involving the young person, their family, and the local services, including education, as holistically and actively as is possible.

Admission to an inpatient unit usually involves at least one meeting with the referrer to clarify the aims of the admission, followed up by a meeting with the young person and their family, and often a visit to the family home. There is often a visit to the unit by the family, if this is practicable and the admission is a planned one.

Discharge procedures follow the reverse pattern with close liaison between the unit and professional services that will be caring for the young person following discharge.

Although virtually all inpatient services are open units, the use of mental health legislation to detain patients is not unusual and should be considered if the patient meets the appropriate criteria.

The inpatient team

A well functioning multidisciplinary team plays a key role in the success of a unit and of the admissions to the unit. Services should be adequately staffed to provide a broad and intensive treatment package within in a safe and secure environment. The multidisciplinary team should include members from across the CAMHS disciplines. This may include:

- Child and adolescent psychiatrists
- Psychologists
- Social workers
- Nurses with mental health and/or learning disability and/or children's nursing qualifications
- Allied health professionals from speech and language, occupational therapy, dietetics, physiotherapy, etc.
- Family therapists
- Specialist psychological therapists, e.g. CBT and IPT
- Other psychotherapists, including from the creative therapies
- Teachers.

There should be adequate numbers of staff to ensure safe and appropriate care for the task to hand. With too few staff the risks of adverse incidents and staff burn out with high turnover are increased. Staff should have appropriate training in child and adolescent psychiatry, as well as child development and systemic working, and should be trained in age appropriate breakaway and restraint techniques. There should be robust arrangements for dealing with both psychiatric and medical emergencies. Strong leadership and management facilitate good coherent team working and, in this respect, the unit's consultant and charge nurse play pivotal roles.

The physical environment is also important and should provide age-appropriate facilities with access to education and a range of local leisure facilities. It should be accessible for families visiting and have strong ties with community CAMHS in the area that it serves.

Specialist inpatient services

Specialist inpatient services are currently rare, but likely to increase in the future as the evidence base for inpatient treatment expends. At present these include services for:
- Eating disorders
- Learning disability
- Forensic patients.

Possible adverse effects of inpatient admission

- Impact on the family
- 'Learning' of new symptoms from other disturbed young people
- Dislocation from a familiar environment and peer group
- Loss of education if the unit is not well supported educationally
- Institutionalization if admission is prolonged with subsequent dependency.

Specific challenges of inpatient treatment

- Assessment, including physical assessment, and close observation
- Consent to treatment—this might include appropriate use of mental health legislation, but in any case must involve assessment of the young person's capacity to consent to their treatment plan
- Good treatment planning, including the setting of goals and involvement of parents and family
- Being able to adapt treatments normally delivered in an outpatient setting to an inpatient unit. This is particularly important when a young person is far from their local services and treatment begun in an inpatient unit may be disrupted on transfer back to their local area.

Day services and intensive outreach

Day services

Day services vary considerably and even more so than inpatient services. The variety of tasks and configuration of day services ranges from intensive assessments to specific behavioural and education-based programmes for younger children to a 'day hospital' for older adolescents with serious psychiatric disorder with an ethos similar to that found in adult psychiatry. Most day services are aimed at a particular patient group determined either by age, presenting problem, or degree of disturbance. Many day services are situated in proximity to inpatient units, and this allows a sharing of values and philosophies, staff expertise, and resources. These non-residential treatment units have the advantage of allowing the child or young person to remain within their own community, and especially their own family with the potential for greater family involvement in the treatment package.

Maintaining a comprehensive treatment and assessment programme alongside a full educational curriculum within a limited time slot is challenging for most day services, and many fall short of being able to keep up a full academic input for their patients, whilst at the same time fulfilling their core clinical tasks.

Many of the other challenges inherent in inpatient settings apply equally to day services and these are complex units to run successfully requiring adequate staffing and resources for a small number of often intensely complex young patients. Staffing of a day service should mirror that already detailed for inpatient services and should cover the whole range of CAMHS professionals. Leadership is a key issue and many day services are nurse-led units with nurses providing the principal leadership roles.

Intensive outreach services

In recent years there has been an increasing emphasis on intensive outreach approaches to treatment with care being delivered in the patient's home, rather than a day service or inpatient unit. This is, at least in part, driven by the move away from extended and expensive inpatient stays. It allows assessment and treatment to take place as close to the child's natural environment as possible, with the family and other local systems being encouraged to be more intimately involved in the process than is otherwise possible. Staff in these treatment programmes need to be of sufficient seniority and experience to act autonomously when required, and the staff/skill mix needs to be adequate to provide an appropriately broad range of therapies. Care plans are tailored to the individual and 24-h access to emergency care is often provided.

Factors associated with positive outcomes in inpatient, day-patient, and intensive outreach treatments

- Well planned evidence-based treatment programmes
- Emotional disorder as opposed to behavioural problems
- Well co-ordinated and high quality aftercare
- A positive therapeutic alliance between the patient, family, and unit.
- Higher intelligence of patients
- Healthy family functioning prior to admission.

Consultation to other services

Consultation to other services and professionals plays a key role in the delivery of comprehensive mental health services to children and young people. All of the strategy documents produced in the last few years recognize the value of using a consultation model to increase the skill base of workers in 'universal services', as well as supporting workers in Tiers 1 and 2 to manage complex cases.

Whilst consultation is often seen as being provided by Specialist CAMHS to frontline workers the HAS Report proposed a model, whereby primary mental health workers would, as part of their role, provide a significant proportion of consultation work around both individual cases and organizations working with children and young people.

Most contemporary CAMHS embrace both of these models.

The aims of consultation

Regardless of who is providing the consultation, a number of different general aims can be identified. Any one consultation service may encompass all, several, or only one of these within its scope. These aims include:

- Promoting general awareness and understanding of the mental health needs and problems of children and young people
- Assisting a whole system, e.g. a residential school, to better understand those for whom they have a care and to respond to them in a more helpful way
- Helping contain anxiety in an individual, or system caring for or providing treatment for a child or young person
- Identifying and facilitating appropriate referrals to specialist CAMHS.

The context of consultation

- The process should be led by the person seeking consultation
- A clear framework of expectations should be established from the outset. These may include:
  - Frequency of consultation
  - Aims and objectives
  - Who will be attending
  - Framework of confidentiality, etc.
- The tasks of the consultation should be clearly stated and understood by all parties. For example, is it aimed at increasing knowledge and skills, assisting with complex cases, deciding on the appropriateness of a referral, etc.
- Adequate resources need to be available to support the consultation process
- The consultation should be provided by the appropriately qualified and experienced member of staff
- Clear lines of accountability should be established
- Regular monitoring and evaluation are required.

Theoretical frameworks for consultation

If any particular consultation is to be successful and productive for the consultee, it needs to take place within a clear theoretical framework otherwise it is likely to become simply a problem-sharing session. Equally, consultation is clearly different from supervision, although there may be an element of the latter in the former. From the consultant's point of view, their approach to consultation will depend on their own training and theoretical framework. However, it is important that the consultant's theoretical approach is acceptable to the consultee and appropriate to the agreed task.

Medical model

The consultant, usually a doctor, uses their expertise to assist in the assessment and understanding of children and young people being cared for. This often involves meeting with the young people and their families, gathering information in a traditional way, and presenting the findings to staff. Whilst many CAMHS clinicians will not see this as true consultation, it can satisfy the needs of an institution for understanding of children with complex problems.

Systems approach

A style used frequently by clinicians trained in systemic practice that focuses on the whole system looking after a child/children, including aspects of the institutions' functioning. Attempts are made to encourage changes within the system that will benefit the child/children.

Solution focused

The consultant does not act as expert, but rather encourages those to whom they are consulting to think creatively and find solutions that will work for them. This approach does not concentrate on finding explanations for or understanding of problems, but focuses on what works.

Training model

Here, the consultant is explicitly the expert, imparting knowledge and offering training in a variety of therapeutic techniques. Within a consultation contract this may be a part of the consultant's role alongside other tasks.

A successful consultation relationship will often embrace one or more of these models and an experienced consultant will choose the approach that best meets the needs of the consultee, whether it is an individual or an institution.

Recommended reading

Health Advisory Service (1995) *Together We Stand*. HAS, London.

National Assembly of Wales (2001) *Everybody's Business*, Strategy Document. National Assembly of Wales, Cardiff.

Scottish Executive. (2004) *Children and Young People's Mental Health: A Framework for Promotion, Prevention and Care*. Scottish Executive, Edinburgh.

Williams R, Kerfoot M. (2005) *Child and Adolescent Mental Health Services*. Oxford University Press, Oxford.

Management and consultant issues

Management

Management of child and adolescent mental health services can be considered under the broad headings of *Operational* and *Strategic*. Although these two are interlinked, operational describes the day to day running of a service, whilst strategic addresses the broader issues of service design and development. In a successful CAMHS, these two will overlap with a high degree of commonality. Indeed the same personnel are often responsible for delivery of both operational and strategic management within any one service. It is, however, likely that a wide range of staff, often including workers from outside the service, will be concerned with the development of a Strategic Plan.

The appropriate positioning of CAMHS within the broader healthcare system has been the matter of much debate and arrangements vary across the UK. Some are managed alongside paediatric services within an organization delivering acute care, while at the other end of the spectrum there are others managed as part of a Community Care Trust or Community Health Partnership. Some co-exist within the same management system as adult mental health services, whilst having little contact with these services. The particular arrangements matter less than the understanding and support for CAMHS within the wider organization. Close working relationships with partners such as Social Work, Education, and the Voluntary Sector are key, and a direct relationship with Health Commissioners is essential in taking forward the strategic vision of a service.

One of the consequences of the myriad of ways by which CAMHS have developed over the last few decades is a lack of consistency in the ways services have been delivered and, indeed, there has been great variability as to what has been available in different parts of the UK. This has made it difficult for commissioners to understand what is good CAMHS practice, and there is now a drive in all jurisdictions of the UK to look towards national strategic planning with agreement about what constitutes good practice and what can be developed within an inevitably limited resource pool.

Characteristics of a 'healthy' CAMHS

- A clear sense of purpose
- A clear commissioning strategy
- Secure resourcing
- Good relationships with referrers with clear referral pathways
- Strong internal management
- Staff all being aware of both their roles and their responsibilities
- Respect between workers both within the service and between the service and their partners
- Clinical practice that is evidence-based and consistent with current best practice
- Room for innovation and experimentation within a safe environment
- A clear governance arrangements
- Open and clear communication within the service, and with patients and other professionals
- A willingness to audit, evaluate, and examine both clinical and management practice
- Members of staff who all have a sense of ownership of and involvement in the planning and delivery of care.

Planning a service

Most CAMHS were, until recently, largely unplanned and current services have often been left with a legacy that does not necessarily lend itself to the delivery of modern evidence-based care. However, this situation is changing and there is now an opportunity for more coherent service planning. Issues that have to be considered in this planning include:
- Conducting a needs assessment of the population
- The available resources including funding and staff
- The local context including geography, deprivation indices and management structures
- Equity of access to services for all, including disabled patients
- Defining the boundaries of the service: age cut-offs, ability, etc.
- Defining the range of services to be delivered
- The evidence base for the treatments to be delivered
- Clarity around transition to other services, e.g. adult psychiatry
- Sufficient built-in flexibility to respond to changes in demand
- Commissioning arrangements
- Partnership working with other agencies
- Involvement of users and carers in service planning and evaluation
- Is the planned service consistent with agreed good practice models of care?

Although there are a variety of ways that services can be configured, most work either with teams covering a defined geographical patch or with a disorder-based teams. For example, there are a number of developmental neuropsychiatry, attention deficit hyperactivity disorder (ADHD) and autism services providing services for children and young people in a wider population area. Similarly, there are now teams working with defined populations, such as looked after children. How services are configured will depend on local needs and resources, and as yet there is no clear evidence to support the 'best way' to plan a CAMHS.

Multidisciplinary teams: understanding the team system

The concept of the multi-disciplinary team is not new in CAMHS. The understanding of team working has, however, changed and CAMHS have moved away from a somewhat authoritarian model, with the consultant psychiatrist assuming team leadership, towards a more functional model. Teams may consist of a number of different professionals with different training and backgrounds, working together to meet the needs of the patient group. These professionals may or may not be managed within the same organization. So, for example, social workers may be managed by local authorities, clinical psychologists may come from a general psychology department and only devote part of their work to CAMHS. On the other hand, there are integrated services, where management is overarching. The key to making teams work in a CAMHS environment is to focus on the work and not on the team relationships. Agreement about what the task is and how it should be accomplished will help to dispel difficulties around rivalry and competition, which can be so destructive in team settings.

In a functional team, members accept responsibility for the work of the team and not only their own contribution. Thus, it is no longer any one person's responsibility to ensure that patients are seen and treated effectively. Team members need to know each other's functions and contributions to the care of patients, so that care can be planned most effectively, but they do not necessarily need to develop close personal relationships as might have been assumed in the past. There must be a balance between flexibility and structure. Teams need to be able to respond to changing demands, but a structure that is too open will lead to loss of direction and ineffectiveness.

The way a team functions also has to make sense to users of the service. Most people in contact with mental health services want to feel that they have been heard and understood. It therefore makes little sense for teams to be structured in such a way as to inhibit a flexible response to the needs of their patients. In this respect, patients have little tolerance, quite rightly, for the cross-referral and passing from one person to another for endless assessments. Teams should work together in such a way that their barriers are not obvious to patients and that care is seamless.

Excellent communications within the team, between different teams, and with organizations outside the service are essential. Amongst other things, they can help others, not least managers and commissioners understand the value of team working in child and adolescent mental health practice.

The ethos of team working is particularly important when dealing with complex cases where there may be multiple systems involved. Seriously ill psychiatric cases, such as anorexia nervosa, complex neurodisability cases, and child protection situations are good examples of this. When dealing with cases like these, a well functioning team can provide not only the best care for their patients, but also support for parents and the wider system, better containing anxiety and providing good information. In addition, workers in such a team are better supported and generally have access to more regular supervision.

The role of supervision in a CAMHS team

Supervision has a key role in CAMHS teams and is one of the factors that allow teams to contain high levels of anxiety. All members of a team should have access to supervision (although the trend is for more experienced practitioners, such as consultant psychiatrists, to have little or no access to supervision). Nevertheless, the standard should be aspired to.

Supervision can take many different forms and may be, for example, case-based or based around a therapeutic modality. It may include purely clinical content, or can be expanded to include career development and other personal issues. Supervision is generally delivered by more experienced clinicians, but managers also have a role in delivering case management supervision to those whom they manage. As with consultation, there are different models of supervision. There are, however, common factors that can help make supervision successful:

- Clear, consistent arrangements, e.g. time, duration, frequency
- Who is to attend
- Agreement about what is to be discussed
- Led by the supervisee(s)
- Confidentiality
- The keeping of a record.

Multidisciplinary teams: managing leadership issues

In traditional CAMHS, leadership of a multi-disciplinary team was usually devolved to the consultant psychiatrist. This would be true regardless of their experience; thus, a newly appointed consultant could find themselves expected to lead a team of very experienced clinicians. Leadership was given rather than earned with all the possible attendant problems that this could raise. In a modern CAMHS team, the question of leadership will tend to be more open. It need not be automatically assumed that the consultant psychiatrist will lead the team; indeed, some teams function with very little medical input at all, other than for supervision, and it would therefore be unacceptable to expect the psychiatrist to lead such a team.

In order to resolve issues of leadership, the team must first agree on what the task/role of the leader is to be. There should then be a greater possibility of avoiding conflict and reaching consensus as to who would be the best person to fulfil this role. The authority of leadership will thus be given by the team. It is immeasurably better if this can be done openly and explicitly to avoid residual envy and rivalries which are likely to undermine both the leader and the work of the team. If the leadership role is to be one that has a significant administrative function, then there may be agreement that the position of leader should be a rotating one, which spreads the burden, and allows more team members to gain experience and understanding about the role of a team leader. If, however, there is an expectation that the leader will deal with difficult clinical questions, and liaise directly with practitioners outside the service, then there may be a need to consider clinical experience and expertise.

Whatever the outcome of a leadership question within a team, all clinical members of the team retain responsibility for their own work, and it is no longer the case that the consultant psychiatrist would be expected to carry case responsibility for a large number of patients seen by other team members.

Ethical and clinical responsibilities

Whilst it is clear that responsibility for the patients whom one is treating remains with the individual clinician, the practice of child and adolescent mental health, involving as it does multi-disciplinary working, and working closely with children, young people, and their families, raises a variety of complex ethical considerations. The days when a consultant psychiatrist was held responsible for all cases referred to the team in which they were working are gone. However, consultants do have a responsibility, as described by the General Medical Council (GMC), to satisfy themselves that appropriate arrangements are in place for the management of referrals and patient care.

Doctors and other professionals working in healthcare do so within clear frameworks of professional guidance. For the medical profession in the UK this stems from the GMCs guidance on 'Good Medical Practice', which forms the basis for consultant appraisal and will be the foundation of revalidation in the future. For psychiatrists, this is further delineated in the *Good Psychiatric Practice* guidance issued by the Royal College of Psychiatrists. Other professionals have their own regulatory bodies, such as the Nursing and Midwifery Council, which produce similar guidance, and set standards in the same way as the Medical Council and Royal Colleges.

Hence, within the UK, there is an increasing amount of guidance regarding proper and safe clinical practice and responsibility. Within the practice of child and adolescent mental health, there are a number of additional ethical issues that deserve closer consideration.

Capacity to consent

This is particularly an issue when treating children and young people under the age of 16, and in the UK has been the subject of legislation and judicial review. The contentious issue is whether or not a young person under the age of presumed adulthood can consent or refuse treatment without, or against, their parents' agreement. In the UK, the age of reaching adulthood is itself inconsistent with young people being able to marry without parental consent or join the armed forces at 16, but not permitted to vote or purchase alcohol until 18. In England and Wales the concept of 'Gillick competence' as defined by the House of Lords ('As a matter of Law the parental right to determine whether or not their minor child below the age of sixteen will have medical treatment terminates if and when the child achieves sufficient understanding and intelligence to understand fully what is proposed; Lord Scarman) provides guidance. In Scotland, the 1991 Age of Legal Capacity (Scotland) Act, further reinforced by the Children (Scotland) Act 1995, made provision that a young person under the age of 16 could consent or withhold consent to any medical, surgical, or dental procedure as long as they had the necessary intelligence, comprehension, and insight to understand the procedure and the implications of it.

Confidentiality

Because of the multi-disciplinary and multi-agency nature of much of CAMHS work, confidentiality is a key issue for most services. Nowhere is this more important than in the area of child protection, where clarity of communication is paramount. GMC guidance states that child patients are entitled to the same level of confidentiality as any other patient, consistent with their capacity to consent and make decisions. Nevertheless, there are occasions when the patient's desire for confidentiality conflicts with the professionals' responsibility to protect their patient from harm or, indeed, protect the public. National guidance and local guidelines are clear that, where a patient or other children are at risk of serious harm, then a breach of confidentiality is justified. Nevertheless, it is good practice to make every attempt to persuade patients to include their parents in decision making about their treatment, where this is clinically appropriate.

Maintaining boundaries

Children and young people are entitled to the same dignity as all other patients, and it is the clinician's responsibility to maintain proper boundaries with their young patients and their families. Children are naturally inquisitive and it can be difficult to establish the degree to which personal information can be shared. Clinicians must maintain awareness of their powerful position as adults in relation to their patients and take special care to ensure that this is not abused.

In the current climate of emphasis on child protection, clinicians need to be aware of potential risks in seeing young people on their own when both parties may be vulnerable to misinterpretation of the situation. Disclosure checking, i.e. using formal checking of police records to detect any prior convictions of professionals goes some way to providing reassurance to patients and families, as well as organizations.

Making video and audio recordings

The use of video or audio recordings in CAMHS practice has a long history both in clinical practice and within training. Recordings may only be made with the explicit consent of the patient and all others involved. The subsequent recordings should be treated as part of the medical records unless specifically otherwise agreed, e.g. where a recording is explicitly made for teaching purposes. There is clear guidance on this issue provided by the GMC and in a Council Report from the Royal College of Psychiatrists.

Research with children

Research in CAMHS is vital in establishing the evidence base for service provision, and yet clinicians are sometimes reluctant to involve children and young people in research because of the complex ethical issues involved. Clinicians are required to ensure that children and young people taking part in research are afforded the highest levels of protection of their physical, mental, ethical, and emotional wellbeing. Matters of informed consent and capacity, as well as the position of parents, especially in regard to younger children need to be taken into account.

Assessment in potential child protection situations

When assessing families with regard to care and protection of children, it is necessary to consider the impact on parents and other carers, e.g. foster carers. The best way to accomplish this is by open communication about any concerns at an early stage so that all share an understanding of the process and possible consequences.

Access to medical records

The guidance here is similar to that governing capacity. That is to say that, if a young person is deemed to have capacity, then he or she is entitled to have access to their medical record, and to allow or refuse others, including their parents, to have access. It would, however, be considered good practice to share medical information with children and help them to understand it within their ability to do so, provided that the information contained therein is not confidential to a third party or that its disclosure would be harmful to them.

Clinical examples

Case 1

James was a 10-year-old boy who had been referred for assessment of ADHD. The diagnosis was confirmed and, at the subsequent treatment planning session, James and his mother were offered the option of medication treatment with methylphenidate. James was keen to take the treatment because he was always getting into trouble at school for interrupting his teacher. His mother, however, did not wish medication at this point. They were offered a behavioural package, including parent training, input to education, and psychoeducation. At review 6 months later, although things had improved, James still had significant symptoms and was still getting into trouble at school. Once again, medication was discussed and, on this occasion, James' mother agreed that he should have a trial. Although James was an intelligent 10-year-old, because of his age, he would not be considered to have capacity to consent and, therefore, his parents had the right to make decisions for him.

Case 2

Lisa was 14 and seriously depressed. She had undergone 3 months of treatment with cognitive behavioural therapy, but was not making progress and was becoming increasingly suicidal. Her team considered medication, although they knew that neither Lisa nor her parents were keen for this treatment. After a lengthy consultation with the family, Lisa decided that she would take treatment with an antidepressant, although neither of her parents wished this. It was explained to her parents that Lisa had the capacity to make this decision for herself and she was prescribed the medication despite their disagreement. Lisa's parents remained involved in her care, but continued to express their disappointment about their daughter's decision.

Recommended reading

General Medical Council (2008) *Guidance for Doctors*. Available at: http://www.gmc-org/guidance (accessed on 18 March 2008).

Royal College of Psychiatrists (2000) *Guidance for the Use of Video Recording in Child Psychiatric Practice*, CR79. RCP, London. Available at: http://www.rcpsych.ac.uk/publications/collegereports/cr/cr79.aspx (accessed 29 March 2008).

Royal College of Psychiatrists (2004) *Good Psychiatric Practice*, 2nd edn, CR125. Available at: http://www.rcpsych.ac.uk (accessed on 18 March 2008).

Williams R, Kerfoot M. (2005) *Child and Adolescent Mental Health Services*. Oxford University Press, Oxford.

Further reading

The following list of recommended texts was compiled by the Faculty Education and Curriculum Committee of the Child and Adolescent Faculty of the UK Royal College of Psychiatrists. It is designed to cover the range of academic subjects that would be expected to be covered in the syllabus of a higher training academic programme for Child and Adolescent Psychiatrists.

General texts

Goodman R, Scott S. (2005) *Child Psychiatry*, 2nd edn. Blackwell Publishers, Oxford.

Graham P, et al. (1999) *Child Psychiatry: a Developmental Approach*, 3rd edn. Oxford University Press, Oxford.

Rutter M, Taylor E. (2002) *Child and Adolescent Psychiatry*, 4th edn. Blackwell, Oxford.

Skuse D. (2003) *Child Psychology and Psychiatry: an Introduction*. Medicine Publishing Company.

Developmental psychiatry, paediatrics, and chronic illness

Eiser C. (1990) *Chronic Childhood Disease: an Introduction to Psychological Theory and Research*. Cambridge University Press, Cambridge.

Hall DMB, Hill P. (1996) *The Child with a Disability*, 2nd edn. Blackwell, Oxford.

Hay D, et. al. (1996) *Development Through Life: a Handbook for Clinicians*. Blackwell, Oxford.

Kliegman RM, et al. (2003) *Nelson's Textbook of Paediatrics*, 17th edn. W.B. Saunders Ltd.

Treatment

Carr A. (2006) *Family Therapy: Concepts, Process and Practice*. John Wiley and Sons Ltd, Harlow.

Freedman J, Coombs G. (1996) *Narrative Therapy: the Social Construction of Preferred Realities*. WW Norton and Company, New York.

Friedberg RA, McClure J. (2002) *Clinical Practice of Cognitive Therapy with Children and Adolescents: the Nuts and Bolts*. Guildford Press.

Graham P. (ed.) (2004) *Cognitive Behaviour Therapy for Children and Families*. Cambridge University Press, Cambridge.

Herbert M. (1990) *Toilet Training, Bedwetting and Soiling*. BPS Blackwell.

Herbert M. (2002) *ABC of Behavioural Methods*. BPS Blackwell.

Home A, Lanyado M. (1999) *Handbook of Child and Adolescent Psychotherapy*. Routledge.

Jones E. (2000) *Family Systems Therapy: Developments in the Milan-Systemic Therapies.* John Wiley and Sons Ltd, Harlow.

Kutcher S. (2004) *Practical Child and Adolescent Psychopharmacology.* Cambridge University Press, Cambridge.

March JS, Mulle K. (1998) *OCD in Children and Adolescents: a Cognitive-Behavioral Treatment Manual.* Guilford Press, New York.

Martin A, Scahill L, Charney DS, Leckman JF (eds). (2003) *Paediatric Psychopharmacology: Principles and Practice.* Oxford University Press, Oxford.

Mash E, Barkley R. (2006) *Treatment of Childhood Disorders*, 3rd edn. Guildford Publications, New York.

Pote H, Stratton P, Cottrell D, Boston P, Shapiro D, Hanks H. (2003) *Systemic Family Therapy Manual.* Leeds Family Therapy and Research Centre School of Psychology, University of Leeds. Available at: http://www.psyc.leeds.ae.uk/researeh/lftre/SFT%20Manual%20from%20LFTRC.doc (The manual can be used as a framework for training and supervision, in developing skills for SpRs.)

Reinecke MA, *et al.* (2003) *Cognitive Therapy with Children and Adolescents: a Casebook for Clinical Practice.* Guildford Press, New York.

Remschmidt H. (2001) *Psychotherapy in Children and Adolescents.* Cambridge University Press, Cambridge.

Roth A, Fonagy P. (2005) *What Works For Whom? A Critical Review of Psychotherapy Research*, 2nd edn. Guildford Press, New York.

Stahl SM, Grady MM, Muntner N. (2004) *Essential Psychopharmacology: the Prescriber's Guide.* Cambridge University Press, Cambridge. (Has an adult focus, but provides an excellent overview of basic psychopharmacology.)

Stallard P. (2002) *Think Good—Feel Good: a Cognitive Behaviour Therapy Workbook for Children and Young People.* John Wiley & Sons, Harlow.

Research and audit

Bell J. (1999) *Doing Your Research Project: a Guide for First Time Researchers in Education, Health and Social Science.* Open University Press, Maidenhead.

Green J. (2004) *Qualitative Methods for Health Research.* SAGE.

Howell D. (2007) *Statistical Methods for Psychology*, 6th edn. Wadsworth, Conneticut.

National Institute for Clinical Excellence. (2002) *Principles for Best Practice in Clinical Audit.* Radcliffe Medical, Oxford.

Forensic

Adcock M, White R. (eds) (1998) *Significant Harm: its Management & Outcome.* Significant Publications, New York.

Ashford M, Chard A. (1997) *Defending Young People in the Criminal Justice System.* Legal Action Group, London.

Bailey S, Dolan M. (eds) (2002) *Adolescent Forensic Psychiatry.* Hodder Arnold, London.

Black D, et al. (1998) *Child Psychiatry and the Law*, 3rd edn. Gaskell, London.

Brophy J. (2001) *Child Psychiatry and Child Protection Litigation*. Gaskell, London.

Newble D, Cannon R. (2001) *A Handbook for Medical Teachers*, 4th edn. Kluwer Academic Publishers.

Reder P, et al. (2003) *Studies in the Assessment of Parenting*. Brunner-Routledge.

(1988) *Competency to Stand Trial Evaluations: a Manual for Practice*. Professional Resource Exchange.

Teaching

Cantillon P, et al. (eds) (2003) *ABC of Learning and Teaching in Medicine*. BMJ Publishing Group, London.

Newble D, Cannon R. (2001) *A Handbook for Medical Teachers*, 4th edn. Kluwer Academic Publishers.

Management and service development issues

Young AE. (2003) *The Medical Manager: a Practical Guide for Clinicians*, 2nd edn. BMJ Books, London.

Bhugra D, Burns A. (1995) *Management for Psychiatrists*, 2nd edn. Gaskell. (Includes chapters on audit, time management, and stress management.)

Richardson G, Partridge I. (eds) (2003) *Child and Adolescent Mental Health Services: an Operational Handbook*. Gaskell.

Williams R, Kerfoot M. (eds) (2005) *Child and Adolescent Mental Health Services: Strategy, Planning, Delivery and Evaluation*. Oxford University Press, Oxford.

Whitney D. *The Power of Appreciative Inquiry: a Practical Guide to Positive Change*. Berrett-Koehler.

Reference

Carr A. (ed.) (2000) *What Works with Children and Adolescents? A Critical Review of Psychological Interventions with Children, Adolescents and their Families.* Brunner-Routledge.

Fonagy P, et al. (eds) (2002) *What Works for Whom? A Critical Review of Treatments for Children and Adolescents.* Guildford.

Rutter M. (1996) *Multiaxial Classification of Child & Adolescent Disorders: The ICD-10 Classification of Mental and Behavioural Disorders in Children and Adolescents.* Cambridge University Press, Cambridge.

Scott A, Shaw M, Joughin C. (2001) *Finding the Evidence: a Gateway to the Literature in Child and Adolescent Mental Health,* 2nd edn. Gaskell.